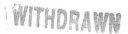

Jack Rothman, PhD
Edwin J. Thomas, PhD
Editors

Intervention Research: Design and Development for Human Service

Pre-publication
REVIEWS,
COMMENTARIES,
EVALUATIONS . . .

"**P**rofessors Jack Rothman and Edwin Thomas represent and define the current meaning of 'intervention research.'

This is a remarkable book in that it engages you in the process of intervention research. As I read the book, I was constantly challenged by perspectives and questions which are not routine research issues. And, intervention research is not research as usual. Frankly, NO ONE SHOULD ATTEMPT TO CONDUCT INTERVENTION RESEARCH BEFORE READING THIS BOOK."

Siri Jayaratne, PhD
Assistant Dean for Research and Professor, School of Social Work, University of Michigan

More pre-publication

REVIEWS, COMMENTARIES, EVALUATIONS . . .

"The topic of joining practice and research in a fruitful marriage usually inspires no more than exhortation or lament. Fortunately, *Intervention Research: Design and Development for Human Service* and the many distinguished contributing authors do neither. The architects of this book, Professors Rothman and Thomas, are among the few scholars in the human services who have pursued this topic systematically and diligently for several decades. *Intervention Research*, using cogent examples from many thoughtful investigators, provides AN INTEGRATED BLUEPRINT FOR DEVELOPING SYSTEMATICALLY USABLE, PRACTICABLE KNOWLEDGE FOR THE HUMAN SERVICES."

Stuart A. Kirk, DSW
Professor, Columbia University School of Social Work

"It's a delight to see that Rothman and Thomas, the two major innovators in intervention research, are working together. The results of their collaboration are this excellent book, A CUTTING-EDGE DEVELOPMENT that sets the stage for advances in research that truly have potential to affect practice. I recommend this book for other researchers, for students, and for practitioners who are concerned with the orderly advancement of knowledge–and the effectiveness–of social work practice."

Joel Fischer, DSW
Professor, School of Social Work, University of Hawaii

The Haworth Press, Inc.

Intervention Research
Design and Development for Human Service

HAWORTH Social Work Practice
Carlton E. Munson, DSW, Senior Editor

New, Recent, and Forthcoming Titles:

Management and Information Systems in Human Services: Implications for the Distribution of Authority and Decision Making by Richard K. Caputo

The Creative Practitioner: Creative Theory and Method for the Helping Services by Bernard Gelfand

Social Work Theory and Practice with the Terminally Ill by Joan K. Parry

Social Work in Health Settings: Practice in Context by Toba Schwaber Kerson and Associates

Gerontological Social Work Supervision by Ann Burack-Weiss and Frances Coyle Brennan

Group Work: Skills and Strategies for Effective Interventions by Sondra Brandler and Camille P. Roman

If a Partner Has AIDS: Guide to Clinical Intervention for Relationships in Crisis by R. Dennis Shelby

Social Work Practice: A Systems Approach by Benyamin Chetkow-Yanoov

Elements of the Helping Process: A Guide for Clinicians by Raymond Fox

Clinical Social Work Supervision, Second Edition by Carlton E. Munson

Intervention Research: Design and Development for Human Service edited by Jack Rothman and Edwin J. Thomas

Forensic Social Work: Legal Aspects of Professional Practice by Robert L. Barker and Douglas M. Branson

Now Dare Everything: Tales of HIV-Related Psychotherapy by Steven Dansky

Intervention Research
Design and Development for Human Service

Jack Rothman, PhD
Edwin J. Thomas, PhD
Editors

The Haworth Press
New York • London • Norwood (Australia)

The Haworth Press, Inc., 10 Alice Street, Binghamton, NY 13904-1580

Library of Congress Cataloging-in-Publication Data

Intervention research : design and development for human service / Jack Rothman, Edwin J. Thomas, editors.
    p.   cm.
Includes bibliographical references and indexes.
ISBN 1-56024-421-6 (acid free paper).
   1. Social service–Research. 2. Human services–Research. 3. Helping behavior–Research. 4. Operant behavior–Research. I. Rothman, Jack. II. Thomas, Edwin J. (Edwin John), 1927-
HV11.I57   1993
361.3–dc20   92-44915
                                                                       CIP

CONTENTS

EVALUATION AND ADVANCED DEVELOPMENT

DISSEMINATION

ABOUT THE EDITORS

Jack Rothman, PhD, holds a faculty position at the distinguished level at UCLA, where he has headed the Research and Development Program of the Center for Child and Family Policies Studies. He is nationally and internationally known for his significant work in systems intervention ("Three Models of Community Organization Practice") and intervention research (*Social R&D: Research and Development in the Human Services*). Other areas of interest include research utilization, organizational innovation and diffusion of innovations. He is author of some fifteen books, several in multiple editions, as well as numerous monographs and journal articles. His most recent research has been on persistently mentally ill, runaway and homeless youth, and health promotion in minority communities. Professor Rothman has received the Gunnar Myrad Award for Distinguished Human Services Research of the Evaluation Research Society and more recently, the first Annual Award for Life Time Contributions to Community Organization of the Association for Community Organization and Social Administration. He has been granted two Fulbright Senior Research Fellowships for International studies, and is a member of various editorial boards of journals emphasizing professional practice, research and research utilization.

Edwin J. Thomas, PhD, is Fedele F. Fauri Professor of Social Work and Professor of Psychology at the University of Michigan. As a founding faculty member, Dr. Thomas has headed the University of Michigan Doctoral Program in Social Work and Social Science, has chaired its supervising committee, and directed its post-doctoral training program in intervention research. He is nationally and internationally known for his seminal work on behavioral science and social work (*Behavioral Science for Social Workers*), behavioral intervention in social work, and more recently, developmental research for human service (*Designing Interventions for the Helping Professions*). Other areas of special interest include marital and family therapy, empirical practice, alcohol abuse, and assessment and research methods. He has been a Senior Fulbright Scholar and visiting professor, one year in England and another in Australia, and has published some 140 articles, book chapters, and books. As Director of the Marital Treatment Project, he is currently conducting research to develop and evaluate unilateral family therapy for alcohol abuse.

ABOUT THE CONTRIBUTORS

Fabricio E. Balcazar, PhD, is a senior research specialist at the University Affiliated Program in Developmental Disabilities and a Courtesy Assistant Clinical Professor in the Department of Psychology at the University of Illinois in Chicago. He was a research associate for four years at the Research and Training Center of Independent Living at the University of Kansas, where he also earned his doctorate degree. Dr. Balcazar is the coauthor of over 20 articles and publications.

Yolanda Suarez-Balcazar, PhD, is an assistant professor of psychology at Loyola University of Chicago, where she also serves on the Undergraduate Steering Committee and the Minority Affairs Committee. Dr. Suarez de Balcazar is currently chair of the International Development Committee of the Association for Behavioral Analysis. She has been a guest editor for several journals and has coauthored articles and book chapters.

Katherine A. Blanchard, MA, resides in Beaumont, Texas. While working as a graduate student research assistant at the University of Kansas Research and Training Center on Independent Living, she evaluated strategies for teaching vocational rehabilitation clients how to recruit help in achieving personal goals.

Patrick W. Corrigan, PsyD, is assistant professor of clinical psychiatry at the University of Chicago, where he directs the Center of Psychiatric Rehabilitation. He also supervises several funded research projects at the center. Dr. Corrigan has published more than 40 articles, books, and chapters.

William N. Dunn, PhD, is professor of public management and policy and information science in the Graduate School of Public and International Affairs and the School of Library and Information Science at the University of Pittsburgh. He has written and co-written journal articles on the methodology of policy analysis and the utilization of the social sciences.

Melody G. Embree, MA, is a doctoral candidate at Michigan State University in the Ecological-Community Psychology Program. She is editor of the women's issues column in *The Community Psychologist* and a representative on the Executive Committee of the Society for Community Research and Action of the American Psychological Association. She has published several journal articles and is the author of a chapter in a book currently in press.

Stephen B. Fawcett, PhD, is professor of human development and director of the Work Group on Health Promotion and Community Development of the Schiefelbusch Institute for Life Span Studies at the University of Kansas. He has twice been honored as a Fellow of the American Psychological Association, is the coauthor of three books, and has served on the editorial board or as a consulting editor of numerous journals. Dr. Fawcett has been a consultant to a variety of organizations including the U.S. Commission on National and Community Service.

Steven R. Forness, EdD, is professor of psychiatry and biobehavioral sciences and principal of the Inpatient School at the University of California at Los Angeles Neuropsychiatric Hospital. His research interest is in direct classroom observation of children with learning or behavioral problems.

Walter M. Furman, MPhil, is the administrator of the Center for Child and Family Policy Studies and a lecturer in the School of Social Welfare at the University of California at Los Angeles. He was formerly the director of program evaluation for the New York State Office of Mental Health.

Yeheskel Hasenfeld, PhD, is professor of social welfare in the School of Social Welfare at the University of California at Los Angeles. He has published and edited several books and many articles in the field of social welfare. Dr. Hasenfeld's main research focus has been in the organization of human services with special emphasis on the impact of the environment and on client-organization relations.

Robert M. Hayes, PhD, is professor emeritus at the University of California at Los Angeles after having served 15 years as dean of the UCLA Graduate School of Library and Information Science. From 1949 until he joined the faculty of UCLA in 1964, Dr. Hayes worked in government and industry and founded a small consulting and research company. From 1969 to 1974, he was Vice President of Becker & Hayes, Inc.

Steven Kapp, MSW, is clinical evaluator at Boysville of Michigan, a large multiservice agency meeting the needs of vulnerable youth and families in Detroit and other Michigan communities.

Kenneth Kavale, PhD, is professor in the Division of Special Education at the University of Iowa. Dr. Kavale received his doctoral degree from the University of Minnesota. His research interests are in learning disabilities and meta-analysis.

Robert Paul Liberman, MD, is director of the NIMH-funded Clinical Research Center for Schizophrenia and Psychiatric Rehabilitation in Los Angeles. He has published over 200 articles, books, and chapters, has served on national and international organizations and committees, and has received numerous awards for his work in schizophrenia, chronic mental illness, and psychiatric rehabilitation.

Sally J. MacKain, PhD, is assistant professor of psychology at the University of North Carolina at Wilmington. She has published a number of research articles and book chapters in the area of psychiatric rehabilitation and has conducted over 40 workshops around the country at state hospitals, correctional facilities, and community mental health centers.

John Mooradian, MSW, is consultant at Boysville of Michigan, a large multiservice agency meeting the needs of vulnerable youth and families in Detroit and other Michigan communities.

Edward J. Mullen, MSW, is professor and associate dean of the School of Social Work at Columbia University. He is also director at the Center of the Study of Social Work Practice, which is sponsored by Columbia University and the Jewish Board of Family and Children's Services, and director of the Mental Health Services

Research Doctoral Program, funded by the National Institute of Mental Health. Dr. Mullen has authored and coauthored numerous articles and books in social work research.

Edward Overstreet, MSW, is associate executive director at Boysville of Michigan, a large multiservice agency meeting the needs of vulnerable youth and families in Detroit and other Michigan communities.

Adrienne L. Paine, PhD, is associate director of the Work Group on Health Promotion and Community Development and research associate with the Schiefelbusch Institute for Life Span Studies at the University of Kansas. Dr. Paine is primarily interested in research that promotes community development, enhances community integration and social support, and works to empower marginal groups. She is the coauthor of several articles in the areas of self-help, community development, and health promotion.

William J. Reid, DSW, is professor and chair of the PhD program in the School of Social Welfare at the State University of New York at Albany. He has conducted many research studies on short-term treatment and is known for his role in the development of the task-centered model of social work practice. Dr. Reid has published over 125 works, his most recent being *Task Strategies* published by Columbia University Press in 1992.

JoAnn Damron-Rodriguez, PhD, is director of education and evaluation, VA, West Los Angeles Geriatric Research Education and Clinical Center. She was previously at the Pacific Geriatric Education Center and at the University of Southern California. She received her doctorate in social welfare from the University of California, Los Angeles, where she was a University Fellow and received the Gold Fellowship for the Study of Aging.

Ronald H. Rooney, PhD, is associate professor in the School of Social Work at the University of Minnesota at Minneapolis. Dr. Rooney has conducted intervention research in a training package for child welfare staff and supervised two intervention research dissertations.

Edmond Shenassa, MA, is currently researching smoking prevention for the Center for Populations Studies for Cancer Prevention at the University of California, San Diego. He has also participated in a study of case management for the Center for Child and Family Policy Studies in the School of Social Welfare at the University of California, Los Angeles.

Elizabeth M. Tracy, PhD, is assistant professor at the Mandel School of Applied Social Sciences at Case Western Reserve University where she teaches social work practice courses and coordinates the school's concentration in children, youth, and families. Dr. Tracy has provided training and consultation on social support assessment and intervention to a number of family preservation programs.

Tony Tripodi, MSW, ACSW, DSW, is coordinator of the PhD program in social welfare at Florida International University. He has served as a research and evaluation consultant for national and international organizations, including the European Common Market and the Zancan Foundation in Padova, Italy. Dr. Tripodi is currently a member of the National Research Advisory Committee, Boysville, Michigan. Previously editor in chief of *Social Work Research and Abstracts*, he serves on the book committee of the National Association of Social Workers and on the editorial boards of several professional journals.

Anita Tumblin, MA, MS, PhD, is currently working in the Psychological Services Division of Secondary Schools Support, Los Angeles Unified School District. She earned her graduate degrees from the Department of Psychology at Memphis State University and conducted postgraduate work at the UCLA Neuropsychiatric Institute Center for the Health Sciences.

Glen W. White, PhD, is training director of the Research and Training Center on Independent Living and research associate with the Sciefelbusch Institute for Life Span Studies at the University of Kansas. Dr. White, a paraplegic since 1964, has been involved in the rehabilitation and independent living field for over 20 years. The author or coauthor of numerous books, articles, and book chapters, he was recently appointed by President Bush as a board member of the Commission on National and Community Service.

James K. Whittaker, PhD, is professor of social work at the University of Washington where he teaches in the area of child and family services. Dr. Whittaker has authored or coauthored numerous articles and seven books on child welfare and social treatment, which have been translated into five languages.

Foreword

The human service professions are in dire need of a research methodology that links knowledge and practice. This is cogently illustrated in social work. The Task Force on Social Work Research, sponsored by the National Institute of Mental Health, recently completed a three-year study in which it examined the current status of research in social work, one of the key professions that employs social and psychological interventions for the purpose of helping people solve problems of growth and adaptation (*Building Social Work Knowledge for Effective Services and Policies: A Plan for Research Development,* Report of the Task Force on Social Work Research, David Austin et al., National Institute of Mental Health, November, 1991). Among the chief observations made by the task force are these: more researchers are required to do research that informs social work practice; there is a lack of integration of research methods and findings with social work practice; and there are deficits in the structural arrangements of research, i.e., a paucity of structures to facilitate collaborative efforts between universities and social agencies. It is further noted that the Council on Social Work Education has reaffirmed its position that schools of social work, to be accredited, must provide instruction that teaches students how to evaluate the effectiveness of their practice.

With respect to these considerations and in reference to the state of the art of research in the social professions, this volume on Intervention Research is most important and most timely for social work and allied disciplines that use interventions in their practice. Three fundamental themes can be abstracted from the book: a conceptualization of intervention research is presented that allows social theoreticians and researchers to distinguish intervention research from other modalities; a new model of research on the design and development of interventions is specified; and guidelines are provided for conducting intervention research in direct practice with individuals and families, as well as in community organizations.

In Chapter 1, Thomas and Rothman conceive intervention research, which is focused on the development of knowledge about interventions, as being comprised of Intervention Knowledge Development, Intervention Knowledge Utilization, and Intervention Design and Development. Intervention Knowledge Development employs conventional social research strategies to produce knowledge from the social and behavioral sciences that can be applied to social practice; and Intervention Knowledge Utilization employs a variety of procedures, such as meta-analysis, marketing strategies, and demonstrations, to package and disseminate knowledge about innovative interventions. Intervention Design and Development is the heart of intervention research because it focuses on the development of new interventions as well as on the requirements for adapting previously used interventions to changing conditions such as population demographics, new social problems, reduced resources, etc. It is the methodology and practice of Intervention Design and Development that provides the uniqueness of intervention research. Paradoxically, the design and development of interventions that are effective has long been a favorite rallying cry for human service practitioners seeking relevant knowledge; yet, it is that research that has been most neglected.

The model of Intervention Design and Development that forms the focus of this book combines and integrates the essential features of two pioneering efforts in the field: *Social R and D: Research and Development in the Human Services*, by Jack Rothman (1980, Englewood Cliffs, NJ: Prentice-Hall) and *Designing Interventions for the Helping Professions*, by Edwin J. Thomas (1984, Beverly Hills, CA: Sage Publications). This integrated model is comprised of six phases: problem analysis and project planning; information gathering and synthesis; design; early development and pilot testing; evaluation and advanced development; and dissemination. The chapters of the book focus on various aspects of these phases and provide a clear view of the creativity that is necessary to develop relevant interventions that achieve practice goals. The reader may form an impression that design and development can be time consuming and complex, and so become disinclined to engage in this type of research. This would be a serious mistake and would reinforce the observation of the Task Force on Social Work Research that research directly related to social work practice is often neglected. Moreover, intervention-oriented researchers must conceive of research on serious social problems as involving possibly more than research by one individual; i.e., research may be programmatic, involving inter- as well as intra-disciplinary efforts by teams of researchers. The conception of Thomas and Rothman presented here is useful for either individual or team research. In addition, researchers can carry out research on various aspects of the model as applied to the development of particular interventions. This is exemplified in several chapters in which specific guidelines and methodologies are discussed and presented.

There is no one particular research technique that is employed in Intervention Design and Development. Both quantitative and qualitative research modalities are used in relation to the particular type of intervention that is being produced. The research experiences that are described help the reader to develop a conceptual and methodological stance for conducting various aspects of intervention research. In addition, they provide a useful frame of reference for theoreticians, instructors, supervisors, and practitioners. We are thus helped in how to think about the meaning of interventions and in what is involved in their development, prior to testing for their effectiveness.

Useful observations and guidelines for intervention research are provided in all of the chapters. Several selected examples serve to illustrate this point. Steven R. Forness emphasizes that meta-analyses should be conducted by those who are familiar with the literature that is being synthesized. One should not simply combine and summarize effect sizes without understanding the details of the studies that are summarized. James K. Whittaker and Elizabeth M. Tracy show how research can be focused on the design of practice guidelines for the use of network interventions with high risk youth and families. They illustrate the importance of designing interventions that are compatible with the philosophy, values, and goals of community agencies and social programs; and they demonstrate the value of their research, noting that it is time consuming.

William J. Reid develops a strategy for the research development of a single intervention, the family problem-solving sequence. His strategy involves the initial development and modification of an intervention through single case studies; the aggregation and further analysis of those studies; and the construction of a more rigorous design. This strategy promises to be especially useful in clinical research efforts.

Intervention Research needs to be conducted in practice settings. A researcher may be engaged in a design and development project in which he or she creates the practice environment in a laboratory-type situation; for example research sponsored by a federal agency, such as that described by Edwin J. Thomas in evaluating and further developing a unilateral family therapy approach with spouses of alcoholics. Or, the research may be conducted by outside research- ers who use the social agency as a laboratory, as in the illustration of the research by James K. Whittaker and Elizabeth M. Tracy. Or, further still, the research may be reflective of collaborative efforts by university researchers and agency personnel. Currently, there is increased federal funding available for collaboration in the areas of mental health and child welfare. There is much in this volume that is helpful for researchers who are engaged in these activities. Of particular importance is the discussion by Yeheskel Hasenfeld and Walter M. Furman who analyze three collaborative research and development projects from the perspective of interorganizational exchange, and offer guidelines for facilitating interorganizational collaboration. Employing concepts such as power balance, structur- al centrality, structural stability, linkages, and motivational compati- bility, the authors provide many useful insights and ideas.

Ronald H. Rooney discusses strategies for enhancing profession- al education. He believes the model of intervention research could be disaggregated so that relevant research could be performed with- in various phases of the model; and, among his suggestions, he advocates more instruction about intervention research in graduate courses and more use of the practice of intervention research in doctoral education. This is very timely because the introduction of intervention research methodologies and issues in doctoral educa- tion most clearly should be given the highest priority.

In summation, this is a book that provides a wealth of ideas about Intervention Design and Development. It offers conceptual schemes, results from recent design and development studies, guidelines, strategies, and methodologies. There is important material in each chapter, which should be read by students, scholars, practice theoreticians, and researchers in the social professions and related disciplines. The contents are provocative and should lead to discussion and further research that will inform practitioners about effective practice innovations at the individual and system levels.

Tony Tripodi
Florida International University

Preface

"I wish those university researchers would just once in a while come up with something concrete that I could use in my work." This hope, and implied condemnation, is muttered almost every day in front line human service agencies. Simultaneously, young application-minded behavioral scientists struggle for some way to make the results of their efforts more immediately "relevant" and socially useful.

What is remarkable is that in the last fifteen years a new approach and methodology has developed that satisfies these requirements, but it has remained outside of the social science mainstream, largely unknown or ignored and rarely employed. The purpose of this book is to describe and explicate intervention research, in particular intervention design and development, a means of creating reliable, practical tools of social intervention in user-ready form.

Although still in its early stages, intervention research sets forth systematic procedures for designing, testing, evaluating, and refining needed social technology, and for disseminating proven techniques and programs to professionals in the community. This formulation has evolved from work by the editors of this volume in developmental research and social R&D, as well as the efforts of others, many of whom have contributed original chapters to this book.

The editors began to integrate their extensive independent investigations in the area by joining in a proposal to the National Institute of Mental Health to support doctoral training in intervention research at the University of Michigan. This materialized in an advanced seminar commencing in 1985, together with stipends for pre- and post-doctoral students and collateral research internships. While the editors had given graduate seminars in aspects of the subject, this was perhaps the first formal training program with a specialized focus on intervention research.

A further step toward convergence was through a National Conference on Intervention Research, held in Los Angeles in March of 1989, under the sponsorship of the Center for Child and Family Policy Studies at UCLA. The conference, which the editors collaborated in planning, brought together scholars from diverse disciplines who were active in varied aspects of intervention research, such as Edward Mullen and William Reid (Social Work), Steven Fawcett (Psychology), Robert Liberman (Psychiatry), Robert Hayes (Information Sciences), and Everett Rogers (Sociology). Through an intensive exchange of ideas, these scholars identified areas of consensus and established a more common terminology, while they also noted variations in emphasis. This volume contains a number of the papers that were presented, and subsequently refined, together with others that were commissioned to achieve a more comprehensive treatment of the subject. The book provides an overview of the main features of the intervention research approach, with illustrations and elaborations by those who have performed cutting-edge research and made important conceptual contributions. It does not, however, comprise a formal text or an exhaustive methodological compendium.

The introductory section of the book sets forth the intervention research paradigm, which provides the framework for the overall presentation. An orienting chapter by the editors establishes the parameters of intervention research and delineates the phases of its core process, design and development (D&D). The phases of D&D are further elaborated and illustrated by Fawcett and his associates as part of the introduction.

These phases constitute the structure of the book, and all chapters have been orchestrated to expressly and consistently reflect the dynamic of the paradigm. All of the material is newly written for this purpose. A flow diagram depicting the paradigm is introduced at the outset and is used as a conceptual guide to visually lead the reader through the various sections of the book. The course of the presentation is as follows:

> *Explication of the D&D paradigm*–Thomas and Rothman; Fawcett and associates;
> *Identification of Pertinent Problems and Project Planning*– Dunn; Rothman;

Information Retrieval and Synthesis–Hayes; Forness and Kavale; Rothman, Damron-Rodriguez, and Shenassa;

Designing Interventions–Mullen; Whittaker and Tracy and associates;

Pilot Testing and Early Development–Rothman and Tumblin; Reid;

Evaluating Effects and Advanced Development–Thomas; Hasenfeld and Furman;

Disseminating Developed Intervention Tools–Corrigan, Mac-Kain and Liberman; Rooney.

Every effort has been made to create an integrated book that reflects a common conceptual and methodological thrust. The editors and authors in this work are seeking to present salient aspects of a community of thought, rather than a set of independent or competing ideas. The contributions are meant to speak for themselves within a defined and embracing conceptual frame.

D&D is a distinct and in some ways innovative formulation. It provides a kind of road map for the serious researcher/practitioner who is interested in applying the methods of research and social science to the needs of practice and policy. It is, however, a composite that amalgamates many existing methodologies to form its substance. Intervention research draws from such areas as evalution research, behavioral assessment, technology assessment, technology transfer, simulation and modeling, meta-analysis, knowledge utilization, practice technology, and systems engineering. It is the configuring of these methodological elements into a phased system of action that harnesses their potential to generate practical interventive innovations. This approach holds the promise of making the production of innovative tools of practice more orderly and responsive to the plaint of human service professionals that was voiced at the beginning of these comments. It may be the single most appropriate model of research for the applied social professions because it serves to create the fundamental means through which those professions attain their societal mission.

Jack Rothman
Edwin J. Thomas

CONCEPTUAL OVERVIEW

Chapter 1

An Integrative Perspective on Intervention Research

Edwin J. Thomas
Jack Rothman

For some time, researchers in human service areas such as social work, mental health and public health have sought approaches to research which yield results that can be put to practical use by practitioners, administrators, and policymakers. They have addressed such questions as how to search out and make appropriate use of available research findings which have potential application, how research methodology may be used to design and develop human service technology, and, more generally, how research for practical use in human service differs from conventional behavioral and social science research.

Varied approaches have been employed to address the practice application of research. There appear to be three main types of endeavors that reflect that intent: (a) empirical research to extend knowledge of human behavior relating to human service intervention (here referred to as Intervention Knowledge Development–KD); (b) the means by which the findings from Intervention Knowledge Development research may be linked to, and utilized in, practical application (referred to as Intervention Knowledge Utilization–KU); and (c) research directed toward developing innovative interventions (referred to as Intervention Design and Development–D&D).

Although there are critical differences in their objectives and methodologies, these three endeavors have a dual commonality: they are in the genre of applied research and they have a specific intervention mission. As applied research, all three are directed toward shedding light on or providing possible solutions to practical problems. The intervention characteristic is more specific and salient for our discussion. This is because most of the questions about practical use addressed in such research involve some aspects of intervention. For example, concerns involving intervention include social and personal problems of those who might need assistance, how to produce change in conditions affecting the problems, what interventions may be appropriate to produce change, what the effects are of such interventions, and how to develop new interventions having general application. It is this common focus on questions of intervention that provides a basis for bringing together these three types of research and inquiry as facets of what will here be called *intervention research.*

The purpose of this analysis is to present intervention research as an integrative perspective for human service research. In so doing, the interventional aspects of the constituent types of intervention research will be highlighted along with some of their relationships when considered from this perspective.

CONTEXT AND OVERVIEW

The three facets of intervention research are depicted in Figure 1 along with some of their possible interrelationships. Intervention Knowledge Development is shown in the figure as an aspect of applied research and of general social and behavioral science research. KD and more conventional research, whether basic or applied, have clear similarities and both may provide knowledge having potential practical application. Their methods of study are identical, as would be the behavior of these researchers, as viewed by an outside observer. An important difference, however, is the purpose of the activities. In KD, there is a distinct effort to create findings that will apply to the understanding and/or solution of practical problems. That is, the questions asked in KD are more instrumental and practical, and the phenomena studied are generally more closely related to interventive problems than is typically the case with more basic research. The findings of KD research generally provide fuel for further phases of intervention research or other

FIGURE 1. Facets of intervention research and some of their interrelationships.

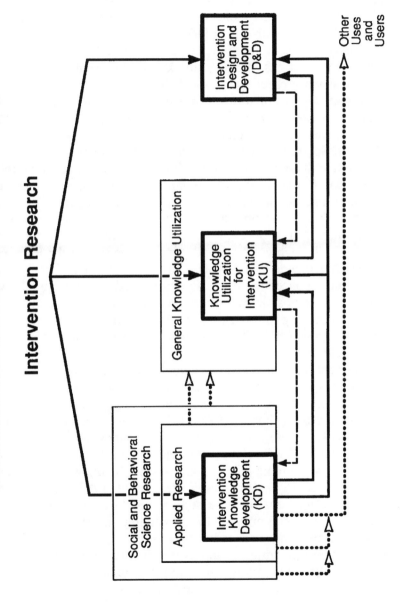

practical use. However, as a facet of intervention research, KD is a distinctive activity with its own objectives, methods, and outcomes (Table 1). As Figure 1 indicates, KD may or may not be carried out as a linked effort with KU or D&D.

The activities of KU have been recognized for some time as consisting of means of converting knowledge from the theory and empirical research of social and behavioral science to knowledge having an application thrust. Carol Weiss has shown that there are a number of alternative meanings and models of knowledge utilization reflected in the literature (Weiss 1979). For example, in the Problem-Solving Model the researcher provides a policymaker with knowledge that will assist in forming a given decision. In the Interactive Model the researcher brings his knowledge to a broader decision-making forum, such as congress, and competes with others bringing different information and views. The Enlightenment Model assumes that knowledge is utilized not in linear fashion, but indirectly through concepts and perspectives that in the long-term eventually come to have impact on those who use knowledge. Closer to home conceptually, Weiss describes the Knowledge-Driven Model, which postulates a somewhat linear effect of knowledge on action by moving through a series of phases from research to development to application. This formulation is consistent with intervention research.

Intervention Design and Development embraces several different approaches that seek to construct a systematic methodology for evolving human service interventions. Among these are developmental research (Thomas 1978a, 1978b, 1984), social R&D (Rothman 1974, 1980a), experimental social innovation (Fairweather 1967), and model development research (e.g., Paine, Bellamy, and Wilcox 1984), among others (e.g., Fawcett, Matthews, and Fletcher 1980; Mullen 1978, 1981, 1983; Reid 1979, 1983). Although the specific orientations of these approaches differ in some respects, they also share common features, including, in particular, a set of steps of interconnected activities that are intended to guide researchers and practitioners to develop innovative interventions for effecting change in problem situations that relate to human service.

D&D likewise has its own objectives, methods, and results, as is indicated in Table 1. This facet of intervention research can be

TABLE 1. Summary of selected differences between Knowledge Development, Knowledge Utilization, and Design and Development in intervention research.

Areas of difference	Facets of intervention research		
	Knowledge Development (KD)	Knowledge Utilization (KU)	Design and Development (D&D)
Objectives	To contribute knowledge of human behavior	To apply knowledge of human behavior	To evolve new human service technology (e.g., treatment methods, programs, service systems, or policies)
Methods	Conventional social and behavioral science research methods	Transformation and conversion of available knowledge into application concepts and theories relevant to given target populations, problems, and intervention methods	Emerging methods include the means of problem analysis, intervention design, development, evaluation and dissemination and related techniques
Outcomes	Information about human behavior in the form, for example, of concepts, hypotheses, theories, and empirical generalizations	Such applications as changes in the understanding or practices relating to populations, problems, or interventions in human service	Such technical means of achieving human service objectives as assessment and intervention methods; and service programs, systems, and policies

carried out as an independent enterprise, except for the KU that generally occurs in the formative stages of most D&D projects. Further, the process of designing and developing interventions of D&D typically involves drawing on many sources of information (e.g., related technology, legal policy, practice innovations, and personal and professional experience) (Thomas 1978a, 1984). However, D&D can be directly linked to a specific KU activity beforehand, with or without that KU enterprise being likewise preceded by a related and linked KD effort.

Each type of intervention research thus has its own integrity and distinctness, yet each is a facet of intervention research, inasmuch as the objects of concern in each relate to an aspect of human service intervention. As indicated above and in Figure 1, the facets may be independent in how they are carried out by researchers and practitioners or they may be conducted so that they are interrelated purposely and systematically in a linked sequence. The arrows with solid lines in Figure 1 indicate such purposely sequenced steps; arrows with broken lines represent indirect or emergent linkage.

FACETS OF INTERVENTION RESEARCH

In discussing the components of intervention research more substantively, we will begin with intervention D&D. D&D is paramount in the process: it is the point at which innovative human service interventions are evolved, and it is often a culminating activity that the other facets precede and lead up to. Following that presentation, KD will be examined more closely, and then KU.

INTERVENTION DESIGN AND DEVELOPMENT

In recent years, D&D has emerged as an explicit paradigm, largely out of frustrations with the inability of conventional research methods to guide the generation of human service interventions. The D&D approaches (e.g., Social Research and Development [R&D], developmental research, model development research) have evolved up to this point largely through independent and concurrent efforts that have been based upon different D&D enterprises and have taken somewhat different form. However, considering the shared objectives of D&D approaches and their methodological similarities within the broader context of intervention research, these seeming differences between D&D formulations can be viewed instead largely as parallel means to achieve common D&D goals.

Accordingly, we present an integrated model of D&D based on an endeavor by the authors to bring together some of the important common features in developmental research, social R&D, and related approaches. In this integration, there are six main phases of intervention D&D: (a) problem analysis and project planning; (b) information gathering and synthesis; (c) design; (d) early development and pilot testing; (e) evaluation and advanced development; and (f) dissemination. Although performed in a stepwise sequence, some or many of the activities associated with each phase continue after the introduction of the next phase (see Figure 2 for a diagrammatic depiction). Also, though ideally stepwise and linear, there is sometimes looping back to earlier phases, as difficulties are encountered or new information is obtained.

Each phase has distinctive activities that need to be carried out in order to complete the work of that phase. For example, in the first phase of problem analysis and project planning, key problems are identified and analyzed, a broad state-of-the-art review is initiated to provide general orientation to the problem, and the feasibility of the D&D project is determined. The phase of information gathering and synthesis consists of the identification and selection of more particular existing types and sources of information relevant to the delineated development task, the establishment of retrieval procedures, along with the gathering, processing, and synthesizing of informational data. Additional activities for these and the other phases of D&D are indicated in some detail in Figure 2. Each listed activity may thus be thought of as a step in the sequence of activities required to complete the work for a given phase, which provides the basis for entering into the next phase. There is ordinarily some flexibility in the process, but the basic pattern proceeds as described. Elaboration regarding phases and aspects of selected constituent activities can be found elsewhere (e.g., Rothman 1980a,

FIGURE 2. Phases and selected activities of intervention design and development (D&D).*

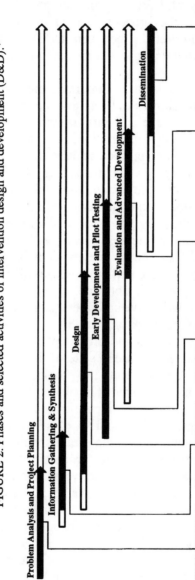

Identify and analyze key problems	Identify and select relevant existing types of information (e.g., empirical research, related practice and technology, social innovation)	Identify design problems and intervention requirements	Develop plan for trial use in a pilot test	Plan evaluation in light of the degree of interventional development	Assess needs and points of access of potential consumers
Initiate state-of-the-art review	Identify relevant information sources (e.g., journals, abstracts, indexes, computerized data bases)	Specify boundaries of the domain of D&D	Create a limited operational model of the intervention for trial use in the pilot test site	Select evaluation methods (e.g., experimental, non-experimental, procedures, and techniques)	Formulate dissemination plan
Determine feasibility (e.g., technical, financial, organizational, political, etc.)	Establish retrieval procedures	Determine design participants (e.g., a design team, including role of users)	Determine the developmental research medium and/or procedure	Conduct pilot evaluation	Design and develop appropriate implementation procedures
Prepare project plan	Gather, process, and store data	Select a D&D site (e.g., laboratory, agency, university)	Determine developmental and monitoring instruments (e.g., developmental logs)	Carry out systematic evaluation	Prepare user-ready innovation for potential consumers
Set a development goal	Collect and analyze original data, as appropriate	Use disciplined problem solving and creativity	Identify and address design problems	Revise intervention, as necessary	Develop means and media to reach potential consumers
	Synthesize data and formulate conclusions	Generate, select, and assemble solution alternatives	Revise intervention, as necessary		Test use of innovation in a "test market"
		Formulate an initial intervention or other innovation model	Continue proceduralization and implementation of model		Monitor and evaluate use
		Initiate proceduralization	Plan field test and select a site		Revise (or reinvent) innovation as necessary
			Expand the trial field test as informed by the pilot		Develop and conduct large scale dissemination, as appropriate
			Implement field test and revise intervention, as necessary		Repeat above steps, as necessary

Legend: Primary emphasis of phase is solid, with open space lines for the secondary emphasis of the phase.

*This schema combines selected elements of Rothman's Social Research and Development Model and Thomas' Research Paradigm

1989; Thomas 1978a, 1984) and in subsequent chapters in this volume.

D&D may be conceptualized as a problem-solving process for seeking effective interventive and helping tools to deal with given human and social difficulties. But unlike many other types of problem solving, D&D is a process that is systematic, deliberate, and immersed in research procedures, techniques, and other instrumentalities. In its aim to produce workable human service technology, rather than generalizable knowledge *per se* (although it may achieve the latter), the methods of D&D are more akin to the field of engineering than to the traditional behavioral sciences. At the same time, it borrows from and exploits these sister fields. Instead of emphasizing the interrelationships of variables, as in conventional research, the primary focus throughout D&D is on the interventive technology to be evolved–for example, an assessment instrument or intervention technique for addressing given individual problems; a service system or policy to deal with problems of a large cohort of individuals; or a legislative program to remedy a structural defect in a social system.

In this connection, a key difference is that D&D takes as its original point of departure a given real-world problem and practical goal, rather than a hypothesis to be tested or a theory to be explored. Thus, at the very inception, the fundamental perspectives of D&D and the basic social sciences diverge. The identification of the problem to be addressed does not necessarily fall to the D&D research team. The focal problem may be identified by agency staff, clients, agency administrators, grassroots citizens, or combinations of these groupings: Rothman (1989) presents a case study involving agency staff problem identification, while Seekins and Fawcett (1987) describe a process in which local residents determine the goals and agenda of D&D. The process may also be driven by knowledge breakthroughs in the scientific realm, but, as studies at industrial R&D show, it is more frequently stimulated by expressions of consumer need and demand (Roberts and Frohman 1978). In any case, it has a mission-oriented, problem-solving cast.

In the information-gathering phase, varied types of data serve as the basis for intervention development. These include basic and applied research, the main contributions of KD research, which are the customary sources of information in knowledge utilization. Other types, however, are also relevant, as indicated earlier, and include scientific technology, allied technology, legal policy, indigenous innovation, practice, personal experience, and professional experience (for further details, see Thomas 1978a, 1984). The researcher may also carry out original research that is topic- or locality-specific to shed light on the subject, such as a needs assessment, survey of practitioners concerning the current state of practice, a Delphi conference, etc.

One or more types of information may be relevant to any particular design task, although there is often a primary type of information with possible supplementary sources. Since the information (or resource) of a given type cannot generally be used in its raw form in design, the information (or resource) must somehow be transformed so that the results or products may be incorporated directly in the design process. Transformation may be thought of as generation processes that involve application of knowledge, such as research findings (e.g., see Rothman 1974, 1978; Thomas 1980), as well as application of legal policy, of professional or personal experience, and the transfer and adoption of already developed technology (for further details, see Thomas 1978a, 1980, 1984).

The process of development is interlaced with the realities of practitioners and clients in close, intensive interaction with one another and researchers. It is only in the context of such real-world encounters, including practitioner and client reaction to proposed intervention designs, that meaningful helping behavior can be explicated and evaluated for eventual general use. D&D methodology in all approaches inherently requires explicit, sensitive involvement with the kinds of people, termed *users*, who will be implicated in the practice implementation of the intervention. This is the case whether the work is performed in natural open settings or structured lab-like conditions. The early development phase includes an initial pilot testing stage to explore the feasibility of an intervention design and to refine it. In the process of interventional refinement, such methods as proceduralization and developmental practice can be particularly useful (see Thomas 1985, 1990).

Evaluation has a defined place in the D&D model because of its critical contribution to appraising the outcomes, including the effectiveness of the intervention. Although there is often some evaluation of aspects of the intervention during early development, particularly its ease of use and implementation, systematic outcome evaluation is typically not undertaken nor should it be carried out until an advanced phase has been achieved when the intervention has been sufficiently well developed to merit rigorous outcome appraisal through use of suitable experimental research methods.

D&D activity has certain characteristics in common with evaluation research, and includes most of evaluation research as a tool and component. In general, evaluation methods in D&D include much of the already established research methodology of social science and program evaluation. However, it is important to emphasize that the purpose for using research methods for outcome evaluation in advanced development is to yield outcome information as an integral part of a technological innovation process: evaluation follows early development, contributes to further design and development as necessary, and precedes and eventually leads to dissemination of the now tested and evaluated intervention.

The dissemination phase has a relatively strong body of literature to inform the process of diffusion and adoption (e.g., see Backer, Liberman, and Kuehnel 1986; Paine, Bellamy, and Wilcox 1984; Rogers 1983; Stolz 1981). There are at least four components here. One involves designing the intervention for usability from the outset, long before dissemination (e.g., see Backer, Liberman, and Kuehnel 1986; Paine 1984). A second entails the packaging or fabricating of the intervention in a form that is easily accessible and applicable by the user, or, put another way, it should be "user-ready" (Rothman 1980b; Rothman, Teresa, and Erlich 1978). The third involves recognition of the need to give attention to the process of "reinvention" as evidenced by adaptations of the innovation made through use (Rice and Rogers 1980; Rogers 1983). A fourth entails use of modes of persuasion, influence, opinion change, and social marketing to motivate users to employ innovative practice tools (e.g., see Rothman et al. 1983).

INTERVENTION KNOWLEDGE DEVELOPMENT

KD research provides important foundation knowledge for understanding aspects of the intervention and for carrying out subsequent D&D. Areas of particular interest in intervention KD include learning more about *the relevant target behavior of potential clients and client systems* (e.g., depression, anxiety, substance abuse, family disorganization, organizational dysfunction), *relevant intervention behavior* (e.g., therapist warmth, empathy, social support, social networks, advocacy, coalition building), and the *relevant behavioral, social, contextual, and environmental conditions* (e.g., supportive, organizational, and community structures). For example, if alcohol abuse were the target behavior of interest, KD research could involve examining the correlates and predictors of excessive alcohol consumption, the variables that bear a relationship to effective intervention methods with alcohol abuse, the effects and effectiveness of alcohol intervention programs, as well as the social, cultural, and environmental correlates of drinking behavior (e.g., personal predispositions, effects of alcohol tax legislation, etc.). The methodology of KD research consists largely of the research methods and techniques of conventional behavioral and social science research, as indicated, including particular applications of these methods, such as those to be found in conventional social welfare research, evaluation research, single-case experimentation, and needs assessment.

The complementary relationships between research and technology have long been recognized in science and industry and, more recently, in selected areas of applied behavior analysis and social research (e.g., see Azrin 1977; Baer, Wolf, and Risley 1968, 1987; Deitz 1978; Paine, Bellamy, and Wilcox 1984; Rothman 1980). There are several ways in which KD research may be performed in the context of intervention research. In the first, *KD is conducted as an independent activity* separate from any KU or D&D that may occur subsequently. For example, many years of earlier research on reinforcement and motivation processes made it possible later to conduct KD research on such applied motivational technologies as token economies (e.g., see Ayllon and Azrin 1965, 1968; Staats 1968) and point systems (e.g., see Phillips et al. 1971). These studies, in turn, made it possible to develop the highly successful Teaching-Family Model, a group home treatment program for troubled predelinquent youths that has been extensively field tested, evaluated, and widely disseminated. In the Teaching-Family system, the youths have been shown to make important changes in their home, educational, and delinquency-related behavior as a consequence of participating in the point system of the group home (Blase, Fixsen, and Phillips 1984). Such KD research, although independent in its conduct from subsequent KU and D&D, may nonetheless be viewed as a facet of intervention research inasmuch as it is indirectly related to eventual KU and D&D carried out by others.

At the macro level, the basic intervention strategy of the Mobilization for Youth, the widely noted Office of Economic Opportunity program in the Lower East Side of Manhattan, was based on prior independent research in differential opportunity theory. The strategy assumed that the most efficacious means for aiding youth development and preventing delinquency was to provide open channels for upward mobility to low-income youth. Previous independent research had shown that a prime cause of delinquent and predelinquent behavior stemmed not from internal personality deficits, but rather from blocked access to opportunity within the social structure. The medium of intervention was thus designed to be structural rather than personal (Cloward and Ohlin 1960).

A second type of KD is *purposely linked to KU and D&D*, as is suggested by the solid lines connecting KD, KU, and D&D in Figure 1. An example of such planned interconnectedness can be found in the work of Fairweather and his associates (Fairweather 1967; Fairweather and Tornatzky 1977). The researchers began with the problem of long-term confinement of patients in mental hospitals and the objective of finding ways to reintroduce them into the community more quickly. Initially, a series of knowledge development activities were undertaken. This included a survey of patients to acquire data about length of hospitalization, a quasi-experiment focused on patients who stayed less than 90 days compared with those with more extended confinement, and an experimental study of four treatment approaches–individual psychotherapy, group therapy, group living, and job training and placement. Based on these and other data, the project moved into a knowledge utilization effort, in which an innovative intervention was designed to address the initiating problem. The intervention involved a Community Lodge concept whereby a small group of patients would live together in a community-based residence on a self-directing basis.

The intervention was then put into development in mental health settings and field-tested. Controlled evaluation was conducted and resulted in a favorable assessment of the approach. At that point, a vigorous diffusion program was undertaken to systematically promote the Lodge model in the mental health field. All the facets of intervention research were carried out within this project through interrelated longitudinal activities. The example illustrates that when this holistic approach is taken, KD and KU overlap the initial stages of D&D.

In their compendium on applying knowledge for practical ends, Glaser, Abelson, and Garrison (1983) describe what is essentially this second type of KU in intervention research in a way that brings forth some of its salient characteristics and assumptions.

> It calls for a rational sequence of activities from research to development to packaging before dissemination takes place. It assumes [substantial] planning. . . . Evaluation is particularly emphasized in this model, in which there is a high initial development cost and which anticipates a high payoff in terms of the quantity, and quality, of a long-range benefits through the model's capacity to reach a large audience of potential users. (404-405)

A third means of conducting KD consists of KD which is *directly joined with or incorporated into D&D activity*, eliminating the need for an intermediary application or conversion step. For example, in the phase of problem analysis and project planning in D&D, there are many aspects of the problem that need to be analyzed using conventional KD research methodology. If the problem were child abuse, for instance, empirical research could be conducted as an aspect of the D&D work to determine the extent of the difficulty, such as its incidence or prevalence, views and experiences of practitioners and/or clients, the component aspects of the problem, possible causal factors, effects of the problem, and shortcomings of current interventions. In the state-of-the art review, examination of current practice in the intervention area may readily involve gathering fresh data by means of conventional research methods, as could many aspects of a D&D feasibility study. Most aspects of evaluation in the evaluation phase likewise involve applications of conventional research methods. It is in this way that the conventional research methods of KD can contribute knowledge directly applicable to D&D as a closely related adjunct to carrying out the steps and phases of the D&D process.

KNOWLEDGE UTILIZATION

The findings from research generally cannot be applied to practice without some intermediate process to put the knowledge into more usable form. The processes and activities by which knowledge from research may be made practical have come to be known as knowledge utilization. They typically involve disciplined judgment and appraisal augmented occasionally by empirical research methods, such as meta-analysis. The processes of KU range from the selection, retrieval, appraisal, codification, and synthesis of relevant knowledge to formulating generalizations, stipulating practice guidelines, and making them operational (e.g., see Rothman 1974, 1980a; Thomas 1980, 1984; Mullen, Chapter 8). This reflects the previously described Knowledge-Driven Model of KU as identified by Weiss (1979).

Each of the aspects of the KU process involves critical analytical work which may not be immediately evident. For example, in selecting and appraising knowledge from behavioral and social science, a number of selection criteria have been proposed, such as the content relevance of the findings, the power of the knowledge, and the identifiability, accessibility, and manipulability of the knowledge referents (Thomas 1964). Others who have given attention to knowledge appraisal and selection criteria include Bloom (1975), Gouldner (1957), Fischer (1978), Hanrahan and Reid (1984), Tripodi, Fellin, and Meyer (1969), and Zetterberg (1965). Although not as well developed as the conventional research methods of KD, much more attention has been devoted to KU than to D&D (e.g., see Glaser, Abelson, and Garrison 1983; Havelock 1973; Rogers and Shoemaker 1971; Rothman 1991).

The processes of KU may lead directly into and be an integral part of the information gathering and design phases of D&D, or they may involve the transformation of knowledge for other uses and users, as is shown in Figure 1. Said another way, the Knowledge Utilization model we have described is always an inherent activity in intervention research, as is the use of other sources of information (e.g., allied technology, professional practices) in developing new human service interventions.

SOME FURTHER IMPLICATIONS

Although not proposed as a new paradigm, intervention research is an integrative perspective that provides a view of research that has important implications for the conduct of research and practice, as well as for their relationship. First, the intervention research perspective offers one provisional answer to the oft-repeated question of what type or types of inquiry and research are relevant to human service. From this perspective of intervention research, the answer is KD, KU, and D&D, the three modes of inquiry just described. Bringing them together as facets of intervention research makes explicit that they are parts of a larger enterprise and that they have distinct connections to each other. Considering the interests of human service as they relate to furthering understanding of the human problems it faces and the practical means of addressing these problems, what is needed is not merely more research or research-related practice, but more research that is intentionally interventive in focus in the form of one or another of the three facets of intervention research described here–namely, KD, KU, and D&D. Although, of the three, D&D is the newest on the research scene and to date has been least employed, it is a critical component of intervention research, inasmuch as it is through D&D that new human service interventions may be designed, developed, and evaluated.

In addition to conducting intervention research independently on one of the three facets, the linkages between the facet modes of inquiry suggest ways to conduct research to enhance the immediacy and relevance of the research to interventive interests. Thus, instead of conducting KD without also carrying out subsequent D&D, KD may be conducted with KU activities directly following. KU can be performed with a subsequent D&D project, and KD, KU, and D&D can be conducted as an ordered sequence as they are so often accomplished, for example, in scientific and industrial R&D.

In the training for research in human service and related areas, emphasis in the past has been largely on providing instruction in conventional methods of behavioral and social science research, and not on the applied and technology-oriented research of D&D (e.g., see Thomas 1978b). D&D provides a critically important additional area of research training for all human service researchers. The intervention research specialist must be capable of carrying water, methodologically speaking, on both shoulders. Likewise, in teaching research to practitioners, they should be familiarized with at least some aspects of one or another facet of intervention research, depending upon which facet(s) would be most relevant in their practice and the priority given to research-related training. Training programs in human service presently vary greatly in how much training is provided in any kind of research, with few programs providing much attention as yet to D&D. D&D provides a critically important additional area of training for all human service practitioners. Such training would make it possible for practitioners to participate more effectively in designing, developing, and evaluating the interventive methods upon which direct practice and policy depend.

CONCLUSIONS

The purpose of this analysis was to offer a perspective on research relating to human service intervention that integrates several important contemporary research modalities. This endeavor has encompassed two different foci of integration: different facets of intervention research and different approaches to D&D. In the first instance, research modes have been identified as Intervention Knowledge Development, Knowledge Utilization, and Intervention Design and Development, each of which is viewed as a facet of intervention research. Each type of research has a separate and established methodology, the integrity and distinctness of which should not be affected by viewing it also as part of intervention research. However, by grouping these types together in this way, their relevance to interests involving intervention in human service is emphasized, along with relationships between and among the facets that might otherwise not be as evident.

The same applies to approaches to D&D (particularly developmental research and social R&D) that have been brought together in the Intervention Design and Development facet of intervention research work. Nonspecialists have often viewed these to be separate and different, but we have tried to demonstrate that they, indeed, can be fitted comfortably under one conceptual roof. We trust that the integration achieved by assembling these otherwise divergent or only loosely coupled approaches to research will stimulate further advances along these lines. We are also hopeful that this effort will make available to human service researchers and practitioners a more coherent, authentic, and useful frame of reference for conducting productive research to enhance working tools in the human services.

REFERENCES

Ayllon, T., and N. H. Azrin, 1965. The measurement and reinforcement of behavior of psychotics. *Journal of Experimental Analysis Behavior, 8,* 357-383.

Ayllon, T., and N. H. Azrin, 1968. *The Token Economy: A Motivational System for Therapy and Rehabilitation.* New York: Appleton-Century-Crofts.

Azrin, N. H. 1977. A strategy for applied research: Learning based but outcome oriented. *American Psychologist, 32,* 140-149.

Backer, T. E., R. P. Liberman, and T. G. Kuehnel, 1986. Dissemination and adoption of innovating psychosocial interventions. *Journal of Consulting and Clinical Psychology, 54,* 111-118.

Baer, D. M. , M. M. Wolf, and T. R. Risley. 1968. Some current dimensions of applied behavior analysis. *Journal of Applied Behavior Analysis, 1,* 91-97.

Baer, D. M., M. M. Wolf, and T. R. Risley. 1987. Some still current dimensions of applied behavior analysis. *Journal of Applied Behavior Analysis, 20,* 313-329.

Blase, K., D. Fixsen, and D. Phillips. 1984. Residential treatment for troubled children: Developing service delivery systems. In *Human Services that Work: From Innovation to Standard Practice,* edited by S.C. Paine, G. T. Bellamy, and B. L. Wilcox. Baltimore, MD: Paul H. Brookes Publishing Co.

Bloom, M. 1975. *The Paradox of Helping: Introduction of the Philosophy of Scientific Practice.* New York: John Wiley.

Cloward, R. A., and L. E. Ohlin, 1960. *Delinquency and Opportunity: A Theory of Delinquent Gangs.* New York: The Free Press.

Deitz, S. M. 1978. Current status of applied behavior analysis: Science versus technology. American Psychologist, *33,* 805-813.

Fairweather, G. 1967. *Methods for Experimental Social Innovation.* New York: John Wiley & Sons.

Fairweather, G., and L. G. Tornatzky. 1977. *Experimental Models for Social Policy Research.* Elmsford, NY: Pergamon Press.

Fawcett, S. B., R. M. Matthews, and R. K. Fletcher, 1980. Some promising dimensions for behavioral community technology. *Journal of Applied Behavior Analysis, 13,* 505-518.

Fischer, J. 1978. *Effective Casework Practice: An Eclectic Approach.* New York: McGraw-Hill Book Co.

Glaser, E. M., H. H. Abelson, and K. N. Garrison. 1983. *Putting Knowledge to Use.* San Francisco, CA: Jossey-Bass Publishers.

Gouldner, A. W. 1957. Theoretical requirements of the applied social sciences. *American Sociological Review, 22,* 92-103.

Hanrahan, P., and W. J. Reid. 1984. Choosing effective interventions. *Social Service Review,* 244-258.

Havelock, R. G. 1973. *Planning for Innovations through Dissemination and Utilization of Knowledge.* Ann Arbor: Institute for Social Research, University of Michigan.

Mullen, E. J. 1978. The construction of personal models for effective practice: A method for utilizing research findings to guide social interventions. *Journal of Social Service Research, 2,* 45-65.

Mullen, E. J. 1981. Development of personal intervention models. In *Social work research and evaluation* edited by R. M. Grinnell. Itasca, IL: F. E. Peacock Publishers, Inc.

Mullen, E. J. 1983. Personal practice models. In *Handbook of Clinical Social Work* edited by A. Rosenblatt and D. Waldfogel. San Francisco, CA: Jossey-Bass Publishers.

Paine, S. C. 1984. Models revisited. In *Human Services that Work: From Innovation to Standard Practice* edited by S. C. Paine, G. T. Bellamy, and B. L. Wilcox. Baltimore: Paul H. Brookes Publishing Co..

Paine, S. C., G. T. Bellamy, and B. Wilcox. 1984. *Human Services that Work: From Innovation to Standard Practice.* Baltimore, MD: Paul H. Brookes Publishing Co.

Phillips, E. L., E. A. Phillips, D. L. Fixsen, and M. N. Wolf. 1971. Achievement place: Modification of behavior of free delinquent boys with a token economy. *Journal of Applied Behavioral Analysis, 4,* 45-49.

Reid, W. J. 1979. The model development dissertation. *Journal of Social Service Research, 3,* 215-225.

Reid, W. J. 1983. Research developments. In *1983-84 Supplement to the Encyclopedia of Social Work,* 17th edition, edited by S. Briar. New York: National Association of Social Workers.

Rice, R. E., and E. M. Rogers. 1980. Re-invention in the innovation process. *Knowledge: Creation, Diffusion, Utilization, 1,* 449-515.

Roberts E. B., and A. L. Frohman. 1978. Strategies for improving research utilization. *Technology Review, 80*(5), 32-39.

Rogers, E. M., and F. F. Shoemaker. 1971. *Communication of Innovations: A Cross Cultural Approach.* New York: Free Press.

Rogers, E. 1983. *Diffusion of Innovations,* 3rd ed. New York: The Free Press.

Rothman, J. 1974. *Planning and Organizing for Social Change: Action Principles from Social Science Research.* New York: Columbia University Press.

Rothman, J. 1978. Conversion and design in the research utilization process. *Journal of Social Service Research, 2,* 117-131.

Rothman, J. 1980a. *Social R&D: Research and Development in the Human Services*. Englewood Cliffs, NJ: Prentice-Hall.

Rothman, J. 1980b. *Using Research in Organizations: A Guide to Successful Application*. Beverly Hills, CA: Sage Publications in cooperation with the Institute for Social Research, University of Michigan, and the National Institute for Social Work.

Rothman, J. 1989. Intervention research: Application to runaway and homeless youths. *Social Work Research and Abstracts, 25*(1), 13-18.

Rothman, J. 1991. *Runaway and Homeless Youth: Strengthening Services to Families and Children*. White Plains, NY: Longman.

Rothman, J., J. Teresa, and J. L. Erlich. 1978. *Fostering Participation and Innovation*. Itasca, IL: Peacock Publishers.

Rothman, J., J. G. Teresa, T. L. Kay, and G. C. Morningstar. 1983. *Marketing Human Service Innovations*. Beverly Hills, CA: Sage Publications.

Seekins, T, and S. B. Fawcett. 1987. Effects of a Poverty-Clients' Agenda on Resource Allocations by Community Decision Makers. *American Journal of Community Psychology*, (15) 305-320.

Staats, A. W. 1968. A general apparatus for the investigation of complex learning in children. *Behaviour Research and Therapy, 6*, 45-50.

Stolz, S. B. 1981. Adoption of innovations from applied behavioral research: "Does anybody care?" *Journal of Applied Behavior Analysis, 14*, 491-505.

Thomas, E. J. 1964. Selecting knowledge from behavioral science. *Building Social Work Knowledge: Report of a Conference*. New York: National Association of Social Workers, 38-48.

Thomas, E. J. 1978a. Generating innovation in social work: The paradigm of developmental research. *Journal of Social Service Research, 2*, 95-116.

Thomas, E. J. 1978b. Mousetraps, developmental research, and social work education. *Social Service Review, 52*, 468-483.

Thomas, E. J. 1980. Beyond knowledge utilization in generating human service technology. In *Future of social work research*, edited by D. Fanshel. Washington, DC: National Association of Social Workers, 91-103.

Thomas, E. J. 1984. *Designing Interventions for the Helping Professions*. Beverly Hills, CA: Sage Publications.

Thomas, E. J. 1985. Design and development validity and related concepts in developmental research. *Social Work Research and Abstracts, 21*, 50-58.

Thomas, E. J. 1990. Modes of practice in developmental research. In *Advances in Clinical Social Work Research*, edited by L. Videka-Sherman and W. J. Reid. Silver Spring, MD: National Association of Social Workers.

Tripodi, T., P. C. Fellin, and H. J. Meyer. 1969. *The Assessment of Social Research: Guidelines for the Use of Research in Social Work and Social Science*. Itasca, IL: F. E. Peacock.

Weiss, C. H. (1979). The many meanings of research utilization. *Public Administration Review, 39*(5), September-October, 426-437.

Zetterberg, H. L. 1965. *On Theory and Verification in Sociology*, 3rd rev. ed. Totowa, NJ: Bedminster Press.

Chapter 2

Conducting Intervention Research– The Design and Development Process

Stephen B. Fawcett
Yolanda Suarez-Balcazar
Fabricio E. Balcazar
Glen W. White
Adrienne L. Paine
Katherine A. Blanchard
Melody G. Embree

One important aim of intervention research is to create means for improving community life, health, and well-being. A form of applied research, it examines relationships between conditions identified by clients as important–such as drug abuse or discrimination–and personal or environmental factors that contribute to such conditions. Intervention researchers attempt as much as possible to fuse the dual purposes of applied science in the same endeavor: promoting understanding of individual and community conditions and contributing to their improvement.

There are five related traditions that are particularly useful in

Thanks are extended to the clients of our intervention research efforts and to those professional colleagues who helped the authors to understand these lessons. Grants from the National Institute on Disability and Rehabilitation Research (NIDRR) to the Research and Training Center on Independent Living (Grant #G0085C3502) helped to support the case study reported in this chapter. The authors also gratefully acknowledge grant support from the Kansas Health Foundation of Wichita, Kansas to the Work Group on Health Promotion and Community Development of the Schiefelbusch Institute for Life Span Studies (Grant #9004041) that helped support development of this manuscript.

conducting intervention research: experimental social innovation, social research and development, developmental research, model development research, and behavioral community research. The paradigm of experimental social innovation (Fairweather 1967; Fairweather and Tornatzky 1977) uses quasi-experimental designs to evaluate the effects of treatment programs and other innovations designed to address social problems. Social research and development (Rothman 1980) applies an engineering model from the physical sciences to characterize the process of developing intervention programs relevant to human services. Developmental research (Thomas 1984) incorporates applied research methods, empirically oriented practice, and other action research strategies to design interventions for the helping professions. Model development research examines how human services proceed from innovation to standard practice (Paine, Bellamy, and Wilcox 1984). Finally, behavioral community research uses concepts and methods of behavior analysis and community psychology to design and implement interventions relevant to community change (Fawcett 1990, 1991; Fawcett, Mathews, and Fletcher 1980; Fawcett et al. 1984; Fixsen, Phillips, and Wolf 1978).

Thomas and Rothman, in Chapter 1, outline a general model of intervention research consistent with these overlapping paradigms. The intervention design and development aspect has six phases: (1) problem analysis and project planning; (2) information gathering and synthesis; (3) design; (4) early development and pilot testing; (5) evaluation and advanced development; and (6) dissemination. This model integrates key features of existing paradigms in its interrelated steps (see Figure 2 in Chapter 1).

The purpose of this chapter is to highlight operations required to implement each phase of intervention design and development. These operations are analogous to what Thomas and Rothman term "activities." Some of the operations overlap the activities and others are in addition to the noted activities. The operations that are discussed reflect the involvement and emphasis of the Work Group on Health Promotion and Community Development at the University of Kansas, and supplement previously discussed activities rather than conflict with them.

PHASES AND OPERATIONS
OF INTERVENTION RESEARCH

Figure 1 outlines critical operations within each phase of the intervention research process that help to ensure success. The phases follow the formulation for intervention design and development undergirding this book. Although the phases are outlined linearly, they often merge in practice as investigators respond to opportunities and challenges in the shifting context of applied research. For each phase, key operations for implementation will be described in the discussion to follow. There will then be a case illustration to show how the operations were carried into action in a specific intervention research project.

PROBLEM ANALYSIS AND PROJECT PLANNING

In our work, several operations have been particularly critical to the problem analysis and project planning phase: identifying and involving clients, gaining entry and cooperation from settings, identifying concerns of the population, analyzing identified problems, and setting goals and objectives. Each operation involves collaboration between researchers and clients, helping gain the cooperation and support necessary for conducting intervention research. We will describe the methods and orientation employed in our approach to intervention research.

Identifying and Involving Clients

Intervention researchers choose a constituency or population with whom to collaborate, such as people who are at risk for heart disease or adolescent pregnancy or those who are low-income or have disabilities. We select a population whose issues and problems are of current or emerging interest to clients themselves, researchers, and society. In collaboration with the project's clients, researchers identify the specific targets and goals of the intervention. Research that addresses the critical strengths and problems of important constituencies has a greater chance of receiving support

FIGURE 1. Phases and operations of intervention research.

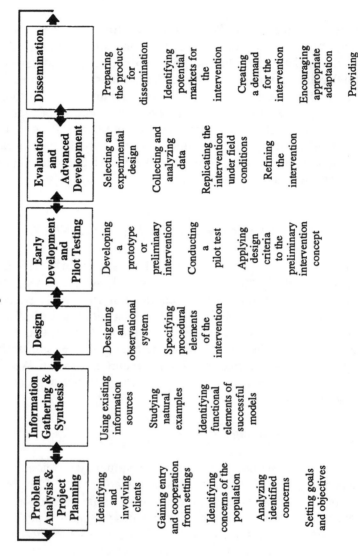

Problem Analysis & Project Planning	Information Gathering & Synthesis	Design	Early Development and Pilot Testing	Evaluation and Advanced Development	Dissemination
Identifying and involving clients	Using existing information sources	Designing an observational system	Developing a prototype or preliminary intervention	Selecting an experimental design	Preparing the product for dissemination
Gaining entry and cooperation from settings	Studying natural examples	Specifying procedural elements of the intervention	Conducting a pilot test	Collecting and analyzing data	Identifying potential markets for the intervention
Identifying concerns of the population	Identifying functional elements of successful models		Applying design criteria to the preliminary intervention concept	Replicating the intervention under field conditions	Creating a demand for the intervention
Analyzing identified concerns				Refining the intervention	Encouraging appropriate adaptation
Setting goals and objectives					Providing technical support forr adopters

from the target population, professional community, and general public.

Gaining Entry and Cooperation from Settings

Key informants can explain local ways to researchers and introduce them to gatekeepers who control access to the setting (Agar 1980). Before approaching an agency or group, investigators should know something about its clients, goals, policies, staff, and programs. Conversations with key informants help researchers understand what they have to offer and how to articulate the benefits for potential participants and members of the group or organization.

Successful intervention researchers form a collaborative relationship with representatives of the setting by involving them in identifying problems, planning the project, and implementing selected interventions (Fawcett 1991). Collaboration helps provide a sense of ownership of the investigation. By working together with those who can facilitate access, researchers gain the cooperation and support necessary to conduct intervention research.

Identifying Concerns of the Population

Intervention researchers must avoid imposing external views of the problem and its solution. Once they have access to the setting, applied researchers attempt to understand the issues of importance to the population. Researchers use informal personal contact (Biddle and Biddle 1968), ethnographic or qualitative research methods (Agar 1980), and surveys and community forums (Fawcett et al. 1982; Rothman 1989).

We have developed the Concerns Report Method to identify the concerns of a variety of people of relative disadvantage who might define the community of interest. Concerns Report applications have involved poverty families (Seekins and Fawcett 1987), residents of low-income neighborhoods (Schriner and Fawcett 1988), institutionalized psychiatric patients, clients of public health services, youth, and people with physical disabilities (Fawcett et al. 1988). The Disabled Citizens' Concerns Report Method has been used by more than 17,000 people with disabilities from 450 different communities in 12 states (Suarez de Balcazar, Bradford, and Fawcett 1988).

Researchers talk with key informants, such as "natural" leaders, advocates, and service providers, to obtain information about local problems and strengths. Researchers may use individual contexts, such as door-to-door canvassing, or group contexts, such as community forums, to clarify dimensions of identified issues and to understand the scope and magnitude of given concerns. By providing an opportunity for clients to identify issues and weigh their importance, control of the research agenda–what is studied and acted upon–is extended to those most affected (Fawcett 1990).

Analyzing Identified Problems

A critical aspect of this phase is analyzing those conditions that people label as community problems. Some key questions help guide the process of problem analysis. What is the nature of the discrepancy between "ideal" and "actual" conditions that defines the problem? For example, if the problem is adolescent pregnancy, what is its actual incidence and prevalence and how does this compare with the normal or ideal incidence for this community? Whose behavior (or lack of behavior) "caused" the conditions that people label as the problem? Whose behavior (or lack of behavior) "maintains" the problem? This analysis helps to frame societal problems in terms of the behavior of key actors and the resulting outcomes or conditions that people label as problems.

For whom is the situation a problem? What are the negative consequences of the problem for affected individuals? What are the negative consequences of the problem for the community? Who (if anyone) benefits from conditions as they are now? How do they benefit? These questions explore the consequences that help explain why the problem exists and why interventions have not succeeded or been attempted.

Who should share the responsibility for "solving" the problem? What behaviors (of whom) need to change for clients to consider the problem solved? What conditions need to change to establish or support needed change? What is an acceptable level of change? This analysis shines the lantern beyond those typically blamed for the problem to others in the immediate or broader environment.

At what level should the problem be addressed? Does the problem reside in the behavior of key individuals, in the immediate physical or social environment, with broader structural conditions such as chronic unemployment, or with governmental or business policies? Is this a multi-level problem requiring action at a variety of levels of change? Is it feasible (technically, financially, politically) to make changes at each identified level? Answers to these and other related questions help guide the choice of intervention research goals.

Setting Goals and Objectives

A final operation in this phase is setting goals and objectives. Goals refer to the broad conditions or outcomes that are desired by the community of interest. A substance abuse initiative, for instance, might cite the following as one of its goals: "Within two years, to reduce the incidence of alcohol use among teen-age youth in the county by 20 percent." Broad goals specify the outcomes, such as risk reduction or goal attainment, that are the end points of intervention efforts.

Objectives refer to those more specific changes in programs, policies, or practices that are believed to contribute to the broader goal. A substance abuse initiative for youth might set several objectives, including: (a) "Within 12 months, to implement training programs on peer refusal of drugs in all classrooms in the school" (program); (b) "Within two years, to pass a city ordinance establishing increased fines for selling alcohol to minors" (policy); and (c) "Within two years, to arrange for peer-led support groups during advisory period in all middle schools in the county" (practice).

In this phase, a careful problem analysis yields potential targets for change and possible elements of the intervention. Stating broad goals and more specific objectives clarifies the proposed ends and means of the intervention research project. These refined purposes help to structure the next phase of knowledge to gathering and synthesis.

INFORMATION GATHERING AND SYNTHESIS

This phase might be subtitled "Not Reinventing the Wheel." When planning an intervention research project, it is essential to discover what others have done to understand and address the problem. Knowledge acquisition involves identifying and selecting relevant types of knowledge and using and integrating appropriate sources of information. Particularly useful sources are existing forms of archival information and natural examples of successful practices of individuals or organizations. The outcome of this phase is a list of apparently functional elements that can be incorporated into the design of the intervention.

There are several key aspects of this phase: using existing information sources, studying natural examples, and identifying functional elements of successful models.

Using Existing Information Sources

A literature review usually consists of an examination of selected empirical research, reported practice, and identified innovations relevant to the social or health concern. Computerized data bases, such as PSYCHLIT or MEDLINE, may be particularly helpful in retrieving possible sources of information.

Intervention researchers must, however, look beyond the literature of their particular fields. This is essential since societal problems do not confine themselves neatly to the disciplines of psychology, social work, architecture, education, public health, or other bodies of knowledge or practice. Thus, intervention research must contribute to both the "scholarship of discovery"–the generation of new knowledge about behavior-environment relations–and the "scholarship of integration"–establishing new linkages between concepts and methods of various disciplines (Boyer 1991).

Studying Natural Examples

A particularly useful source of information is observing how community members faced with the problem, or a similar problem, have attempted to address it (Wolf and Ramp 1991). Interviews with people who have actually experienced the problem, such as clients, or those with knowledge about it, such as service providers, can provide insights into which interventions might or might not succeed, and the variables that may affect success. Studying unsuccessful programs and practices may be particularly valuable, since nonexamples help us to understand methods and contextual features that may be critical to success.

Identifying Functional Elements of Successful Models

Once information is gathered, researchers analyze the critical features of the programs and practices that have previously addressed the problem of interest. Some questions to ask are: Is there a model program, policy, or practice that has been successful in changing targeted behaviors and outcomes? What made a particular program, policy, or practice effective?

Is there a model program, policy, or practice that was unsuccessful? What caused it to fail?

Which events appeared to be critical to success (or failure)? What conditions (e.g., organizational features, client characteristics, broader environmental factors) may have been critical to success (or failure)?

What specific procedures were used in the program, policy, or practice? Was information provided to clients or change agents about how and under what conditions to act? Were modeling, role-playing, practice, feedback, or other training procedures used? What positive consequences, such as rewards or incentives, and negative consequences, such as penalties or disincentives, helped establish and maintain desired changes? What environmental barriers, policies, or regulations were removed to make it easier for the changes to occur?

By studying successful and unsuccessful models of programs that have attempted to address the problem, researchers identify potentially useful elements of an intervention. This synthesis of existing knowledge helps to guide design and development activities.

DESIGN

This and the next section outline operations in the particularly interrelated phases of design and early development and pilot testing. Two types of products result from intervention research: (1) the research data that may demonstrate relationships between the intervention and the behaviors or outcomes that define the problem of interest, and (2) the intervention–which may include a strategy, technique or program; informational or training materials; environmental design variables; a motivational system; a new or modified policy; or other procedures.

There are two particularly important operations during this phase: designing an observational system and specifying procedural elements of the intervention.

Designing an Observational System

Researchers must design a way of observing events related to the phenomenon naturalistically, a method system for discovering the extent of the problem and detecting effects following the intervention. This is critical to pilot testing. The observational system is closely linked to the process of designing an intervention; it serves as a feedback system for refining early prototypes. Clients, especially those most affected by the issue, should be involved in specifying the behaviors and environmental conditions that need to be changed (and observed).

Once the focus of change is identified, it is necessary to define these behavioral events in ways that can be observed (Baer, Wolf, and Risley 1968; Bijou, Peterson, and Ault 1968). The observational system consists of three working parts. First, definitions of the behaviors or products associated with the problem are defined in operational terms. For example, in a substance abuse prevention initiative, the key behaviors that compose peer refusal skills might be specified and defined. Second, examples and nonexamples of the behaviors or products are provided to help discriminate occurrences of the behavior or product. Third, scoring instructions are prepared to guide recording of desired behaviors or products. Relevant behaviors and outcomes may be measured using direct observation by independent observers or self-monitoring or self-reporting for events that may be difficult to observe directly (Barlow, Hayes, and Nelson 1989).

This strategy–also known as functional analysis–helps to establish relationships between environmental changes and behaviors related to the problem. Skinner (1969) emphasized the importance of observing environmental conditions present before the behavior to be changed occurs (antecedent conditions), the response to these antecedent conditions (behavior), and what changes in the environment occur following the behavior (consequences or outcomes). Intervention research using such measurements can help to establish general statements about behavior-environment relationships and the conditions under which they are applicable.

For instance, in an intervention research study designed to promote courteous treatment of clients by receptionists of human service agencies, researchers measured whether receptionists' greetings and other statements showing courtesy (the behavior) occurred when clients entered the agency (antecedent conditions) (Johnson and Fawcett 1988; in press). Results suggested that courteous treatment (the behavior) could be increased by a combination of training, feedback, and incentives (the intervention) and that these effects may generalize to increased client satisfaction with the agency after training (consequences or outcome).

The type of measurement system chosen depends on many factors, including how many individuals and behaviors must be observed, the length of the observation sessions, the size of intervals within the session, and the availability of trained observers (Cooper, Heron, and Heward 1987). The reliability and validity of the observations are affected by observer training and experience and by the complexity and obtrusiveness of the measurement system. Preliminary results from the observation system help to guide the selection of procedures and their refinement.

Specifying Procedural Elements of the Intervention

By observing the problem and studying naturally occurring innovations and other prototypes, researchers can identify procedural elements for use in the intervention. These procedural elements–including use of information, skills, and training for their acquisition, environmental change strategies, policy change or enforcement strategies, or reinforcement or punishment procedures–should be specified in enough detail so that they can be replicated by other typically-trained change agents (Fawcett, Fletcher, and Mathews 1980). For instance, researchers evaluating an agency-based registration procedure to encourage voter registration among poverty clients specified in detail the change in registration site, informational signs, verbal requests to register, and praise for registering to vote that composed the intervention (Fawcett, Seekins, and Silber 1988). The embryonic observational system and intervention are refined in the next phase of intervention research.

EARLY DEVELOPMENT AND PILOT TESTING

During the early development and pilot testing phase, a primitive design is evolved to a form that can be evaluated under field conditions. This phase includes the important operations of developing a prototype or preliminary intervention, conducting a pilot test, and applying design criteria to the preliminary intervention concept.

Developing a Prototype or Preliminary Intervention

By this stage in the design process, preliminary intervention procedures are selected and specified. To develop a prototype for use in pilot testing, researchers may also need to establish and select a mode of delivery, such as workshops, telephone consultation, peer-mediated instruction, or other ways of communicating the intervention to intended users. For example, researchers attempting to reduce violations of handicapped parking spaces developed a protocol to encourage local merchants to install upright handicapped parking signs and police officers to enforce existing ordinances (Suarez de Balcazar, Fawcett, and Balcazar 1988). Feedback from consumers and implementers should be obtained to help refine and simplify the prototype for the intervention.

Conducting a Pilot Test

Pilot tests are designed to determine whether the intervention will work–"to see if the beast will fly." Pilot tests are implemented in settings convenient for the researchers and somewhat similar to ones in which the intervention will be used. When access to real settings is difficult, researchers sometimes test prototypes in analog situations, such as initially testing a training program for low-income peer counselors by using actors to play the role of actual clients (Whang, Fletcher, and Fawcett 1982). The observational system that was devised is instrumental here. These pilot tests help to determine the effectiveness of the intervention and identify which elements of the prototype may need to be revised.

Applying Design Criteria
to the Preliminary Intervention Concept

The design process is informed by common guidelines and values for intervention research. There is considerable agreement about standards for appropriate community intervention in the related fields of behavioral psychology (Baer, Wolf, and Risley 1968, 1987), behavioral community psychology (Fawcett, Mathews, and Fletcher 1980; Fawcett 1990, 1991), and social welfare (Thomas 1984). Relevant questions include: Is the intervention effective? Is it replicable by typical end-users? Is it simple to use? Is it practical? Is the intervention adaptable to various contexts? Is it compatible with local customs and values?

Although such criteria do not suggest how to optimize these standards, they do help to guide the design of interventions that are subjected to pilot testing and formal evaluation.

EVALUATION AND ADVANCED DEVELOPMENT

Intervention research is distinguished from pure activism by its use of research methods to examine how and why a change program does or does not work. Using pilot tests and field replications to test and refine the intervention sets intervention research apart from mere program evaluation.

There are four major aspects of the evaluation and advanced development phase: selecting an experimental design, collecting and analyzing data, replicating the intervention under field conditions, and refining the intervention.

Selecting an Experimental Design

Experimental designs, whether single-subject or between-group designs (Hersen and Barlow 1984; Cook and Campbell 1979;

Thomas 1984), help demonstrate causal relationships between the intervention and the behaviors and related conditions targeted for change. Factors affecting design choice include the goals and magnitude of change sought by clients, the types of behaviors and the desired immediacy of changes, the stability of the setting or context, and the goals of the research.

Single-subject designs, such as the interrupted time-series design (Cook and Campbell 1979) or multiple baseline design (Baer, Wolf, and Risley 1968), are particularly valued in intervention research. These designs control for historical artifacts that could be misinterpreted as changes due to an implemented intervention. Such designs also rule out other threats to internal validity (Campbell and Stanley 1968). With these designs, repeated measures of the target behavior are obtained before and after an intervention that is staggered across individuals, groups, or communities. Visual inspection is usually sufficient to detect changes or discontinuities following intervention. Since demonstrations of experimental control require larger effects with single-subject designs, they are particularly appropriate to the usual goal of intervention research: producing socially (not only statistically) significant results.

Collecting and Analyzing Data

During a pilot test and more formal evaluations of an intervention, data are collected and analyzed continuously. Ongoing graphing of the behavior and related outcomes helps to determine when initial interventions should be implemented and whether supplemental procedures are necessary.

Using two or more independent observers to collect data at the same time helps to ensure the reliability or replicability of the findings. As a general rule, levels of interobserver agreement of 80 percent or higher throughout the research suggest that the instrumentation is consistent over time. Such reliability assessments help readers to judge whether the measurement system will yield similar results if used by others.

Replicating the Intervention Under Field Conditions

A primary goal of intervention research is to develop interventions that are effective in a variety of real-life contexts with those who actually experience the problem. Replication under various field conditions helps to assess the generality of the effects of the intervention.

Additional testing under actual field conditions is necessary if initial evaluations are conducted with analog participants, under simulated situations, or implemented by other than the eventual users. By the time the intervention has reached this stage, instructions, manuals, and other tangible forms of the prototype will have been developed, tested, and revised.

Refining the Intervention

Errors are instructive: the results of full field testing are used to resolve problems with the measurement system and intervention. For example, a substance abuse prevention program designed to encourage peer support among adolescents may be effective with middle-income, but not low-income, youths or vice versa. Adaptations in the language, content, and intervention methods may produce desired behavior changes and outcomes for the full range of intended beneficiaries. Repeated tinkering with the intervention helps to ensure that it will reliably produce intended effects.

DISSEMINATION

Once the community intervention has been field tested and evaluated, it is ready to be disseminated to community organizations and other target audiences. Several operations help to make the process of dissemination and adaptation more successful: preparing the product for dissemination, identifying potential markets for the intervention, creating a demand for the intervention, encouraging appropriate adaptation, and providing technical support for adopters.

Preparing the Product for Dissemination

In preparing the intervention for dissemination, several issues emerge: choosing a brand name, establishing a price, and setting standards for the intervention's use (Seekins and Fawcett 1988).

Choosing a Brand Name

A brand name helps differentiate an intervention from other similar ones at the point of adoption and while in use. For example, the brand names "Teaching-Family Model" (Phillips et al. 1971) or "Community Lodge Model" (Fairweather 1967) enable potential adopters to distinguish these group home programs from other residential interventions for predelinquent youths and adults with psychiatric disabilities. Adopters come to recognize brand names for community interventions; they associate the name with certain values such as effectiveness, dependability, or efficiency.

Establishing a Price

Choosing the right price for the intervention is important when attempting to penetrate a market segment, such as staff or administrators of particular types of health or human service organizations. When the goal is widespread adoption with little necessity for ongoing technical support, such as for a simple training procedure, the price might be set low to reflect the modest development and production costs and the limited discretionary budget of potential adopters. When the goal is slower diffusion to adopters who may require extensive technical support, such as in the case of a comprehensive treatment program for vulnerable populations, the price (in terms of money, staff time, and organizational requirements) might be set at an appropriately higher level.

Setting Standards for Use

By establishing guidelines for using community interventions correctly, researchers provide the basis for maintaining the integrity of the product. For example, the Concerns Report Method (Fawcett et al. 1982) uses an established protocol for conducting needs assessments and community forums. Specifications about the conditions of local sponsorship under which it can be used, the procedures for involving clients, and other features help to assure the integrity of the process and the quality of the product.

Identifying Potential Markets for the Intervention

In defining a market of potential adopters for a community intervention, researchers should ask several questions. Which people can benefit personally from the intervention? Who (with the use of the intervention) could contribute most to solving the problem? Is the goal of dissemination broad-based adoption (i.e., saturation of the market) or more restricted use by selected adopters? Which market segments–types of health or human service organizations– would most likely adopt and benefit from the intervention if they were aware of it? Which media approach–public service announcements, direct mail, or other strategies–would be most appropriate and feasible to inform the targeted market segment?

It may also be helpful to identify potential "early adopters" whose use of the product may encourage others in the selected market segments to adopt the intervention. Researchers disseminating the Concerns Report Method, for example, targeted opinion leaders in the independent living movement as sponsors for early applications of this needs assessment process (Fawcett et al. 1988). Rogers and Shoemaker (1971) suggest that early adopters' potential influence may be associated with their relatively greater resources, sophistication, education, and willingness to try innovative practices. Perhaps such characteristics put them in more frequent contact with their colleagues, increasing the chances that these potential adopters will see firsthand the benefits of using the innovation.

Creating a Demand for the Intervention

Disseminators must convince potential purchasers that they will really benefit from the intervention. Seekins and Fawcett (1988) identified several strategies used in marketing of innovations, including modeling of the innovation, arranging sampling of the innovation and its benefits, and advertising.

Modeling

Models–including experts, celebrities, or others with whom the selected market segment can identify–are shown using the innovation and deriving benefits from its use. Similar modeling strategies are commonly used to "sell" socially useful ideas, practices, and products. Consider, for example, the widespread use of public service advertisements featuring professional athletes on inner-city streets telling kids why they should not use drugs.

Sampling

The effects of modeling can be further enhanced by offering opportunities for potential purchasers to sample relevant products. For example, researchers interested in disseminating training materials for leaders of self-help groups (see the case study to follow) provided information, demonstrations, and opportunities to review materials at national and regional conferences. If sampling results in positive consequences for the targeted adopter and ultimate client, the likelihood of adoption and continued use of the intervention is increased.

Advertising

These modeling and sampling strategies can be supplemented by advertising campaigns that prompt potential adopters to obtain and use the product. Advertising highlights desirable features of the intervention such as its effectiveness relative to other products, low cost, and decreased time and effort for users. For example, printed brochures for a Consumer Involvement Training Program (Balcazar et al. 1989; Seekins, Balcazar, and Fawcett 1986) featured testimonials from early adopters that highlighted the product's effectiveness and utility. The advertising campaign may also include other incentives to encourage adoption, such as a description of support services available with the purchase of the innovation. Ultimately, such strategies for enhancing demand will succeed if the product provides adopters with such benefits as effectiveness, low cost, and less user time relative to other similar interventions currently on the market.

Encouraging Appropriate Adaptation

Adaptation–sometimes known as "reinvention" (Rice and Rogers 1980)–of an innovation occurs when adopters modify the intervention to fit local conditions after its original development by others. Elements of interventions, such as the content and format of an educational program, may be modified or deleted, and new elements may be added (Seekins and Fawcett 1991). There is, of course, a tension between permitting reinvention (adaptation) and preserving the quality of the intervention (model fidelity). Encouraging adaptation may accelerate the rate of adoption, but some changes may result in a loss of effectiveness, dependability, or other valued attributes of the innovation (Seekins and Fawcett 1988). Disseminators are challenged to permit (and even encourage) necessary adaptation while collecting ongoing measures of process and outcome to determine whether the intervention continues to meet established standards.

Providing Technical Support for Adopters

Intervention researchers and program staff, as the innovation's designers and implementers, are the primary knowledge experts concerning the intervention. Adopters may require support personnel from the research or program team to assist with troubleshooting or adapting the intervention to meet their specific needs (Ramp 1984). For example, adopters of the Concerns Report Method (Fawcett et al. 1982) for setting client improvement agendas received technical assistance that included help in establishing working groups, preparing surveys, conducting data analysis, and implementing community forums. As private sector enterprises with a reputation for excellence have discovered, technical support may be critical in implementing the product (Peters and Waterman 1982). This is important since those innovations that reliably produce the intended consequences are more likely to maintain long-term client satisfaction.

A CASE STUDY OF INTERVENTION RESEARCH: DEVELOPING A STRATEGY TO ENHANCE SELF-HELP GROUPS THROUGH LEADER TRAINING

This general model of intervention research is illustrated in a case study. The phases of the process–problem analysis and project planning, information gathering and synthesis, design, early development and pilot testing, evaluation and advanced development, and dissemination–are depicted in the case example. The case study features a training program for peer leaders of self-help groups.

Self-help groups are a common form of support for an estimated 15 million people (Riessman 1982). These groups exist for people who experience many types of problems in living (e.g., spouse abuse), health conditions (e.g., AIDS), and disabilities (e.g., parents of children with spina bifida). These groups are formed by people who come together to share their experiential knowledge about common concerns (Borckman 1976). The power of mutual-aid groups lies in the giving and receiving of support for personal concerns.

This case study describes the design and development of a strategy of facilitative interaction, and of a training program for leaders of self-help groups to aid them in using it. It notes how support is provided when group members share experiences with common problems and how leader training can enable members to be better resources for each other.

Intervention Research Process

Problem Analysis and Project Planning

This project developed in response to concerns by self-help clearinghouse staff and self-help group leaders about the need for a means of improving the functioning of self-help groups and for sharpening leadership skills. Self-help group leaders have experiential knowledge that enables them to help others, yet there are aspects of group leadership in which they may benefit from some support or training.

The researchers conducted phone interviews with self-help group leaders to identify the goals of their support groups and any problems with group functioning (Suarez de Balcazar et al. 1989). Leaders reported group goals to include emotional-peer support, information, and problem solving. The problems in group functioning reported by leaders included a lack of participation by group members, limited setting of personal goals, minimal sharing of information and advice, and inequitable distribution of group responsibilities.

Consultations with local group leaders, peer counselors, and directors of self-help clearinghouses further confirmed the need for leadership development to address the concerns of peer group leaders and professionals assisting self-help groups. Consultations also provided information about what effective group leaders and members do during meetings and the leadership skills that may help encourage members to participate more fully.

The broad goal of this intervention research project was consistent with goals of self-help group leaders: to enhance the ability of self-help groups to establish a supportive environment for group members. One instrumental objective was to develop a handbook that provides modeling and prompting techniques used to establish effective leadership skills. An evaluation objective was to examine the effects of such procedures on supportive transactions in self-help groups.

Information Gathering and Synthesis

An extensive review of the literature (Suarez de Balcazar 1986) yielded a preliminary list of behaviors related to the construct of support. It also suggested the need for an objective measurement system for recording behaviors that demonstrate support among group members. Consultations with self-help clearinghouse directors, peer counselors, and self-help group leaders–and observations of group meetings–helped refine the list of support activities and critical leadership skills. These behaviors were incorporated into the training program for leaders.

Researchers approached a nonprofessional staff member of a poverty agency about the possibility of starting a peer-led self-help group for low-income women. The staff person acknowledged the need for the group and agreed to be the leader. She had worked for the agency for approximately 18 years and had personal experience as a client of public assistance programs. The researchers expressed their interest in learning about support groups and in collaborating with the group leader and members to develop a leader's handbook.

Researchers also approached the leader of a Multiple Sclerosis self-help group about collaborating with the research project. The researchers solicited and responded to feedback from group leaders and members about the importance of identified leadership skills and the acceptability of leader training methods and materials.

We obtained permission from the group leaders and members to audiotape group meetings. Audiotapes of each meeting were transcribed and analyzed to identify and define the behaviors involved in leading and participating in group meetings.

The literature review and study of different types of naturally occurring self-help groups helped to pinpoint what may be a critical feature of well-functioning groups–something we have termed "supportive transactions" (Paine et al. 1992). A supportive transaction refers to when a member's disclosure about a personal problem is followed by one or more types of support (e.g., emotional support, information about alternatives, supportive disclosure by another member). Well-functioning groups may ensure that members who disclose personal problems receive at least some form of support. This assumption helped to guide the design and early development and pilot testing phases.

Design

At one level, the researchers designed an intervention strategy for encouraging facilitative interaction among members of self-help groups. Researchers also designed the tools to implement the strategy: a leader training handbook (Paine et al. 1990) and an observational coding system for assessing support in self-help groups (Paine, Suarez de Balcazar, and Fawcett 1988). Their design involved several steps. First, an extensive literature review on social support yielded a list of behaviors of self-help group members such as emotional support, information about alternatives, modeling, goal setting, and tangible assistance (Suarez de Balcazar 1986). Second, audiotapes of actual group meetings permitted analysis of the activities of members and leaders, expanded the list of behaviors, and helped to refine their definitions. Third, consultations from experts in the area of social support and self-help further refined the list of behaviors and definitions. An observational coding system, the Self-Help Behavior Assessment Instrument (Paine, Suarez de Balcazar, and Fawcett 1988), included definitions, scoring instructions, and examples and nonexamples of self-help group behaviors such as disclosure, emotional support, information about alternatives, prompting, and other behaviors of leaders and members of self-help groups. Finally, the researchers specified the procedural elements of the intervention, including modeling, role-playing, and feedback on the use of skills for promoting supportive interactions.

Early Development and Pilot Testing

The *Leader's Handbook* (Paine et al. 1990) was designed to be effective, easy to read, complete, and practical. The training format used in the prototype consisted of traditional methods of behavioral instruction–clear descriptions of target behaviors, rationales, examples, practice, and feedback (Borck and Fawcett 1982; Fawcett and Fletcher 1977). Each handbook chapter contained a description of and rationale for each leadership skill, examples and written exercises, and role-play situations to practice each skill. Training with the handbook took approximately eight to ten hours of reading the text (or hearing the content presented orally), discussing the examples and exercises, and role-playing. The prototype for the handbook was first pilot tested with university students in a simulated group support situation. Feedback from the initial pilot test suggested that the training showed some effects with supportive transactions, but might be shortened and simplified to meet the time demands and learning requirements of leaders.

Evaluation and Advanced Development

The initial evaluation of the leader training was conducted in collaboration with the leaders of two mutual-aid groups: one for low-income women and another for people with multiple sclerosis (Paine et al. 1992). A multiple baseline design across groups, also known as an interrupted time series design with switching replications (Cook and Campbell 1979), was used to evaluate the effectiveness of leader training in increasing the percentage of supportive transactions. Observations of group members' and leader's behaviors were recorded from transcripts of audiotaped group meetings. Researchers recorded the frequency of support activities (e.g., disclosure, emotional support), the percentage of supportive transactions that included each type of support (e.g., information about alternatives, emotional support), and the frequency of leader prompts to encourage support.

Training with the low-income women's group was conducted during several one- to two-hour sessions between two of the group's biweekly meetings. Comments and suggestions from the group leader helped to clarify unclear sections of the handbook and led to substantive modifications. For example, the low-income women's group leader did not feel comfortable with the suggested format for asking direct questions about what members planned to do outside the meeting, and this method of prompting was modified accordingly. The handbook was then used with the leader of the multiple sclerosis self-help group. Although the training procedures remained essentially the same as with the low-income women's group leader, they were also modified to accommodate leader concerns. For example, suggestions to encourage group members to set personal goals were largely eliminated in accordance with this group's norms.

The results of this study indicated that the training procedures may have increased the percentage of occurrence of certain types of supportive transactions: those including statements of information about alternatives, for the low-income women's group; and statements of supportive disclosure, for the multiple sclerosis self-help group (Paine et al. 1992). Consistent with the project's goals, its evaluation focused on the process of supportive transactions in self-help groups. Since group leaders did not endorse a particular outcome for participants, an assessment of group effectiveness was deemed inappropriate.

These findings suggest that the handbook may help sharpen leadership skills and that different parts of the handbook may be useful for different types of groups. The handbook was refined in field testing. The content was modified to reflect experiences and learning styles of additional users. Further replications of the training procedures under controlled conditions will help refine the methods and establish the generality of these findings.

Dissemination

The researchers conducted workshops for group leaders using the *Leader's Handbook* and developed a workshop leader's guide to assist in dissemination. Conference presentations and brochures announcing the availability of workshops for group leaders helped to promote awareness of this training program. Additional brochures describing what support groups do and what a group member should expect to give and receive at group meetings were widely distributed and served as an indirect promotional activity.

The handbook was designed for use by self-help group leaders. Markets for the handbook include staff of self-help clearinghouses, independent living centers, and other health, education, and human service agencies that provide workshops for self-help group leaders and members. Approximately 200 handbooks were distributed on a national basis in the first two years of dissemination. As materials are adopted within different cultural contexts, we would expect them to be adapted or redesigned to fit culturally defined modes of support. Adopters may use different parts of the handbook or workshop guide and adapt particular sections to meet their own needs.

Summary

This intervention research project resulted in new knowledge about self-help group functioning and a training program for self-help group leaders. The intervention, a facilitative interaction strategy, and related *Leader's Handbook,* helped to establish a more supportive environment. This resulted from providing members and leaders with an opportunity to develop their skills in sharing personal experiences and obtaining needed support and information. This facilitation of self-help group functioning may contribute to feelings of personal empowerment for group members and an enhanced capacity to cope (and helping others to cope) with problems in living.

GENERAL CONCLUSION

This chapter described a model of intervention research that attempts to enhance our understanding of community conditions and, in particular, the effectiveness of interventions intended to improve them. The model is interactive, assuming a dynamic interplay between clients, researchers, and eventual purchasers and users of interventions. Collaboration between researchers and clients in all phases–from identifying community problems to adapting the innovation in context–helps to assure more effective products in the intervention research paradigm.

Several challenges must be addressed by intervention researchers. First, intervention design and development takes a long time, with a given project usually exceeding the expected lengths of commitment for a graduate student's thesis or dissertation. Accordingly, it is often necessary (and appropriate) to arrange shorter-term rewards for graduate student collaborators, such as publications of pilot research or descriptive reports about the project and interim findings. Second, intervention research is labor-intensive, requiring the involvement of many junior research colleagues whose work must be supported through both course credit and grants or other funding.

Third, the work of intervention research is complex, demanding a variety of research and interpersonal skills, ranging from collecting and analyzing data to puzzling through how to embed an intervention in a politically sensitive context. Fourth, the methodological challenges of conducting research in real-world contexts and the presumption that applied work cannot be scientific make the professional rewards uncertain. Intervention research requires an ability to see possible natural experiments and to balance rigor and relevance (Fawcett 1991). Finally, the length of intervention research projects, often three or more years, requires an educated hunch about what society will be concerned about in the future and a strategy for sustaining support for the endeavor beyond usual cycles of grant funding. When these challenges are overcome, researchers can experience the satisfaction of product-oriented, collaborative research.

Innovations that result from intervention research can serve as powerful tools for community change. By developing methods relevant to the concerns of disadvantaged and marginal populations, scientist-practitioners can contribute to understanding of and attention to the inequities that contribute to their problems in living. By involving clients as collaborators, design and development efforts build upon the experiential knowledge of those affected. When effective methods of addressing community problems are widely adopted, the effects of intervention research are multiplied. As such, intervention researchers can blend the roles of scientist and change agent as they attempt to understand and improve local communities and their organizations and initiatives.

REFERENCES

Agar, M. H. 1980. *The Professional Stranger: An Informal Introduction to Ethnography.* New York: Academic Press.

Baer, D. M., M. M. Wolf, and T. R. Risley. 1968. Some current dimensions of applied behavior analysis. *Journal of Applied Behavior Analysis,* 1, 91-97.

Baer, D. M., M. M. Wolf, and T. R. Risley. 1987. Some still current dimensions of applied behavior analysis. *Journal of Applied Behavior Analysis,* 20, 313-327.

Balcazar, F. E., T. Seekins, S. B. Fawcett, and B. L. Hopkins. 1989. Empowering people with physical disabilities through advocacy skills training. *American Journal of Community Psychology,* 18(2), 281-296.

Barlow, D. H., S. C. Hayes, and R. O. Nelson. 1989. *The Scientist Practitioner: Research and Accountability in Clinical and Educational Settings.* New York: Pergamon Press.

Biddle, W. W., and L. J. Biddle. 1968. *The Community Development Process.* New York: Holt, Rinehart, & Winston.

Bijou, S. W., R. F. Peterson, and M. H. Ault. 1968. A method to integrate descriptive and experimental field studies at the level of data and empirical concepts. *Journal of Applied Behavior Analysis,* 1, 175-191.

Borck, L. E., and S. B. Fawcett. 1982. *Learning Counseling and Problem Solving Skills.* Binghamton, NY: The Haworth Press.

Borckman, T. 1976. Experiential knowledge: A new concept for the analysis of self-help groups. *Social Service Review,* September, 445-453.

Boyer, E. April 5, 1991. Remarks made during a forum on challenges to higher education at the University of Kansas by the President of the Carnegie Foundation for the Advancement of Teaching.

Campbell, D. T., and J. C. Stanley. 1968. *Experimental and Quasi-Experimental Designs for Research.* Chicago: Rand McNally & Company.

Cook, T. D., and D. T. Campbell. 1979. *Quasi-Experimentation:* Design and Analysis Issues for Field Settings. Chicago: Rand McNally College Publishing Company.

Cooper, J. O., T. E. Heron, and W. L. Heward. 1987. *Applied Behavior Analysis.* Columbus, Ohio: Merrill Publishing.

Fairweather, G. W. 1967. *Methods for Experimental Social Innovation.* New York: John Wiley and Sons.

Fairweather, G. W., and L. G. Tornatsky. 1977. *Experimental Methods for Social Policy Research.* New York: Pergamon Press.

Fawcett, S. B. 1990. Some emerging standards for community research and action. In *Researching Community Psychology: Integrating Theories and Methodologies*, edited by P. Tolan, D. Keys, F. Chertok, and L.E. Jason. Washington, DC: American Psychological Association, 64-75.

Fawcett, S. B. 1991. Some values guiding community research and action. *Journal of Applied Behavior Analysis, 24*, 621-636.

Fawcett, S. B., and R. K. Fletcher. 1977. Community applications of instructional technology: Training writers of instructional packages. *Journal of Applied Behavior Analysis, 10*, 739-746.

Fawcett, S. B., R. K. Fletcher, and R. M. Mathews. 1980. Applications of behavior analysis in community education. In *Behavioral Community Psychology: Progress and Prospects*, edited by D. S. Glenwick and L. A. Jason. New York: Praeger, 108-142.

Fawcett, S. B., R. M. Mathews, and R. K. Fletcher. 1980. Some promising dimensions of behavioral community psychology. *Journal of Applied Behavior Analysis, 13*, 505-518.

Fawcett, S. B., T. Seekins, and L. Silber. 1988. Low-income voter registration: A small-scale evaluation of an agency-based registration strategy. *American Journal of Community Psychology, 16*, 751-758.

Fawcett, S. B., T. Seekins, P. L. Whang, C. Muiu, and Y. Suarez de Balcazar. 1982. Involving consumers in decision making. *Social Policy, 13*, 36-41.

Fawcett, S. B., T. Seekins, P. L. Whang, C. Muiu, and Y. Suarez de Balcazar. 1984. Creating and using social technologies for community empowerment. *Prevention in the Human Services, 3*, 145-171.

Fawcett, S. B., Y. Suarez de Balcazar, P. Whang-Ramos, T. Seekins, B. Bradford, and R. M. Mathews. 1988. The concerns report: Involving consumers in planning for rehabilitation and independent living services. *American Rehabilitation, 14*(3), 17-19.

Fixsen, D. L., E. L. Phillips, and M. M. Wolf. 1978. Mission-oriented behavior research: The teaching family model. In *Handbook of Applied Behavior Analysis*, edited by T. Brigham and C. Catania. New York: Irvington, 603-628.

Hersen, M., and D. H. Barlow. 1984. *Single Case Experimental Designs: Strategies for Studying Behavior Change* (2d Edition). New York: Pergamon.

Johnson, M. D. and S. B. Fawcett. *In press*. Courteous service: Its assessment and modification in a human service organization. *Journal of Applied Behavior Analysis*.

Johnson, M. D. and S. B. Fawcett. 1988. Quality circles: Enhancing responsiveness of service agencies to consumers. *American Rehabilitation, 14*, 20-21.

Paine, S. C., G. T. Bellamy, and B. Wilcox. 1984. *Human Services that Work: From Innovation to Standard Practice*. Baltimore: Paul H. Brooks.

Paine, A. L., Y. Suarez de Balcazar, and S. B. Fawcett. 1988. *The Self-help Behavioral Assessment Instrument*. Lawrence, KS: The Research and Training Center on Independent Living, University of Kansas.

Paine, A. L., Y. Suarez de Balcazar, S. B. Fawcett, and L. Borck-Jameson. 1990. *Self-Help Group Leader's Handbook: Leading Effective Meetings*. Lawrence,

KS: The Research and Training Center on Independent Living, University of Kansas.

Paine, A. L., Y. Suarez-Balcazar, and S. B. Fawcett, and L. Borck-Jameson. 1992. Supportive transactions: Their measurement and enhancement in two mutual-aid groups. *Journal of Community Psychology, 20*, 163-180.

Peters, T. S., and R. H. Waterman, Jr. 1982. *In Search of Excellence: Lessons from America's Best-Run Companies*. New York: Harper & Row.

Phillips, E. L., E. A. Phillips, D. L. Fixen, and M. M. Wolf. 1971. Achievement Place: Modification of behavior of predelinquent boys with a token economy. *Journal of Applied Behavior Analysis, 4*, 45-59.

Ramp, K. K. 1984. Effective quality control for social service programs: One piece of the puzzle. In *Human Services that Work: From Innovation to Standard Practice*, edited by S. C. Paine, G. T. Bellamy, and B. Wilcox. Baltimore: Paul H. Brooks, 261-268.

Rice, R. E., and E. H. Rogers. 1980. Reinvention in the innovation process. *Knowledge: Creation, Diffusion. and Utilization, 1*, 499-513.

Riessman, F. 1982. The self-help ethos. *Social Policy, 13*, 42-43.

Rogers, E. M., and F. F. Shoemaker. 1971. *Communication of Innovations: A Cross-Cultural Approach* (2d ed.). New York: The Free Press.

Rothman, J. 1980. *Social R&D: Research and Development in the Human Services*. New Jersey: Prentice-Hall, Inc.

Rothman, J. 1989. Intervention research: Application to runaway and homeless youth. *Social Work Research and Abstracts, 25*, 13-18.

Schriner, K. F., and S. B. Fawcett. 1988. Development and validation of a community concerns report method. *Journal of Community Psychology, 16*, 306-316.

Seekins, T., F. E. Balcazar, and S. B. Fawcett. 1986. *Consumer Involvement in Advocacy Organizations, Vol. I-IV.* Lawrence, KS: The Research and Training Center on Independent Living, University of Kansas.

Seekins, T. and S. B. Fawcett. 1987. Effects of a poverty clients' agenda on resource allocations by community decisionmakers. *American Journal of Community Psychology, 15*, 305-320.

Seekins, T., S. B. Fawcett. 1988. *Toward an Implicit Technology of Dissemination.* Unpublished manuscript, Department of Human Development and Family Life, University of Kansas, Lawrence.

Seekins, T., and S. B. Fawcett. 1991. *Two Studies Using Procedures to Encourage Re-Invention.* Unpublished manuscript, Department of Human Development, University of Kansas, Lawrence.

Skinner, B. F. 1969. *Contingencies of Reinforcement: A Theoretical Analysis.* New York: Appleton-Century-Crofts.

Suarez de Balcazar, Y. 1986. Review of research conducted with self-help groups and analysis of support behaviors performed by members during group meetings. Unpublished manuscript, Department of Human Development, University of Kansas, Lawrence.

Suarez de Balcazar, Y. B. Bradford, and S. B. Fawcett. 1988. Common concerns of disabled Americans: Issues and options. *Social Policy, 19*(2), 29-35.

Suarez de Balcazar, Y., S. B. Fawcett, and F. E. Balcazar. 1988. Effects of environmental design and police enforcement on violations of handicapped parking spaces. *Journal of Applied Behavior Analysis, 21*, 291-298.

Suarez de Balcazar, Y., T. Seekins, A. L. Paine, S. B. Fawcett, and R. M. Mathews. 1989. Self-help and social support groups for people with disabilities: A descriptive report. *Rehabilitation Counseling Bulletin, 23*(2), 151-158.

Thomas, E. J. 1984. *Designing Interventions for the Helping Profession.* Beverly Hills, CA: Sage Publications.

Thomas E. J., and J. Rothman. In press. *Intervention Research: Creating Effective Methods for Professional Practice.* Binghamton, NY: The Haworth Press.

Whang, P. L., R. K. Fletcher, and S. B. Fawcett. 1982. Training counseling skills: An experimental analysis and social validation. *Journal of Applied Behavior Analysis, 15*, 325-334.

Wolf, M. M., and K. K. Ramp. 1991. Consumer feedback and the teaching-family model: On the *auld art* of keeping dragons away. Unpublished manuscript, University of Kansas, Lawrence.

PROBLEM ANALYSIS AND PROJECT PLANNING

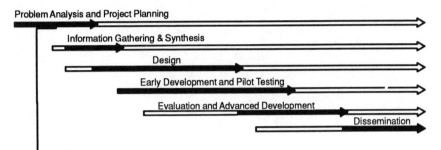

Problem Analysis and Project Planning

Information Gathering & Synthesis

Design

Early Development and Pilot Testing

Evaluation and Advanced Development

Dissemination

Identify and analyze
key problems

Initiate state-of-
the-art review

Determine feasibility
(e.g., technical,
financial,
organizational,
political, etc.)

Prepare project plan

Set a development
goal

Chapter 3

Problem-Centered Intervention Research– Methods of the Second Type

William N. Dunn

INTRODUCTION

In the past twenty and more years there has been considerable progress in intervention theory and research. Early work synthesizing extant research on planned social change (Rothman 1974) presented the general contours of an approach to intervention research. Some of the later work on social R&D (Rothman, 1980a) elaborated this early approach, while others (e.g., Thomas 1984) extended it in useful ways. Intervention research has drawn heavily on knowledge utilization, a rapidly growing field in which a considerable body of literature has accumulated (see Glaser, Abelson, and Garrison 1983; Dunn and Holzner, 1988). In contrast to research on knowledge utilization, which often resembles a spectator sport in its largely passive approach to describing and explaining processes of knowledge transfer to policymakers and practitioners, intervention research employs an active or experimental approach to social problem solving (see, for example, Fairweather 1967; Fairweather and Tornatzky 1977). Here, the primary goal is not conducting research, per se, but utilizing research-based knowledge to design specific tools for improving practice and policy (Rothman 1974; 1980a; 1980b).

Despite notable achievements, the emerging field of intervention theory and research thus far has not acknowledged or addressed a methodological and practical problem facing all the social sciences: Methods employed by practitioners of intervention research are not appropriate for structuring or formulating problems as an essential aspect of their solution.[1] This methodological deficit is often fatal, judging by the large number of systematic studies, case materials, and records of experience which show that applied social scientists fail more often because they formulate the wrong problem than because they choose the wrong solution (see, for example, Ackoff 1974b, Fischhoff 1977, 1986; Hogwood and Peters 1985; Mitroff, Mason, and Barabba 1983; Siebe 1981). To paraphrase John Tukey, we sorely lack methods which yield "an approximate answer to the right question, which is often vague, [rather] than an exact answer to the wrong question, which can always be made precise" (quoted in Rose 1977:23).

This methodological deficit often creates enormous difficulties for intervention researchers and other practitioners of the applied social sciences. Rothman (1989:17), for example, suggests that anticipatory problem formulation may have enhanced the success of the Runaway Adolescent Pilot Project (RAPP):

> In presenting a complete picture of the interventive process, certain organizational obstacles should be pointed out; social research and development cannot be conducted effectively without anticipation of some degree of interorganizational turbulence . . . there were bureaucratic delays, different time expectations, contract difficulties, disruptive turn-over in DCS staff, misunderstandings, executive management problems, reluctance by line staff to fill out forms, and others.

To be sure, every obstacle or problem cannot be anticipated. But problem structuring methods can make a significant contribution to the programmatic foresight necessary in complex practice domains.

In the absence of appropriate problem structuring methods, intervention researchers are hampered in efforts to formulate problems which encompass the most important elements, for example, suit-

---

1. Representative of the negligent stance toward problem structuring in the social sciences is the disclaimer by Cook and Campbell in what many (including this author) regard as one of the most innovative and philosophically reflective methodology texts available to the applied social scientist: "Many topics . . . will only be lightly touched upon, including . . . how to check on the importance of one's guiding research questions . . ." (Cook and Campbell 1979:2).

able project objectives, creative design options, or constraints on the achievement of expected project outcomes. Given a particular formulation of the problem, how can they know when all or most of the important problem elements have been included in the set? How can they know when they have formulated an approximate solution to the right problem, as distinguished from an exact solution to the wrong problem?

When faced with these questions, intervention researchers are in a situation similar to that of the homesteaders described by Morris Kline in *Mathematics: The Loss of Certainty* (1981). The homesteaders, while clearing their land, are aware that enemies lurk in the wilderness which lies beyond the clearing. To increase their security, the homesteaders clear a larger and larger area, but never feel completely safe. They frequently must decide whether to clear more land, or attend to their crops and domesticated animals within the perimeter. The homesteaders do their best to push back the wilderness, knowing full well that the wilderness is always there, and that one day enemies may surprise and destroy them. The homesteaders also are aware that there are enemies within, enemies which may undermine and distort their judgment. They hope that they will not choose to tend the crops and livestock when they should have chosen to clear more land.

THE STRUCTURE OF PRACTICAL PROBLEMS

Intervention researchers, like homesteaders, require methods which enable them to know when they have cleared enough land, that is, to know when they have approximated the proper boundaries of a problem. The bulk of social science research methods available today, however, assume that the boundaries of problems are or have been well defined. Many writings in the applied social sciences posit that practical problems come in relatively well-bounded packages in which there is an explicit statement of some decisionmaker's preferences, a systematic exposition of the alternative actions available, and a model that relates these alternatives to the stated preferences in a manner which permits an efficient choice among the alternatives (see Stokey and Zeckhauser 1978).

This view of practical problems assumes that the boundaries

which circumscribe preferences, alternatives, and their relationships are relatively well defined. In effect, we are faced with what Mitroff (1974:223-24) describes as a structured decision problem, where the relationships between decisionmakers (D_i), preferences or utilities (U_{ij}), alternatives (A_i), outcomes (O_j), and states of nature (S_j) are certain, probabilistic, or uncertain. Structured problems "are problems about which enough is known so that problems can be formulated in ways that are susceptible to precise analytic methods of attack" (Mitroff 1974: 224).

Structured decision problems are properly contrasted with problems which are "ill structured" (Simon 1973), "squishy" (Strauch 1976), or "messy" (Ackoff 1974b). Formally, an ill-structured problem is one for which decisionmakers (D_i), preferences or utilities (U_{ij}), alternatives (A_i), outcomes (O_j), or states of nature (S_j) are unknown or equivocal. In the language of intervention project design, ill-structured problems have several common properties (compare Harmon and King 1985:28):

- *Project Goals*. The goals of a project are ambiguous or unknown, so that determining what goals to achieve is part of the problem. "Our problem is not to do what is right," stated Lyndon Johnson, "our problem is to know what is right" (Wood 1968:v).

- *Project Phases*. The phases through which project goals are to be achieved are indeterminate. Linkages among phases are complex; feedback and feedforward loops may occur at any time. The pattern of phases is more like a tangled river network (Beer 1981:30) than an assembly line, tree, or cycle.

- *Project Alternatives*. The solution alternatives required to achieve goals are ambiguous or unknown. Knowledge about what alternatives work best under which conditions is rudimentary or simply unavailable, making the process of policy-program design uncertain at best (Linder and Peters 1985, 1987).

- *Project Problem Domain*. The domain of potentially relevant goals, phases, and alternatives is unbounded. No exhaustive or even approximate set of goals, phases, and instruments is available. The problem domain thus appears to be unmanageably huge, requiring what Dery (1984:6) calls "a never-ending discourse with reality."

Characterized in this fashion, ill-structured problems are not uncommon; they are pervasive (Simon 1973:186). The pervasiveness of ill-structured problems is primarily a consequence of the fact that conflicting representations of problems are continuously created, maintained, and changed by stakeholders who affect and are affected by an intervention. If one or a few stakeholders were engaged in the cooperative formulation of problems, then it would be feasible and appropriate to invest the bulk of time and effort to solving relatively well-structured problems. The typical case, however, is one in which intervention researchers spend great energy attempting to understand the conflicting problem definitions of large numbers of stakeholders.

In analyzing and formulating social policies in legislative settings, for example, it is not only necessary to address the problem definitions of legislators, but also those of legislative staff, executive agency personnel, and representatives of numerous public interest groups. Seasoned analysts know well that the process of formulating problems occurs throughout the policymaking process; it involves legislators and other immediate clients as well as what Lipsky (1971) calls "street level bureaucrats." The problem definitions of ordinary citizens situated at the "periphery" of the policymaking process must also be understood (Sabatier and Mazmanian 1983:149-151). Thus, the process of formulating problems is not confined, temporally or spatially, to those phases of policymaking conventionally labelled "problem formulation" or "problem analysis." Competing problem formulations are distributed throughout the policymaking process.

Stakeholders situated at various locations in the policy or project cycle actively construct different representations of problems, using different sets of assumptions to interpret external events which Dewey called a "problem situation." These sets of assumptions, which have been variously described as conceptual models (Allison 1971), systems of interpretation (Rein 1976), cognitive maps (Axel-

rod 1976), schema (Taylor and Crocker 1980), frames of reference
(Holzner and Marx 1979), and construction systems (Dunn et al.
1986), differ among stakeholders who construct, for their own interest or survival, competing representations of the same problem
situation. Yet critical elements of a problem situation may lie outside the boundaries of a given construction system; what is unrec-
ognized and unknown cannot be understood or anticipated. Inade-
quately trained technicians at nuclear power facilities may endanger
millions of citizens by searching for air leaks with candles (Fischhoff 1977), warnings placed on cigarette packages may preclude
future opportunities to confront public health problems (Sieber
1981), and the institutionalization of pretrial release actually may
increase the jail population (Nagel and Neef 1976).

A major challenge facing intervention research is to deal effectively with the complexity arising from the mutual construction of
problems. In designing and implementing social interventions, researchers often face a tangled network of competing problem formulations, a problem-of-problems (metaproblem) which is ill structured because the domain of relevant goals, phases, and solution
alternatives is unbounded, that is, unmanageably huge. Here, the
central task is to structure a problem-of-problems, a second-order
entity which is the class of all first-order problems, which are its
members. Unless these two levels of problems are clearly distinguished, we are likely to formulate the wrong problem by confusing
member and class, thus ignoring the rule that "whatever involves
all of a collection must not be one of the collection" (Whitehead
and Russell 1910:37; also see Watzlawick, Weakland, and Fisch
1974:6). To the extent that intervention researchers and other applied social scientists ignore this rule, they can claim approximately
75 years of obsolescence (compare Bateson 1972:279; also see
Hofstadter 1979).

THE PRINCIPLE OF METHODOLOGICAL CONGRUENCE

The distinction between member and class, between second-order and first-order problems, provides a basis for assessing the
appropriateness of different methods now available to the applied
social scientist (see Dunn 1988). Methods can be assessed accord-

ing to what might be called the principle of methodological congruence: The appropriateness of a particular type of method is a function of its congruence with the type of problem under investigation. The principle of methodological congruence is similar to a more general principle which, originally stated by L. A. Zadeh, asserts that conventional scientific methodologies are incompatible with social problems which have exceeded a given threshold of complexity (see Brewer and de Leon 1983:125).

The bulk of methods available to applied social scientists are methods of the first type, that is, methods appropriate for relatively well-structured problems where relationships between decision-makers (D_i), utilities (U_{ij}), alternatives (A_i), outcomes (O_j), and states of nature (S_j) are certain or probabilistic. These first-order methods, well known to users of standard research methods and statistics textbooks, include procedures ranging from questionnaire and survey design to modern multivariate analysis. The principle of methodological congruence asserts, however, that these first-order methods are inappropriate, and therefore should not be used to address second-order problems which have been characterized as squishy, messy, or ill structured. Surveys, for example, are appropriate and useful first-order methods which enable the efficient and reliable collection of answers to questions that researchers believe to be important. But survey design provides no way to determine what questions should be included within the set. This second-order task cannot be accomplished with methods of the first type.[2]

The principle of methodological congruence, in addition to specifying the conditions under which distinct levels of methods are appropriate, helps to remove some of the ambiguities surrounding the definition of Type III errors. In contrast to Type I and Type II statistical errors, Type III errors are typically defined in somewhat vague terms as conceptualizing, formalizing, or solving the "wrong" or "less appropriate" problem (see, for example, Mitroff and Featheringham 1976; Raiffa 1968:264). By drawing on the

---

2. Focus groups, open-ended interviews, brainstorming, and other generative procedures are often used in conjunction with survey and questionnaire design. Although these procedures are methods of the second type, as defined here, the argument below suggests they are essentially ineffective as problem structuring methods.

distinction between member and class we may formulate a more concrete definition of Type III errors: solving the wrong problem by employing a method whose level is incongruent with that of the problem under investigation.

Some of the practical consequences of observing or ignoring the principle of methodological congruence are suggested in Figure 1, which displays a process of problem-centered intervention research. The process of problem-centered intervention research involves several important distinctions:

Problem Sensing and Problem Structuring. Intervention research rarely begins with clearly articulated problems, but with a sense of diffuse worries and inchoate signs of stress (Rein and White 1977:262). These are not problems, but problem situations. Policy problems "are products of thought acting on environments; they are elements of problem situations that are abstracted from these situations by analysis. What we experience, therefore, are problem situations, not problems which, like atoms or cells, are conceptual constructs" (Ackoff 1974b:21).

Problem Structuring and Problem Solving. Intervention research is a multi-level process which includes first-order methods of problem solving as well as second-order methods of problem structuring. Methods of problem structuring are meta-methods, in that they are "about" and "come before" methods of problem solving. The principle of methodological congruence suggests that first-order methods of problem solving are rarely if ever appropriate for structuring second-order problems. When practitioners apply first-order methods to second-order problems they typically make "errors of a third kind: solving the wrong problem" (Raiffa 1968:264).

Problem Resolving, Problem Unsolving, and Problem Dissolving. The terms problem resolving, problem unsolving, and problem dissolving refer to three kinds of error correcting processes (see Simon 1973; Ackoff 1974a). Although the terms "resolving," "unsolving," and "dissolving" stem from the same root (L. *solvere* = to solve or dissolve), these error correcting processes occur at distinct levels (see Figure 1).

Problem resolving involves the reanalysis of a correctly structured problem in order to reduce calibrational errors, for example, errors involving the rejection of the null hypothesis when it is true (Type I error) or accepting the null hypothesis when it is false (Type II error). Problem unsolving, by contrast, involves the abandonment of a solution based on the wrong problem and a return to problem structuring as a means to formulate the right problem. Problem dissolving, on the other hand, involves the recognition and abandonment of an incorrectly formulated problem prior to any effort to solve it.

In summary, methods appropriate at one level are inappropriate at the next. This means that questions of methodological appropriateness cannot be satisfactorily resolved without first considering the level of the problem to which a method is applied. When intervention researchers and other applied social scientists violate the principle of methodological congruence, they are likely to solve the wrong problem, thus committing a Type III error.

METHODS OF THE SECOND TYPE

Methods of the second type, while generally available to the social science community, are seldom included as an integral part of training in applied social research. Textbooks, manuals, and handbooks rarely cover a range of second-order methods which have been expressly designed for structuring second-order problems variously described as squishy, messy, or ill structured. For example, authoritative sources such as the *Handbook of Research Design and Social Measurement* (Miller 1991) contain no references to methods of the second type, such as brainstorming (Osborn 1948), synectics (Gordon 1961), policy capturing (Hammond 1980), the analytic hierarchy process (Saaty 1980), interpretive structural modeling (Warfield 1976), multiple perspective analysis (Linstone et al. 1981), and strategic assumption surfacing and testing (Mason and Mitroff 1981).

Among the hypotheses which might be offered to explain the lack of attention to methods of the second type, it bears notice that

FIGURE 1. Problem-centered intervention research.

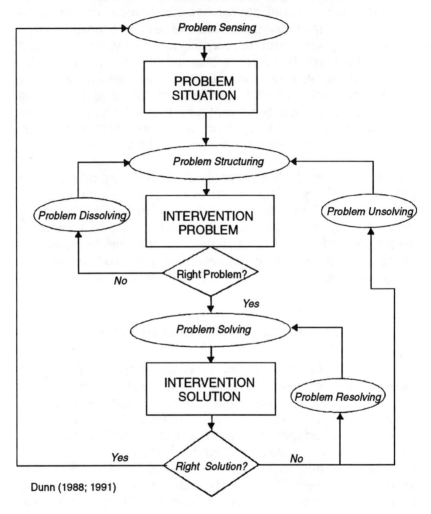

Dunn (1988; 1991)

many who write about research methods have fewer opportunities to work in complex, real-life contexts than practitioners who are the presumed beneficiaries of these methods. Perhaps in response to the rarified incentive systems of academic tenure and professional publishing, those who write about social science research methods may be unaware that policymakers and practitioners spend much of their time structuring policy problems, not solving them. Consequently, there may be considerable time between the emergence of practical needs and efforts to satisfy them through the development of appropriate new methods.

A second plausible hypothesis has to do with the vague or ambiguous character of many methods of the second type. Although there is some recognition that competing perspectives of a problem may assist in the discovery of otherwise hidden policy-program goals, phases, and alternatives, the available guidelines for conducting brainstorming sessions (Osborn 1948), continuous decision seminars (Lasswell 1960), or multiple perspective analyses (Linstone et al. 1981) represent general heuristics which cannot be easily replicated or evaluated. Even when methods of the second type are reasonably well specified and replicable, as is the case with policy capturing (Adelman, Stewart, and Hammond 1975), the analytic hierarchy process (Saaty 1980), and strategic assumption surfacing and testing (Mason and Mitroff 1981), standards for evaluating the extent to which researchers have performed well in structuring a problem are ambiguous or simply unavailable. As Mitroff and Mason acknowledge (1981b:73-86), there is no test which guarantees the completeness of a set of problem representations. Saaty (1980:14) makes much the same point: "there is no set procedure for generating objectives, criteria, and activities to be included in a hierarchy or even a more general system." The ambiguity or absence of performance criteria is closely related to problems of interpreting the results of laboratory and field research on the efficacy of methods of the second type. Understandably, research on the performance of these methods in producing improved problem representations has yielded equivocal or conflicting findings (see, for example, Cosier 1978,1981; Cosier, Ruble, and Aplin 1978; Mason 1969; Mitroff, Barabba, and Kilmann 1977; Mitroff and Mason 1981b; Schwenk and Cosier 1980).

The further development and application of methods of the second type presupposes the identification of explicit criteria for assessing the performance of these methods in structuring problems. A first step in this process is to recognize that all methods of the second type are heuristics which aim at the discovery of elements which define a problem and one or more of their general relationships. Apart from this broad aim, methods of the second type perform functions which are constitutive and regulative (compare Dery 1984:5). Methods designed to discover the elements which define a problem are constitutive, since they answer the question: What elements constitute the problem? Regulative methods, by contrast, aim at the discovery of patterned relations among these elements. Here the question is: How are the elements which define the problem regulated? The distinction between the constitutive and regulative functions of methods calls attention to the fact that the process of problem structuring requires that we test not only our comprehension of patterns believed to regulate a problem, but also the adequacy of our definition of the problem's constituent elements.

Methods of the second type also differ in terms of replicability. Methods with low replicability involve general and ambiguous guidelines, while methods with high replicability involve specific and readily comprehensible prescriptions for performing a defined sequence of operations. As instruments of discovery, such highly replicable methods have been characterized by Landa (1984:39) as algorithmic-heuristics. Nonalgorithmic heuristics, by contrast, are based on imprecise and vague methodological prescriptions, for example, the prescription to examine multiple perspectives of a problem in order to discover its sources and potential solutions.

Methods of the second type may be sorted into four categories (see Table 1) formed by the intersection of types of purpose (constitutive or regulative) and degrees of replicability (high or low). In one category are methods the primary purpose of which is to enumerate or count elements believed to constitute the boundaries of a problem. Although they represent a powerful medium for generating potential policy goals and solution alternatives, these methods tend to be ambiguous and general. Consequently, they cannot be easily replicated by two or more researchers. Methods of the second type, such as brainstorming (Osborn 1948), continuous decision seminars (Lasswell 1960), and multiple perspective analysis (Linstone et al. 1981), belong in this category.

In a second category are methods the purpose of which is to enumerate patterns which regulate elements within the boundaries

TABLE 1. Functions of methods of the second type.

	PURPOSE OF METHOD	
REPLICABILITY OF METHOD	Constitutive	Regulative
Low	ELEMENT ENUMERATION (Multiple Perspective Analysis)	PATTERN ENUMERATION (Interpretive Structural Modeling)
High	ELEMENT ESTIMATION (Policy Grid Analysis)	PATTERN ESTIMATION (Strategic Assumption Surfacing) and Testing)

of a previously defined problem space. Although they are a useful medium for representing a variety of patterned relations among policy goals and alternatives–for example, patterns portrayed by physical and biological metaphors and analogies such as trees, rivers, waterfalls, or epidemics–these methods are, again, so ambiguous and general that they cannot be replicated with the confidence that two or more researchers will reach the same conclusions. Synectics (Gordon 1961) and other forms of analogical reasoning (see, for example, Rein 1976; Schon 1983) belong in this category of methods of the second type.

A third category of methods of the second type includes procedures the purpose of which is to estimate elements which constitute the boundaries of a problem. These methods are highly replicable by virtue of their specificity, precision, and comprehensibility. Presently, there are few methods in this category; the absence of boundary-approximating rules or tests makes it impossible to know whether we have defined the right problem (see Saaty 1980:14; Mitroff and Mason 1981a:73-86). Methods such as policy grid analysis, however, appear to provide replicable estimation procedures (see Dunn and Ginsberg 1986; Dunn 1988; also see Kelly 1955).

In the fourth category are methods of the second type which aim to estimate patterns believed to regulate relationships between previously defined elements, for example, patterns of conflict and cohesiveness, distance and proximity, or consistency and inconsistency among policy actors, policy goals, policy alternatives, and policy outcomes. In this category are highly replicable methods including policy capturing (Adelman, Stewart, and Hammond 1975), interpretive structural modeling (Warfield, 1976), Q-methodology (Brown 1980), the analytic hierarchy process (Saaty 1980), and strategic assumption surfacing and testing (Mason and Mitroff 1981). Singly and in combination, these methods are a powerful medium for creating spatial, geometric, and quantitative representations of the structure of problems. In addition to their replicability, these methods provide tests for estimating the ecological validity (Adelman, Stewart, and Hammond 1975), consistency (Saaty 1980), and plausibility (Mason and Mitroff 1981) of patterns believed to represent the structure of policy problems. Nevertheless, these methods do not permit estimates of the boundaries of a problem.

PERFORMANCE CRITERIA

Our confidence in methods of the second type would be enhanced considerably if explicit criteria were available to assess the performance of researchers in structuring ill-structured problems. In this context, Rescher (1980) has formulated an integrated set of criteria for assessing the plausibility of inductive estimates made under conditions where deterministic and probabilistic conclusions are not possible. These criteria are suitable for assessing the performance of methods of the second type.

Methods of the second type, as noted above, are appropriate under real-life conditions where the researcher does not know and therefore must discover the appropriate decisionmakers (D_i), utilities (U_{ij}), alternatives (A_i), outcomes (O_j) and states of nature (S_j). The function of methods of the second type is to produce plausible estimates of the elements which constitute the problem as well as the patterns regulating these elements (see Figure 2). The plausibility of these estimates—as opposed to their statistical probability or deductive certainty—depends on the extent to which they satisfy requirements of inductive estimates in general (see Rescher 1980:24-26):

Character. An estimate (P*) of a problem (P) must have the same character as its estimanda. An estimate of a length must be a length, not a temperature. In estimating the elements which constitute a problem we typically must estimate elements which are subjective in character, since problems are products of thoughts acting on environments. In turn, estimates of patterns which regulate relationships among elements typically must be systemic, since policy problems are second-order entities composed of the diverse problem formulations of many interdependent stakeholders. In short, any estimate (P*) of a problem (P) must have the character of a representation which is subjectively meaningful in a complex system of stakeholders.

Replicability. The process of producing an estimate (P*) of a problem (P) must be replicable, thus maximizing the likelihood that two or more researchers can obtain similar results in similar circumstances. Without replicable methods researchers are little more than intelligent clinicians who must rely on their own wits and whatever anecdotal knowledge they have acquired through trial and error in the field (Fischhoff 1986:112). The replicability of methods of the second type is a function of their specificity, precision, and comprehensibility.

Coordination. An estimate (P*) of a problem (P) must coordinate with the elements of that problem and their relationships. The closer the process of coordination, the more accurate the estimate. Estimates based on observations of the ways that stakeholders actually construe problems should coordinate more closely than estimates based on the specialized constructs of researchers, for example, constructs such as "rationality," "utility," or "revealed preference."

Cost-Effectiveness. The costs of producing an estimate (P*) of a problem (P) must be reasonable. A method which yields inaccurate estimates at a low cost is less cost-effective than a method which yields accurate estimates at a higher cost, particularly in cases where an inaccurate estimate obscures externalities, sleeper effects, spillovers, and other negative unanticipated consequences. The opportunity costs of defining the wrong problem may be enormous.

Correctness in the Limit. When the information on which an estimate is based becomes increasingly complete, the estimate (P*) of a problem (P) eventually should approximate the true answer being estimated. Although the "true" definition of a problem cannot be known with certainty–indeed, the problem is to estimate the "boundary with ignorance"–increasingly complete information should produce increasingly accurate estimates. In the limit, an estimate (P*) should converge on the true but unknown value of the problem (P).

Methods of the second type now available to the applied social sciences satisfy one or several of these criteria. For example, methods such as multiple perspective analysis and synectics, while they satisfy the criterion of character, do not fare well on criteria of replicability, coordination, and correctness in the limit. Methods such as policy capturing, Q-methodology, interpretive structural modeling, the analytic hierarchy process, and strategic assumption surfacing and testing satisfy in different ways criteria of character, replicability, and coordination. As we have seen, however, these latter methods do not provide any rule or test which permits analysts to assess the completeness of a set of elements defining a problem. In other words, these methods do not satisfy the correctness in the limit criterion. As such, they do not provide plausible estimates (P*) of the elements which constitute a problem (P).

In contrast to these methods of the second type, policy grid analysis (Dunn et al. 1986; Dunn and Ginsberg 1986; also see Mancuso and Shaw 1988) satisfies a performance criterion on which other methods are lacking: correctness in the limit. Apart from meeting the criteria of character, replicability, coordination, and cost-effectiveness, the unique advantage of policy grid analysis is its capacity to estimate the boundaries of a second-order problem composed of the competing problem representations of policy stakeholders.

The method of estimation is precise and readily comprehensible, since it involves a series of three simple steps (Dunn et al. 1986). The first step is saturation sampling, whereby the analyst generates

FIGURE 2. Boundaries of ignorance. Rank by cumulative relative frequency in five knowledge systems.

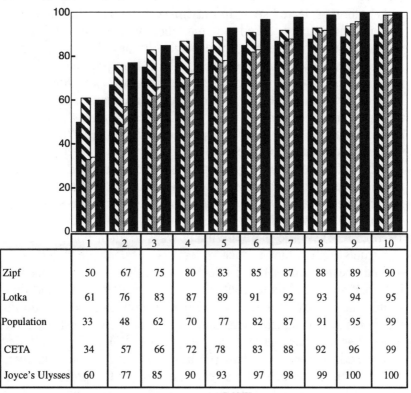

	1	2	3	4	5	6	7	8	9	10
Zipf	50	67	75	80	83	85	87	88	89	90
Lotka	61	76	83	87	89	91	92	93	94	95
Population	33	48	62	70	77	82	87	91	95	99
CETA	34	57	66	72	78	83	88	92	96	99
Joyce's Ulysses	60	77	85	90	93	97	98	99	100	100

BANK

Knowledge Systems
Zipf   Lotka   Population
CETA   Joyce's Ulysses

SOURCES: Zipf (1949), Price (1986), U.S. Bureau of the Census (1989), Dunn (1988), Simon (1972).

a snowball sample of stakeholders who affect or are affected by an existing or proposed intervention. Each person in an initial set of stakeholders, selected so as to maximize differences in issue position and influence, is asked to name others who agree and disagree with one or more existing or proposed solutions. The stakeholders so named are asked to name others, who in turn provide additional names. The process is continued until no new stakeholders are named, at which point "there is no sampling variance, because the total universe has been surveyed, unless one considers the group as some subsample from a super population" (Sudman 1976:211).

The second step involves the elicitation of constructs used by stakeholders to represent a given problem situation. These constructs are the "ideas, basic paradigms, dominant metaphors, standard operating procedures, or whatever else we choose to call the systems of interpretation by which we attach meaning to events" (Heclo 1976:253-54). While there are many ways to elicit policy-relevant constructs (e.g., face-to-face interviews, telephone interviews, mailed questionnaires, computer conferencing), the basic procedure is to ask stakeholders to contrast a range of alternatives and then supply the constructs in terms of which the contrasts were made. At the point when stakeholders can supply no new constructs, the researcher assumes that an accurate estimate (P^*) of the boundaries of the stakeholder's problem (P) has been made. The constructs which form the stakeholder's representation of the problem situation can be subjected to various forms of statistical analysis (see Mancuso and Shaw 1988), although this is not a necessary feature of the process.

The third step in policy grid analysis is second-order boundary estimation. Here the researcher constructs a cumulative frequency distribution of all unique constructs elicited from stakeholders at various stages in the selection of the snowball sample. The various stakeholders are plotted on the horizontal axis; the number of non-duplicative and therefore new constructs is plotted on the vertical axis. As information about the constructs of a gradually expanding sample of stakeholders becomes more complete, estimates of the elements which define the problem space become more accurate. These improvements in the accuracy of estimates represent a continuous transformation of individual problem representations into a systemic or second-order problem representation.

THE BOUNDARIES OF IGNORANCE

The fundamental premise which underlies and justifies all problem structuring methodologies is the principle of bounded ignorance: ignorance is a prerequisite of rationality when dealing with complex problems. The kind of rationality at issue, however, is what may be called *erotetic rationality*. Erotetic rationality, a prerequisite for discovering the boundaries of ignorance, differs from other well-known formulations such as "comprehensive rationality," "bounded rationality," or "economic rationality." In the present period, when many of the most severe social problems involve epistemological uncertainty, it is obviously desirable not only to know *that* we do not know, but also to know *what* we do not know. In this context, there is little promise of knowing what we do not know so long as we visualize problems in terms of (infinitely) open systems or in terms of (infinite) differences in meaning in complex cultural systems. Unbounded ignorance virtually guarantees nonrational or irrational solutions.

The boundaries of ignorance can be approximated, thus meeting the correctness in the limit criterion, by adapting to our purposes work which, initiated by de Saussure in France during the last century, investigated the boundaries and distribution of words in any written text. Work in this area was continued by George Zipf (1949), an American linguist who was also interested in the boundaries and distribution of words in natural languages. Work similar to that of de Saussure and Zipf, although undertaken for different purposes, was also performed in the United States by Lotka (1926) and in the United Kingdom by Bradford (1934). Along with Derek de Solla Price (1986), the latter two were interested in bibliometric problems which involve, as did Zipf's research, large-scale cultural phenomena driving science.

The extraordinary feature of all these investigators is that they discovered, in slightly different forms, law-like regularities within cultural systems with diverse patterns of internal meaning. The same kind of rank-frequency regularities were observed in each of their projects. The rank-frequency law of Zipf states that if the words occurring in a natural language text of sizable length (e.g., Joyce's *Ulysses*) are listed in order of decreasing frequency, then the rank of any given word in the list would be inversely proportional to the frequency of occurrence of the word. Zipf's rank-size law is:

$$r \times f = k$$

where r and f are the rank and frequency of words and k is a constant. In the case of Joyce's *Ulysses*, for example, the words used once and which occupy the first rank occur approximately one-half of the time; the words used twice occur about one-sixth of the time; and one-twelfth occur three times each. Lotka and Bradford found the same pattern in their work on the distribution of scientific productivity and on the redundancy of library holdings.

My own interest in these regularities comes from research using a particular qualitative cognitive mapping method, the policy grid, developed in its original form as the role repertory grid by the American humanistic psychologist George Kelly (1955). After analyzing the distribution of personal constructs elicited from various groups, it was discovered that the distributions approximate Zipf's rank-frequency law. In Figure 2, Zipf's law (series 1) is compared with four additional series including Price's estimate (1986) of the life-time journal productivity of physicists (series 2), my estimate of the rank-population size of the ten largest U.S. cities in 1988 (series 3), the occupational constructs generated during 1983 (Dunn, Cahill, and Kearns 1984) from 135 unemployed workers participating in Comprehensive Employment Training Act (CETA) programs (series 4), and the rank-frequency of uncommon words (see Simon 1972) used in James Joyce's *Ulysses* (series 5). The rank-frequencies for these series are normalized by expressing them as cumulative relative frequencies.

These series show that in each (very different) knowledge system the principles of correctness in the limit and character effectively establish the boundaries of ignorance. Although these results are preliminary, they suggest that it is possible to estimate the boundaries of subjective meanings (the so-called "universe of meaning") in any given knowledge system, thus arriving at approximate knowledge of how much is not known. An important advantage of grid analysis, apart from the bounded ignorance it supplies with respect to complex cultural and cognitive systems, is that the approximate boundaries of a complex system of meanings is frequently reached after 15-25 interviews. It is also possible to transform (logarithmically) both the Zipf and the observed distributions so that they approximate linearity. The deviations of the obtained distribution from the Zipf distribution may be used as an index to estimate the extent to which we have committed errors in defining a policy problem.

By constructing such distributions it is possible to move beyond the notion that meanings are infinite, or so broad that they are simply unmanageable. The experience with these distributions so far strongly indicates that this is not the case.

CONCLUSIONS

Methods of the second type satisfy the requirements for inductive truth estimates in general. When used as a means for furthering the development of intervention research, these methods may contribute to the improvement of our understanding of the complex system of problems typically found in contexts of social policy. Methods of the second type, when aided by knowledge of rank-frequency regularities in knowledge systems, do not only permit us to know how much we do not know about a complex problem for which uncertainties and stakes are high. These methods also call attention to a new definition of (erotetic) rationality on the basis of the principle of bounded ignorance. This may provide some relief to the homesteaders.

REFERENCES

Ackoff, R. L. 1974a. Beyond problem solving. *General Systems, XIX*, 237-239.
Ackoff, R. L. 1974b. *Redesigning the Future: A Systems Approach to Societal Problems*. New York: John Wiley.
Adelman, L., T. R. Stewart, and K. R. Hammond. 1975. A case history of the application of social judgment theory to policy formulation. *Policy Sciences, 6*, 137-159.

Allison, G. T. 1971. *Essence of Decision: Explaining the Cuban Missile Crisis*. Boston: Little, Brown.

Axelrod, R. A. 1976. *Structure of Decision*. Cambridge, MA: Harvard University Press.

Bateson, G. 1972. *Steps to an Ecology of Mind*. New York: Ballantine.

Beer, S. 1981. *The Brain of the Firm*. New York: John Wiley.

Bradford, S. C. 1934. Sources of information on special subjects. *Engineering* 137:85-86.

Brewer, G. D. and P. deLeon. 1983. *The Foundations of Policy Analysis*. Homewood: The Dorsey Press.

Brown, S. R. 1980. *Political Subjectivity: Applications of Q Methodology in Political Science*. New Haven: Yale University Press.

Cook, T. D. and D. T. Campbell. 1979. *Quasi-Experimentation*. Boston: Houghton Mifflin.

Cosier, R. A. 1978. The effects of three potential aids for making strategic decisions on prediction accuracy. *Organizational Behavior and Human Performance, 22*, 295-306.

Cosier, R. A. 1981. Dialectical inquiry in strategic planning: A case of premature acceptance. *Academy of Management Review. 6*. 643-648.

Cosier, R. A., T. L. Ruble, and J. C. Aplin. 1978. An evaluation of the effectiveness of dialectical inquiry systems. *Management Science, 24*, 1483-1490.

Dery, D. 1984. *Problem Definition in Policy Analysis*. Lawrence, KS: University Press of Kansas.

Dunn, W. N. 1988. Methods of the second type: Coping with the wilderness of conventional public policy analysis. *Policy Studies Review. 7*, 4:720-737.

Dunn, W. N., A. G. Cahill, M. J. Dukes, and A. Ginsberg. 1986. The policy grid: A cognitive methodology for assessing change dynamics. In *Policy Analysis: Perspectives, Concepts, and Methods*, edited by W. N. Dunn. Greenwich, CT: JAI Press.

Dunn, W. N., A. G. Cahill, and K. P. Kearns. 1984. Application of the policy grid to work-related frames of reference. Working paper. Pittsburgh: University of Pittsburgh, University Program for the Study of Knowledge Use.

Dunn, W. N. and A. Ginsberg. 1986. A sociocognitive approach to organizational analysis. *Human Relations, 39*(11), 955-975.

Dunn, W. N. and B. Holzner. 1988. Knowledge in Society: Anatomy of an Emerging Field. *Knowledge in Society: The International Journal of Knowledge Transfer*, 1, 1:1-27.

Fairweather, G. W. 1967. *Methods for Experimental Social Innovation*. New York: John Wiley.

Fairweather, G. W. and L. G. Tornatzky. 1977. *Experimental Methods for Social Policy Research*. New York: Pergamon Press.

Fischhoff, B. 1977. Cost benefit analysis and the art of motorcycle maintenance. *Policy Sciences, 8*. 177-202.

Fischhoff, B. 1986. Clinical policy analysis. In *Policy Analysis: Perspectives,*

Concepts, and Methods, edited by W. N. Dunn. Greenwich, CT: JAI Press, 111-128.

Glaser, E. M., H. H. Abelson, and K. N. Garrison. 1983. *Putting Knowledge to Use: Facilitating the Diffusion of Knowledge and the Implementation of Planned Change*. San Francisco: Jossey-Bass.

Gordon, W. J. 1961. *Synectics*. New York: Harper and Row.

Hammond, K. R. 1980. Introduction to Brunswikian theory and methods. *New Directions for Methodology of Social and Behavioral Science*, *3*, 1-12.

Harmon, P. and D. King. 1985. *Expert Systems: Artificial Intelligence in Business*. New York: John Wiley.

Heclo, H. H. 1976. Policy Dynamics. In *The Dynamics of Public Policy*, edited by R. Rose. Beverly Hills: Sage Publications.

Hofstadter, R. 1979. *Godel, Escher, Bach*. New York: Random House.

Hogwood, B. W. and B. G. Peters. 1985. *The Pathology of Public Policy*. Oxford: Clarendon Press.

Holzner, B. and J. Marx. 1979. *Knowledge Application: The Knowledge System in Society*. Boston: Allyn and Bacon.

Kelly, G. 1955. *The Psychology of Personal Constructs*. New York: M. W. Norton.

Kline, M. 1981. *Mathematics: The Loss of Certainty*. New York: Basic Books.

Landa, L. N. 1984. Algorithmic-heuristic theory. In *Encyclopedia of Psychology*, edited by R. J. Corsini and B. D. Ozak. New York: John Wiley.

Lasswell, H. D. 1960. Technique of decision seminars. *Midwest Journal of Political Science*. *4*(2), 213-226.

Linder, S. H. and B. G. Peters. 1985. From social theory to policy design. *Journal of Public Policy*. *4*(3), 237-259.

Linder, S. H. and B. G. Peters. 1987. A design perspective on policy implementation: The fallacies of misplaced prescription. *Policy Studies Review*. *6*(3), 459-475.

Linstone, H. G., A. A. Meltsner, M. Adelson, A. Mysior, L. Umbdenstock, B. Clary, D. Wagner, and J. Shuman. 1981. The multiple perspective concept: With applications to technology assessment and other decision areas. *Technological Forecasting and Social Change*. *20*, 275-325.

Lipsky, M. 1971. Street-level bureaucracy and the analysis of urban reform. *Urban Affairs Quarterly*. *6*, 391-409.

Lotka, A. J. 1926. The frequency distribution of scientific productivity. *Journal of the Washington Academy of Science* 16, 2:317-323.

Mancuso, J. C. and M. L. G. Shaw (eds.) 1988. *Cognition and Personal Structure: Computer Access and Analysis*. New York: Praeger Press.

Mason, R. O. 1969. A dialectical approach to strategic planning. *Management Science*. *15*, 403-414.

Mason, R. O. and I. I. Mitroff. 1981. *Challenging Strategic Planning Assumptions: Concepts, Techniques, and Methods*. New York: John Wiley.

Miller, D. C. 1991. *Handbook of Research Design and Social Measurement*. 4th ed. Newbury Park, CA: Sage Publications.

Mitroff, I. I. 1974. *The Subjective Side of Science.* New York: Elsevier.

Mitroff, I. I., V. P. Barabba, and R. H. Kilman. 1977. The application of behavioral and philosophical technologies to strategic planning: A case study of a large federal agency. *Management Science. 24,* 44-58.

Mitroff, I. I. and T. Featheringham. 1976. Towards a behavioral theory of systemic hypothesis-testing and the error of the third kind. *Theory and Decision. 7,* 205-220.

Mitroff, I. I. and R. O. Mason. 1981a. *Creating a Dialectical Social Science: Concepts, Methods, and Models.* Dordrecht: D. Reidel.

Mitroff, I. I. and R. O. Mason. 1981b. The metaphysics of policy and planning: A reply to Cosier. *Academy of Management Review. 6,* 649-651.

Mitroff, I. I., R. O. Mason, and V. P. Barabba. 1983. *The 1980 Census: Policymaking Amid Turbulence.* Lexington, MA: D.C. Heath.

Nagel, S. S. and M. Neef. 1976. Two examples from the legal process. *Policy Analysis. 2*(2), 356-357.

Osborn, A. F. 1948. *Your Creative Mind.* New York: Charles Scribner.

Price, D. de S. 1986. *Big Science, Little Science—and Beyond.* New York: Wiley.

Raiffa, H. 1968. *Decision Analysis.* Reading, MA: Addison-Wesley.

Rein, M. and S. H. White. 1977. Policy research: Belief and doubt. *Policy Analysis. 3*(2), 239-272.

Rein, M. 1976. *Social Science and Public Policy.* Baltimore: Penguin Books.

Rescher, N. 1980. *Induction.* Pittsburgh: University of Pittsburgh Press.

Rose, R. 1977. Disciplined research and undisciplined problems. In *Using Social Research in Public Policy Making,* edited by C. H. Weiss. Lexington, MA: D. C. Heath, 23-36.

Rothman, J. 1974. *Planning and Organizing for Social Change: Action Principles from Social Science Research.* New York: Columbia University Press.

Rothman, J. 1980a. *Social R&D: Research and Development in the Human Services.* Englewood Cliffs, NJ: Prentice-Hall Publishers.

Rothman, J. 1980b. *Using Research in Organizations: A Guide to Successful Application.* Beverly Hills: Sage Publications.

Rothman, J. 1989. Intervention research: Application to runaway and homeless youths. *Social Work Research and Abstracts. 25*(1), 13-18.

Saaty, T. L. 1980. *The Analytic Hierarchy Process.* New York: McGraw-Hill.

Sabatier, P. A. and D. A. Mazmanian. 1983. Policy implementation. In *Encyclopedia of Policy Studies,* edited by S. S. Nagel. New York: Marcel Dekker.

Schon, D. A. 1983. *The Reflective Practitioner.* New York: Basic Books.

Schwenk, C. R. and R. A. Cosier. 1980. Effects of the expert, devil's advocate, and dialectical inquiry methods on prediction performance. *Organizational Behavior and Human Performance. 26,* 409-424.

Sieber, S. D. 1981. *Fatal Remedies.* New York: Plenum.

Simon, H. A. 1972. The sizes of things. In *Statistics: A Guide to the Unknown,* Edited by J. M. Tanur, F. Mosteller, W. H. Kruskal, R. F. Link, R. S. Dieters, and G. R. Rising. San Francisco, CA: Holden-Day. 195-202.

Simon, H. A. 1973. The structure of ill-structured problems. *Artificial Intelligence. 4*, 181-201.

Stokey, E. and R. Zeckhauser. 1978. *A Primer of Policy Analysis*. New York: Norton.

Strauch, R. E. 1976. A critical look at quantitative methodology. *Policy Analysis. 2*, 121-144.

Sudman, S. 1976. *Applied Sampling*. New York: Academic Press.

Taylor, S. E. and J. Crocker. 1980. Schematic bases of social information processing. In *Social Cognition*, edited by E. Higgins. Hillsdale, NJ: Erlbaum.

Thomas, E. 1984. *Designing Interventions for the Helping Professions*. Beverly Hills, CA: Sage Publications.

Warfield, J. B. 1976. *Societal Systems: Planning, Policy, and Complexity*. New York: John Wiley.

Watzlawick, P., J. Weakland, and R. Fisch. 1974. *Change: Principles of Problem Formation and Problem Resolution*. New York: W. W. Norton.

Whitehead, A. N. and R. Russell. 1910. *Principia Mathematica. 1.* Cambridge: Cambridge University Press.

Wood, R. C. 1968. Foreword. In *The Study of Policy Formation*, edited by R. A. Bauer and K. J. Gergen. New York: The Free Press.

Zeckhauser, R. and E. Shaefer. 1968. Public policy and normative economic theory. In *The Study of Policy Formation*, edited by R. A. Bauer and K. J. Gergen.

Zipf, G. 1949. *The Principle of Least Effort*. New York: Addison-Wesley.

Chapter 4

Planning for Intervention Research

Jack Rothman

Project planning is a basic requirement for any research endeavor, regardless of its purpose or methodological bent. It is necessary to consider such matters as study design, funding, staffing, sampling, data analysis, and the reporting of findings. In intervention research, general considerations such as these pertain, but certain factors receive particular emphasis or unique treatment. This discussion of planning for intervention research assumes that readers are familiar with research planning generally, or can readily access such information in other available published sources. I will focus on the more distinctive features, with special reference to design and development.

The characteristics of intervention research affect the nature of planning for its implementation. There is a dual intended output consisting of a knowledge product, in common with other research, and also a practical product, in the form of an intervention device or method. This involves the researcher in the formulation and actual implementation of a practice or program initiative, a special case of what Perloff (1979) designates "evaluator intervention." The role has also been referred to as "a program advocate . . . someone who believes in and is interested in helping programs and organizations succeed" (Shadish, Cook, and Leviton 1991). The researcher is both creating and studying change-producing social innovations at the same time, in the same arena. Perloff observes that this allies the researcher compassionately with the welfare of those whose benefit is being pursued, but also poses methodological quandaries. From the standpoint of human resources planning, it points to the need for broader than typical staffing competencies within the project. Skills and perspectives encompassing both scientific inquiry and practice application must be included and brought into productive inter-action.

Intervention research thus cannot be performed by a lone investigator who embodies all relevant domains. The research needs to be conducted out of an organizational base that provides diverse resources. Haug (1971) puts it this way:

> The . . . common current format is the 'project,' involving one or more researchers, assistants and clerk-technicians. Such a project may be located temporarily in an agency, as is frequently the case in evaluative research, or it may be housed in a university or research center, in which instance it will do . . . research in one or more agencies on a visiting basis, or focus on some segment of the population without regard to agency affiliation. (198-199)

Because of the need for an organizational infrastructure, according to Haug, bureaucratic factors enter into project planning. Provision must be made for capabilities representing research management. The organization element includes, as implied, acquisition of an applied setting in which innovative interventions-in-the-making can be developed and put to trial use. Twain (1975) addresses this in terms of "sponsorship." He indicates that a variety of methods can be used to obtain and maintain such agency sponsorship and that different forms of sponsorship may be employed. This places additional demands on the planning process.

Because of the complex and multifaceted character of intervention research, it requires a long-term effort consisting of a series of distinct but interconnected phases performed over time. Planning may thus be thought of as encompassing a sequence of sub-studies, each of which is different and substantial in its own right. At the same time, each one has to be planned with reference to what preceded it and what will follow. Initial planning seeks to provide both sufficient structure to project forward through the set of phases and enough flexibility to allow modification of plans based on experiences and results produced along the way.

These orienting considerations will shape the discussion to follow. The concept of phases, which was treated last in the introduction, will be covered first in the body of the analysis.

PHASED ACTIVITIES OVER TIME

The time span for an intervention research project may extend over a five- to ten- year period. My initial work in the Community Intervention Project included a three-year segment for retrieval and synthesis of relevant research literature together with the formulation of intervention designs, another three years for field testing and development of selected designs, and three years for diffusion of a resulting practice handbook. This was a particularly elongated time frame because the methodology of intervention research was tested and shaped while simultaneously being employed in practice. In that sense, the methodology itself was being piloted, requiring extra time. Further experience has shown that a nine-year span can be contracted considerably. For example, in another project, work through intervention design was accomplished within a year. Still, a substantial multi-year outlook is always necessary.

The extensive time-line implicates funding, facilities, staff retention, etc. It is typically impractical to secure funding at the outset to cover the full extent of the work. It most cases, it is necessary to obtain funds for an early segment and to acquire sequential waves of funding as the project proceeds. In addition, since the nature of the work shifts considerably from phase to phase, it is not necessary to hire and maintain a full-complement and consistent staff group throughout. Only a core staff requires tenure–perhaps the director, maybe an assistant, and a trusted secretary-office manager. Twain (1975) observes that: "the provision of long-term funding to maintain institutional support for a core . . . staff is essential. As projects are terminated, successive projects can be worked into the budget" (42). The number of staff members and facility space requirements fluctuates from phase to phase, with the strongest demands coming during the field testing/development period. While "phase funding" (as it is termed by Twain) is less than blanket support, it is a realistic and probably necessary way to proceed and can have successful results. Some anxiety, slippage, and inefficiency can be expected under the circumstances, but even in industrial R&D undertakings that are similarly prolonged, funding materializes in stages based on in-process outcomes and changing market conditions.

With this phased arrangement it is possible to approach different funding sources for different segments of work. Certain governmental agencies or foundations are highly interested in the consolidation and synthesis of knowledge, others respond favorably only to controlled field experiments, and there are those that lean toward the dissemination/utilization of knowledge or of practice innovations. It is possible, if necessary, to frame each phase so as to strike a different, seemingly self-contained pose, while providing continuity and holistic integrity within the project entity. Planning, in this framework, must allow time for further support planning as the work proceeds.

The protracted task environment presents a potential hazard with both academic and practical ramifications. If one assumes that findings and reports in the form of monographs, articles, and books come into being only at the conclusion of the entire lengthy process, this can imperil a faculty member's curriculum vitae and promotion status. For younger faculty members, such marathon-distance publishing can be detrimental to the attainment of tenure.

Fortunately, each of the phases offers rich potential for milestone contributions to knowledge. Project planning should anticipate and prepare for analysis and communication of substantive findings and conclusions. Whatever information gathering and assessment takes place to steer intervention design and development can be structured so as to simultaneously inform the professional and behavioral science literature. It becomes a matter of allocating time to achieve the parallel objectives. If there is no provision for reflection and documentation, but rather a press to move forward to the next activity, the project will have forfeited an opportunity to contribute to knowledge and to provide the means and credentials for the career advancement of members of the staff. These opportunities are readily available in most projects. In the Community Intervention Project one or two books accompanied sequential steps: through design (Rothman 1974); development (Rothman, Teresa, and Erlich 1978; Rothman, Erlich, and Teresa 1976); and dissemination (Rothman et al. 1983).

This issue is discussed by Haug (1971) in terms of the intertwined professional and bureaucratic components of intervention-oriented research. The bureaucratic aspect strives to complete concrete action tasks. The professional aspect wants to pause to integrate ideas. Haug indicates that both those styles are necessary in overlapping "role segmentation" fashion. Accordingly, it is appropriate and necessary to build reflective periods into a project plan. The staff "fluctuates between these modes . . . in sequential segments of time as the major research emphasis changes, and even within each segment is forced to juggle both administrative and contemplative duties at the same time" (201). The matter of accommodating research and publishing activities is elaborated by Ronald H. Rooney in Chapter 15.

USE OF AN APPLIED FIELD SETTING

Intervention tools that are created through design and development must be in a form that can be readily applied by some designated set of ultimate users. For this to occur, the intervention needs to be put into practice and tested in a setting that approximates the environment of the projected user group. For this reason, planning a project necessitates attention to the inclusion of such an applied natural environment. In pilot testing and early development it is possible to use a more artificial and controlled lab-like framework. Thomas and Santa (1982) employed this approach in formulating unilateral family therapy. The service program was established as an independent entity within the university under the supervision of the overall project director. But ultimately, all practice innovations have to be refined and evaluated in natural human service contexts to assure confidence in their feasibility and effectiveness in the "real world."

For a university-based project, this implies an interinstitutional arrangement at some time in the life of the undertaking. Intervention research, from this standpoint, entails administrative and operational involvements between organizations, with all the attendant complications, as alluded to by Yeheskel Hasenfeld and Walter M. Furman, in Chapter 13. Planning must entail the identification of collaborating human service bodies and the establishment of suitable working relationships.

A number of useful guides to such planning have emerged in the literature. For example, criteria for selection of field sites includes such factors as a reasonably favorable agency predisposition toward participation in evaluation, an appropriate range of practice opportunities and staff characteristics, and a commitment by the administration to utilize project results (Alkin, 1985). Weiss (1984) indicates that procedures should be planned with the participation of representatives from the user setting. This helps to ensure feasibility and fit, and also engenders interest in and commitment to the study. Such participation also counteracts administrators' and staff's overexpectation in the agency.

Rossi (1977) makes the point that project results, especially in the short run, may be equivocal and, hence, disappointing to service professionals. Ironically, there is often a high level of skepticism in the practice community about researchers and their undertakings, coupled with a high level of expectation once a substantial research program has been set into motion. The sheer cost and expenditure of energy on non-service-related activities contributes to a predisposition to see practical results. A plan that includes early agency involvement in study decisions, including an appropriate definition of anticipated outcomes, may mitigate against later reactions of discouragement.

It is advisable that understandings and arrangements be specified in tangible form. Positive working relationships customarily are thought of primarily in informal terms. However, when organizations and their interconnecting operations are jointly involved in an activity, a contractional framework provides direction and serves as a safeguard against conflict. Fairweather and Tornatzky (1977) stress the importance of including "administrative agreements" in the project plan. In their view, research for social innovation must include "providing the research staff with the social conditions under which such experiments can be carried out. This usually requires the negotiation of essential 'contracts' with those who will be involved in one way or another in the experiment itself" (123).

The authors hold that the administrative agreement must be in written form and contained in a letter, memo of understanding, or formal contract. It should cover the following factors:

On the Part of the Agency:
1. An understanding that the research budget is to be expended in the manner, and for the purposes, intended in the research proposal;
2. An understanding giving the researchers authority to select and randomly assign persons to the conditions presented in the experimental plan;
3. An agreement to support the experiment when it receives complaints about special treatment, funding, or staffing;
4. Agreements concerning the sharing and/or assignment of personnel, funds, and/or space;
5. An understanding not to interfere with the model in the proposed experimental plan;
6. An agreement not to violate the integrity of the research design nor to participate in procedures designed to curtail a full-time research effort;
7. An agreement not to seek either inflammatory or self-serving publicity.

On the Part of the Project:
1. Not to exceed the dimensions of the agreed-upon experimental program in size, type, or duration;
2. Not to violate any of the existing institutional norms except those agreed upon by all parties as an inherent part of the research;
3. To provide those services proposed in the research proposal;
4. To give periodic progress reports, as appropriate, to all cooperating parties;
5. Not to change any of the agreed-upon procedures without specific permission from cooperating units; upon the emergence of any unforeseen difficulties involving other cooperating units, the experimenters will request a meeting to discuss these problems (136-137).

Service and research activities and perspectives clearly are not identical. If they do not actually clash, at minimum they can be disjunctive. Some degree of disruption of normal patterns in the applied environment can be predicted. If properly planned for, such disruption can be held to a minimum. According to Morell (1979), researchers need to be sensitive to their potential personal intrusiveness and understand well the service mission of the institution they will enter. A plan to train researchers for this role would be salutary. Morell suggests training with regard to organizational and administrative problems of service settings, system theory, communication skills, and the ethics of applied research. There also should be provision for conveying relevant information to agency staff. Morell suggested workshops and seminars as one way to accomplish this.

In addition, the study plan could emphasize the use of procedures that fit most smoothly within the service context. Reliance can be placed on nonintrusive measures that are embedded in the natural operations of the agency. Reid (1978) has advanced the notion of "the social agency as a research machine." Service data are collected routinely by agencies, and computerized information systems have made this data ever more accessible and well organized. Agency disruption can be minimized to the degree that the project plan draws upon such material.

Additional guidelines for planning agency-based research have been drawn from the experiences of a team of intervention researchers (Schilling et al. 1988). Their main points include:

- approach and orient the agency at least six months in advance;
- invite agency suggestions on research objectives and procedures;
- gear operations, if possible, to tangibly benefit the agency program;
- make procedures compatible with agency processes;
- specify costs to the agency openly and clearly;
- indicate practitioner time demands, client risk and potential liability;
- provide ongoing recognition to agency personnel for effort and accomplishments;

- provide ongoing feedback through progress reports;
- help implement intervention products in the agency setting.

Such facilitative actions can easily be overlooked if not explicitly structured into the project operational plan.

PLANNING THE STAFF COMPONENT

Deciding on the composition and organization of the staff poses important and somewhat particularistic problems for intervention research. The work requires a staff group that is typically very diverse and fairly large. Diversity relates to the many different types of tasks involved in the process. People from a range of specializations with differing competencies are necessary, from those with the facility of working close to the margin of science to those with ease in communicating with and understanding the operational problems of practitioners. In addition, a variety of supplementary technical and administrative staff are often involved.

In one project, Fairweather (1967) required a staff of 23 in service, research, and consultation functions. These were drawn from a hospital and a university, and included the involvement of the board of directors of a nonprofit rehabilitation corporation. The range of specializations was great, as Table 1 indicates. Administrative planning problems arise in blending these multiple actors within an organization of considerable scale and complexity.

Another sense of mixed staff composition is conveyed in this report by Klausmeier (1968) of an educational R&D center:

> Execution of the Center programs requires proper interdisciplinary staffing. The Center subscribes to the philosophy that the most productive research and the development of effective instructional systems will derive from teams composed primarily of behavioral scientists, subject-matter specialists, and experts in curriculum and other areas closely related to educational practice. The behavioral scientist contributes his research skills and knowledge of the subject field; the experts in curriculum and other fields contribute knowledge about methodology and other relevant instructional variables. (153)

TABLE 1. Personnel participating in the hospital-community study with their primary institutional affiliation.

hospital		university		nonprofit rehabilitation corporation
Service	*Research*	*Consultants*	*Research*	*Service*
One psychiatrist	One chief social	Legal	One chief social	Board of
One social	innovative	Accounting	innovative	Directors
worker	experimenter	Insurance	experimenter	
Two nurses	(principal	Statistical	(principal	
Four nursing	investigator)	Computer	investigator)	
assistants	One	Medical	Two social	
	experimental	Janitorial	innovative	
	assistant		experimenters	
			Three	
			experimental	
			assistants	

The complexities of staff planning are underlined by the recognition that a vital segment of the staff, particularly in the development phase, is situated outside of the project domain in a community service organization and under the supervision of an external administrator. Control of that staff is secondary and through the community agency's chain of command. An interorganizational administrative agreement or contract is the means by which control is exerted in that circumstance, as previously suggested.

A typical intervention research project focuses on a given problem or objective, readjusting its staffing arrangements as it proceeds. The common organizational form mirrors what Sayles and Chandler (1971) identify as "structure based or work-flow stages." Thus there is likely to be a somewhat different staff configuration for retrieval and design, development, and diffusion. The first phase may require the use of information science specialists, the development phase will certainly draw on evaluation specialists, and the diffusion phase must rely on people with media competency who can create handbooks, videotapes, charts, or other intervention implementation packages.

While most intervention research programs comprise a single project, it is possible to conceive eventually of a large center or institute that includes several different projects working on different problems. In administrative planning under such circumstances one might establish two different organizational formats: project groups and functional groups. Based on the industrial R&D experience, Sayles and Chandler listed the relative advantages of creating one or another arrangement (1971, 185):

PROJECT GROUPS	FUNCTIONAL (SPECIALIST) GROUPS
Advantages:	*Disadvantages:*
Full-time attention of personnel to the project	Part-time attention to any one project
Single focal point for sponsor and contractor for all project matters	No single focal point for a given multidiscipline job
Project visibility	Poor visibility of a given job
Cradle-to-grave responsibility for a given job	Diffused responsibility for a given job
Flexible level of reporting for project	Department reporting level relatively fixed
Tailor-made to fit the job	Must accommodate full range of interest for each specialist
Disadvantages:	*Advantages:*
Personnel experience limited to project experience	Reservoir of personnel skilled in a given functional area
Little interchange with similar functions outside the project; tendency to "reinvent the wheel"	Automatic interchange of ideas and solutions in a given functional area (prevents "reinventing the wheel")
Massive requirements for facilities for short periods	Amortizes large facilities over extended time
Fluctuating manpower levels and skills mix	Work base spread over many projects; therefore, relatively stable manpower level
Job performance very sensitive to organizational structures, skills, and ability of personnel	Overall performance relatively insensitive to structures–largely dependent on quality of personnel

Recruitment of staff for intervention research must be very sensitive to the research/practice mix. It would be useful to find empirical investigators with practice interests or experience, and applied staff with an appreciation of research. Twain (1975) suggests using functionally defined job categories rather than traditional titles in order to attract appropriate personnel. He notes that if the nature of the work and specific tasks are not clearly stated beforehand, staff may attempt to shape the job along conventional lines to make it conform to their own professional self-image and existing abilities.

A colleague recently related a revealing experience in staffing a large innovative research and service effort. Clinical services in an entire Veteran's Administration hospital were assigned to participate in the new program. There would be a clinical director who was to help identify service problems, working in conjunction with a research director. The problems would be presented to the research unit to analyze and process to the point of designing clinical intervention models. These would then be moved into the clinical operation for testing and refinement with patients.

While the overall administrator made every effort to hire top-level professionals to run the research and clinical arms, the experiment was unsuccessful. Recruiting very well-established, highly regarded, creative professionals in their separate fields to direct the two units had backfired. Each professional pursued his own existing narrowly defined set of interests with insufficient regard for the other individual or for the overall project concept. Each made new and impressive professional contributions that built on their previous work, but that did little for the integrative undertaking.

It would have been wiser in this situation to have engaged able midcareer persons who had demonstrated their abilities, but who were not firmly set in their professional ways. Such individuals would have been more amenable to influence and direction from the overall administrator.

A distinct leadership and supervision style is appropriate to design and development. Individuals from divergent backgrounds will expect different types of supervision from those above them in authority. In his studies of R&D lab supervisors, Pelz (1967) found that personnel performance was highest where the supervisor had a leadership style that gave neither complete autonomy nor excessive direction. Frequent interaction with staff and a participatory climate produced the most effective work. Thus, both the extremes of laissez-faire and domination are inappropriate. Dominating supervision results in apathy and resistance; laissez-faire leadership brings about dissatisfaction and low productivity. The preferred leadership calls for both "security" and "challenge," the climate Pelz found conducive to creativity. Pelz notes that it is the existence of *both* security and challenge, not a midpoint between them, that is effective. The challenge to leadership is to find a way to keep a heterogeneous group of people fixed on a predetermined common goal, and at the same time to leave room for individual and group imagination and autonomy. Project leadership must somehow blend freedom and flexibility with structure and bureaucratic expectation.

Gibson (1964) adds that leadership in R&D programs should have competency in both research and practice application: direct application experience, a commitment to high standards of research, imaginative thinking, a capacity to inspire creative effort on the part of others, and the inclination to reward such effort.

Integration of project work cannot rely on top leadership only. Staff need to be recruited who have the capacity to collaborate with other professionals within the project and in field agencies. Skills that might be highlighted in job descriptions have been delineated by Shadish, Cook, and Leviton (1991). These include:

- the ability to function in complex, uncertain, ambiguous situations;
- a programmatic leaning;
- negotiation skills;
- flexibility;
- the capability to respond rapidly to requests;
- communication skills;
- the ability to listen.

Professional and technical capabilities are, naturally, of highest saliency, but without these more personal and human relations attributes among the staff, the entire operation stands a chance of becoming seriously fragmented and aborted.

CONCLUSION

I have noted that intervention research planning contains characteristics that are common to research planning generally, as well as unique characteristics. The focus has been on the unique. To complete the discussion and provide a more holistic overview, basic factors that need to be considered in preparing a project plan are listed below.

- Funding–for the first phase and in general
- Timeline
- Administrative responsibilities, arrangements, lines of authority
- Space requirements
- Staff composition, functions, and size for different phases
- Auxiliary staff needed
- Information sources and retrieval procedures
- Field settings
- Field arrangements, expectations, and limitations
- Contracts with field sites
- Measuring instruments
- Sampling requirements and methods
- Data analysis procedures
- Data processing methods and costs
- Materials handling
- Provision for professional monographs, reports, and articles
- Relationships to funding or sponsoring bodies
- Dissemination of intervention products

There is a danger that a nicely constructed list such as this will convey the notion that the design and development process is contained and predictable. This would be sadly misleading. The environment of this type of work has been characterized elsewhere as "turbulent" (Rothman 1980), containing, as it does, tensions between research and practice, the differential demands of production and reflection, the interplay of varied disciplines and competencies, and the fluctuating requisites of successive task phases. Meticulous planning is essential to keep a project on an even keel, but flexibility is also essential to adjust to shifting tides.

REFERENCES

Alkin, M. C. 1985. *A Guide for Evaluation Decision Makers*. Beverly Hills: Sage.

Fairweather, G. W. 1967. *Methods for Experimental Social Innovation*. New York: John Wiley.

Fairweather, G. W. and L. G. Tornatzky. 1977. *Experimental Methods for Social Policy Research*. Oxford: Pergamon.

Gibson, R. E. 1964. A systems approach to research management. In *Research, Development and Technological Innovation: An Introduction*, edited by J. R. Bright. Homewood, IL: Richard D. Irwin, 34-57.

Haug, M. R. 1971. Notes on the art of research management. In *The Organization, Management, and Tactics of Social Research*, edited by R. O'Toole. Cambridge, MA: Schenkman, 198-210.

Klausmeier, H. J. 1968. The Wisconsin research and development center for cognitive learning. In *Research and Development Toward the Improvement of Education*, edited by H. J. Klausmeier and G. T. O'Hearn. Madison, WI: Dembar Educational Research Services.

Morell, J. A. 1979. *Program Implementation: The Organizational Context*. Oxford: Pergamon.

Pelz, D. July 14, 1967. Creative tensions in the research and development climate. *Science*, 160-165.

Perloff, R. (ed.) 1979. *Evaluator Interventions: Pros and Cons*. Beverly Hills: Sage.

Reid, W. J. 1978. The social agency as a research machine. *Journal of Social Service Research*, 2(1):11-23.

Rossi, P. H. 1977. Boobytraps and pitfalls in evaluation of social actions programs. In *Readings in Evaluation Research* (2nd ed.), edited by F. G. Caro. New York: Russell Sage Foundation, 239-248.

Rothman, J. 1974. *Planning and Organizing for Social Change: Action Guidelines from Social Science Research*. New York: Columbia University.

Rothman, J. 1980. *Social R&D: Research and Development in the Human Services*. Englewood Cliffs, NJ: Prentice-Hall.

Rothman, J., J. L. Erlich, and J. G. Teresa. 1976. *Promoting Innovation and Change in Organizations and Communities: A Planning Manual*. New York: John Wiley and Sons.

Rothman, J., J. G. Teresa, and J. L. Erlich. 1978. *Fostering Participation and Innovation: Handbook for Human Service Professionals*. Itasca, IL: F. E. Peacock.

Rothman, J., J. G. Teresa, T. L. Kay, and G. C. Morningstar. 1983. *Marketing Human Service Innovations*. Beverly Hills: Sage.

Sayles, L. R. and M. K. Chandler. 1971. *Managing Large Systems*. New York: Harper & Row.

Schilling, R. F., S. P. Schinke, M. A. Kirkham, N. J. Meltzer, and K. L. Norelius. 1988. Social work research in social service agencies: Issues and guidelines. *Journal of Social Service Research*, 11(4), 75-87.

Shadish Jr., W. R., T. D. Cook, and L. C. Leviton. 1991. *Foundations of Program Evaluation*. Newbury Park: Sage.

Thomas, E. J. and C. A. Santa. 1982. Unilateral family therapy for alcohol abuse: A working conception. *The American Journal of Family Therapy, 10*, 49-60.

Twain, D. 1975. Developing and implementing a research strategy. In *Handbook of Evaluation Research, Vol. 1*, edited by E. L. Streuning and M. Guttentag. Beverly Hills: Sage, 27-52.

Weiss, C. H. 1984. Increasing the likelihood of influencing decisions. In *Evaluation Research Methods: A Basic Guide*, edited by L. Rutman. Beverly Hills: Sage, 159-190.

INFORMATION GATHERING
AND SYNTHESIS

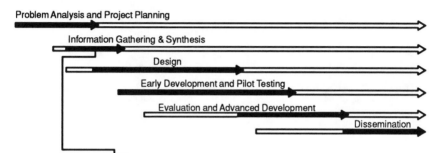

Problem Analysis and Project Planning

Information Gathering & Synthesis

Design

Early Development and Pilot Testing

Evaluation and Advanced Development

Dissemination

Identify and select
  relevant existing
  types
  of information (e.g.,
  empirical research,
  related practice and
  technology, social
  innovation)

Identify relevant
  information sources
  (e.g., journals,
  abstracts, indexes,
  computerized
  data bases)

Establish retrieval
  procedures

Gather, process, and
  store data

Collect and analyze
  original data, as
  appropriate

Synthesize data and
  formulate
  conclusions

Chapter 5

Information Science Methods for Knowledge Retrieval– Basic Approaches and Emerging Trends

Robert M. Hayes

INTRODUCTION

The Objective

The objective in this paper is to discuss the role of information resources in the support of intervention research in the human service field. There is concern about the apparently overwhelming amount of information that might be of value, possibly without adequate means for separating that which is relevant, gaining access to it, or analyzing and organizing it.

The facts, though, indicate that the means are all available for managing the wealth of information; the real problem is that there is differential use of these means. That is, while the means indeed are available for search, access, and processing, all too many investigators are unaware of them, fail to use them, or do not possess the necessary skills to use them. Therefore, the primary objective here is to review the resources that can he used and to highlight their role in intervention research.

There are a number of dichotomies in strategies for information access: one can go it alone or use an information specialist–a librarian or a person with a combination of subject knowledge and expertise in use of information tools; one can use manual indexes or computer data bases, or combinations of them; and one may need current and recent material or retrospective material. The mix of strategies, of course, depends upon the immediate operational needs for information and the resources that are available. This chapter, therefore, will identify the range of tools that are available and discuss the issues involved in choice among the potential strategies. The body of the paper will be analytical and narrative, with extensive annotated references provided at the end.

Historical Context

It is important to note that the issues in information access have been the subject of intensive discussion for at least the past three decades. While the initial focus of concern was for support to the needs of the natural sciences and technology, there has been increasing concern for services to the social sciences, to the arts and humanities, and to the professions.

At UCLA, these concerns led to the establishment of several specialized information centers, among them the Brain Information Service, the ERIC Center on the Community College, and the Water Resources Information Center (Trester 1981). The question at hand requires an orientation that includes the methods of librarianship, of computer-based retrieval, and of administrative agencies for delivery of information services.

Of specific relevance to information services needed in intervention research is a project concerned with UCLA campus-wide strategic planning for information resources to support research, instruction, and public service. At the outset of that project, discussions were held with every dean on campus to assess the requirements of each school and college. Among these were the Schools of Social Welfare and Public Health and the Departments of Psychology and Sociology. There appeared to be many areas in the School of Social Welfare for which such needs could be identified, and it was the intent that a small ad hoc committee of faculty be formed to explore them. Unfortunately, for whatever reason, nothing then happened, but the intervention research framework provides an excellent fulcrum for reactivation.

Generic Needs Identified Across the Campus

Five generic needs have been identified across the campus in the course of the strategic planning project. First, there are almost universal needs for data base development and data base utilization. Faculty need assistance in establishing data bases, in selecting appropriate software, in downloading relevant data from national and campus data sources, and in establishing the means for retrieval and analysis of the data files. On the surface, it would appear that intervention has as much or even more need in this respect as other endeavors on campus. Second, there are increasing needs for "expert system development." This body of techniques for information use attempts to formalize the knowledge of experts in a field. It does so by establishing a "knowledge base," a decision logic structure, and an interface for communication. For the problems in intervention research, expert system development appears to be especially appropriate. Third, there are many areas on campus that are concerned with large-scale projects that require management tools. While these are well established in technological areas, they are quite new to the humanities, the social sciences, and the socially-oriented professions. Solutions to problems in intervention research may well require interinstitutional projects of substantial size, requiring sophisticated tools in project management. Fourth, there are needs for management of "digitized image files" in schools and departments across the entire campus. While such needs in intervention research are not immediately apparent, there is a potential for applications of this kind. Fifth, desktop publishing has become increasingly important as a means for rapid production of quality reports. Intervention research activities on campus or in cooperative projects will certainly involve use of this technology.

THE PARADIGM

The paradigm supporting this book distinguishes several stages in utilization of research in human services: creating the pool of empirical knowledge, developing a suitable set of generalizations, visualizing and applying intervention designs in operational contexts, testing outcomes in practice, and using those products evaluated as successful in broadly based practice. It identifies sequential phases: (1) problem analysis and project planning; (2) information gathering and synthesis; (3) design; (4) early development and pilot testing; (5) evaluation and advanced development; (6) diffusion.

There is a need for continuing evaluation of operational effectiveness.

That paradigm has been exhibited in the structure of this book. By intent, therefore, the role of this chapter would appear to lie in the second of those transition phases–information gathering and synthesis–with emphasis on accessing existing knowledge as the basis for creating new intervention methods. That is an acceptable focus, but it must be noted that information support is a continuing requirement throughout each of the stages, not simply initially, drawing on the pool of knowledge, publications, and data bases.

For example, a typical project might be to seek new and improved ways of reducing teenage pregnancies. Early on, it will be necessary to acquire information on the nature of the problem and the characteristics of those who are involved in it. It will also be useful to obtain data on existing programmatic efforts, particularly those that have been evaluated as more successful. With this information, researchers can formulate a promising intervention design. Later, if the design is tested in field settings, it will be useful to obtain information on the structure and operation of this field of service. Still later, when it is time to disseminate an effective intervention package, information will be necessary regarding marketing techniques that have been successful with human service professionals, particularly those serving adolescents. Intervention research is starved for information from the initiation and construction of projects to the implementation of successful ones in practice.

From the technical standpoint, this implementation requires development of means for ongoing acquisition of information resources, description of information content, search and retrieval procedures, data analysis, and information communication and dissemination. It may also require creation of administrative agencies for management of information resources.

THE GENERIC ISSUES

I will begin by discussing the generic issues, the categories of sources, the problems in accessing them, and the means that have been developed to solve those problems. Then I will turn to specifics related to their use in intervention research.

The World of Information

The world of information, indeed, can appear overwhelming. Obviously there are formal publications–the books and journals specific to a field. But beyond them are the conference proceedings and the informal publications, especially reports; for intervention research there is likely to be special interest in environmental impact reports, government publications, and reports on behavioral research activities.

However, these traditional print publications are being supplemented increasingly and even replaced by data files. For example, national demographic data files, such as the U.S. Census, are being made available in computer form; for some, computer data files are the only form of distribution. National economic data–Bureau of Labor Statistics data, industrial and agricultural production data, and stock and commodity data–are now primarily distributed in computer form. Even at the state and local level, there is an increase in the use of computerized data–social welfare measures, police and fire statistics, and data about hospitals and schools, for example. Typical data would include location of facilities, demographics of surrounding populations, and land usages. Survey data are generally stored in computer data bases, and even though the results of analysis may be published, the data bases are still the primary resources to consult.

Other media–films, audiotapes, videotapes–are also important sources of data. Interviews with parents, school administrators, teachers, and social services personnel are suggestive data sources. Films or videotapes of events of facilities can provide important experiences or ideas in support of research and practice.

Problems in Gaining Access to These Information Resources

It may appear that these information resources are an overwhelming specter rather than a wealth of support. Actually, the real problems lie not in the existence of material but in gaining access to it. First, there is the problem of identifying existence and relevance of information materials of potential importance. Then, one must determine their availability and the means for access to them. In addition, especially for the computer-based information resources, one must have sophisticated means for using them.

The Means for Problem Solution

The library and the specialized information center are the administrative means to solve these problems. Within each of them are technical staff and operating procedures to assist in information acquisition and assembly; in development of tools for description of information resources (vocabularies, thesauri, and classifications); and in indexing, abstracting, and classifying the resources to aid in subsequent retrieval service. Information specialists and brokers can aid in the analysis and synthesis of information. Also, there are means for dissemination and communication, such as desktop publishing and electronic mail, that facilitate use of results.

The library, in particular, serves as the primary collection of materials to support research and instruction. It provides a wide range of reference support services. It provides the catalog, which at UCLA and most other major universities is available in "online, public access" mode (Ferguson et al. 1982). It can provide auto- . mated support to individual faculty and information centers on the campus. It can serve as a means to access reference data bases and services (Kemp 1979). It is beginning to acquire new forms of publication–CD-ROM, in particular–especially of information access tools, such as indexing and abstracting publications (Lambert and Ropiequet 1986).

The library is important not only as the storehouse of information but as the source of professional support in the acquisition and use of the full range of information resources. In particular, the use of computer-based information services is complex and expensive; as a result, the librarian has continued to be an important, even necessary intermediary not only in the formulation of searches but in training users (Whitehall 1986).

The specialized information center serves as an agency with more specialized staff, collections that may be more specific than those of the general library, and special services in data analysis. COSATI (i.e., Committee on Scientific and Technical Information), of the federal government, defined an information center as "a formally structured organizational unit specifically (but not necessarily exclusively) established for the purpose of acquiring, select-ing, storing, retrieving, evaluating, analyzing, and synthesizing a body of information in a clearly defined specialized field. . ." (CO-SATI 1969). Among these defining responsibilities, the unique con-tribution of the information center is in the substantive aspects of "evaluating, analyzing, and synthesizing"; it is in this way that the information center makes the wealth of information accessible and applicable to the needs in application.

Of increasing importance has been the acquisition of numerical data bases by such information centers (National Referral Center 1979). At UCLA, that activity is performed by the Social Science Data Archives, at least as far as the needs in the social sciences and related professional schools are concerned.

THE INFORMATION RESOURCE NEEDS
IN INTERVENTION RESEARCH

What significance does this basic framework have for interven-tion research? This question has four different contexts: the typical academic disciplines, instruction, professional practice, and policy and politics. The information needs and the mechanisms to support them differ among those contexts. The first, the academic research context, and perhaps to some extent the second, instruction, appear to be well served. For these, the problems lie in identification of existing source data. The university library and the social science data archive fulfill the needs in that area; there may need to be a supplementary agency, such as a specialized information center, but there are established means for utilizing such a center in support of academic discipline research and instructional objectives.

The real and largely unmet needs lie in the latter two of the contexts listed: research to create the practical tools for professional practice and policy formulation. There, the needs are much more diffuse, more difficult to define, but of far greater immediacy. The mechanisms for meeting those needs are poorly developed, if they exist at all. The situation in the social sciences is a sharp contrast to that in medicine, supported by a strong national library network centered on the National Library of Medicine, and for the physical sciences and engineering, with a wealth of indexing and abstracting services to support their needs. It is for this reason that emphasis must be given to the necessary role of information resources at every stage of the paradigm and in the acquisition of new and original data. Data are needed that will build consensus, validate practice, and support conversion to broad-based practice.

As one means for solution in the full range of contexts, but especially in the areas of practice and policy, it is of value to consider establishment of an "Intervention Research Information Center," operationally modeled on the ERIC center but with its own focus of subject responsibility (Greenwood 1972; Carroll and Maskewitz 1980). It could be initiated as a support to research and instruction, but from the beginning it should provide information services for applied and technical purposes. Such an information center would serve as the agency for identifying information materials of import to intervention research and practice; it would identify sources for them and, as appropriate, acquire materials of central importance; and it would catalog, index, and abstract relevant information materials to provide ready means for access. All of these are traditional services of libraries and of associated information centers.

The most important services of such a center, though, are substantive in the analysis of the information contained in these materials and preparation of "state of the art" reviews (Kemp 1979; Drazan 1982). Typically, information centers will serve as the focal point for commissioning such studies, publishing the results, and disseminating them to appropriate users. Information is thus made into a dynamic part of professional practice.

As a second means for solution in the full range of contexts, there would be value in developing means to support personal use of information resources. This would require controlling literature on a current basis, and supplementing one's own data files with additional sources. The personal computer is now so inexpensive, so readily available, that the individual researcher and practitioner can easily consider use of it for word processing, data base management, data downloading and access, personal file management, file searching, and personal scheduling. There is a wide range of inexpensive personal file managers that can support these individual needs (several that cost less than $100, as will be identified later, provide a high level of effectiveness). Beyond those individual needs are the means for personal communication–desk top publication, electronic mail, computer-mediated FAX.

SPECIFIC RESOURCES

To provide as much specificity as possible, I will conclude by briefly reviewing the wide range of currently available resources. Many of these will be familiar, but there is value in providing a comprehensive overview. Any reference librarian can readily assemble a listing of this kind, using the standard general and specific reference sources (Gale 1982). I assembled these lists using such subject categories as: gerontology, children and youths, drug abuse, handicapped, family structure, urban and regional research, race, and culture.

Indexing and Abstracting Journals

These are some standard indexing and abstracting journals specific to these fields:

Social Planning, Policy, and Development Abstracts
Social Work Research and Abstracts
Current Literature on Aging
Gerontological Abstracts
Index to Periodical Literature on Aging
Adolescent Mental Health Abstracts
Child Abuse and Neglect Research
Child Development Abstracts and Bibliography
DSH (Deafness, Speech, and Hearing) Abstracts
Rehabilitation and Handicapped Literature
Drug Abuse Bibliography
Sage Family Studies Abstracts
Poverty and Human Resources Abstracts
Human Resources Abstracts
Quarterly Digest of Urban and Regional Research
Sage Urban Studies Abstracts
Urban Affairs Abstracts
Sage Race Relations Abstracts

Also, there is the *Social Science Citation Index*, which is the single most valuable tool for access to current and retrospective literature. While it is by its design broad in coverage, it is exceptionally valuable in even the most narrow fields of study.

Reference Data Bases

Many reference data bases are specific to the field of concern (Hall 1983; Gale 1984; Directory of Periodicals Online 1985; Edelhart 1985; Bowker 1987; Cuadra 1989). Each of them is created by a "source," such as indexing or abstracting journals, usually as part of the process of producing reference publications. Access to them can then be provided in a number of ways. For some, there are CD-ROM versions which can be acquired and mounted on microcomputers; for others, the data base is available in magnetic tapes to be mounted on large mainframe computers for access through local campus online public access catalogs; for most, access is provided by a number of national online access services. The national online access services in the United States include, in particular, BRS, Inc.; Dialog; and WilsonLine. The following lists the relevant data bases that are available online.

NAME	SUBJECT	SOURCE	SERVICE
AgeLine	Gerontology	AARP	BRS
Handsnet	Health care		Connect, Inc.
BIRD	Family	Robert Febre	French service
Child Abuse and Neglect	Children	HEW	Dialog
DHSS-Data	Health care	UK Social Security	British service
DrugInfo	Drugs	Univ. of Minnesota	BRS
Family Resources	Family	National Council	BRS, Dialog
		on Family Relations	BRS, Dialog
National Report	Family	Buraff	Exec Tele
Quality of Worklife	Family	Management Direct	BRS, Exec Tele
Social Sciences Index	Social Sciences	H.W. Wilson	WilsonLine
Social SciSearch	Social Sciences	ISI	BRS, Dialog
Social Work Abstracts	Social Work	NASW	BRS, Dialog
Sociological Abstracts	Sociology	Sociol. Abstracts	BRS, Dialog

NAME	SUBJECT	SOURCE	SERVICE
Alcohol and Alcohol	Alcoholism	NIAAA	
Problems Science			BRS
Alcohol Information for			
Clinicians and Educators	Alcoholism	Project CORK Institute	BRS
Dissertation Abstracts	General	UMI	BRS
DrugInfor	Drugs	Univ. of Minnesota	BRS
ReHabData	Rehabilitation	Naric	BRS
PsychInfo	Psychology	APA	Dialog

Retrieval Software

Each of the data base access services, each CD-ROM publication, and each of the various academic online public access catalogs provides a set of software capabilities–for interfacing with the users, for formulating queries, for efficiently and effectively searching their files, for sequencing and formatting the results of searches, and for downloading those results. Each package of software differs slightly from the others, but the functionalities are all very similar (ERIC 1983; Vigil 1986; Glossbrenner 1987).

The search capabilities provide for combining search terms into queries through the use of Boolean operators (logical AND, OR, and NOT). Comparators ("less than," "greater than," "equal to") allow one to specify ranges of dates or other numerical values. Truncation permits one to specify portions of search terms so that variant forms (such as plurals) of a given word can be covered by a query. Data fields are used to pinpoint the kinds of data on which a search will be performed (such as author, title terms, date of publication, publisher, subject terms, etc.).

The interfaces are designed to assist the user in communicating and interacting with the computer. Some require that the user know the language of the system and specify the structure of the query; others use menus that require or permit the user to select from a set of choices. Some require that the user know the specific vocabulary of subject terms; others permit very flexible use of terms in a natural language fashion.

The searching processes incorporate a variety of techniques, including what is called "hypertext"–linkages between records that permit one to call up a record based not on a specified search but on built-in relationships among the records in the file.

Personal File Management

An especially important requirement is to provide the researcher or analyst with tools that will make access to and use of the data from these sources simple and effective for both data analysis and data presentation. A wide variety of microcomputer-based software is now available to support the establishment and maintenance of personal files. Of special value now is the ability to "download" (i.e., to transfer data from central facilities) from online public access catalogs or from national database access services. In this way, large amounts of data relevant to specific needs can be obtained easily and inexpensively, to be added to a personal file for later retrieval and combination with other sources of data.

There are data base managers (such as dBase, RBase, PC File, and Paradox) to support the file maintenance functions that cost on the order of a few hundred dollars. There are also programs that provide exceptionally rapid access in freetext or hypertext searching modes; many of them cost less than $100 retail, and the "street price" is usually about two-thirds of the recommended retail price (Seymour 1989; Bond 1990).

Name	Typical Retail Price
Active life	$149.00
Agenda (Lotus)	395.00
askSam	295.00
Current 1.1 (IBM)	395.00
Gofer	79.95
Golden Retriever 2.0	99.00
Info Select	99.95
INFO-XL	265.00
Instant Recall	99.95
Memory Lane	99.00
MemoryMate	69.95
PackRat	395.00
Text Collector	69.00
Tornado	99.95
Tracker	99.95
Who-What-When	295.00

They differ in specific functionalities, of course, but basically they each provide effective means for establishing, maintaining, and using personally searchable data files, with full-text retrieval. It is easy to establish relatively large data files (approximately 20 megabytes) from national data bases and university catalogs which can then be accessed to meet specific needs by these kinds of packages.

CONCLUSION

This chapter highlighted the array of tools available to support researchers and practitioners in the field of intervention research in their needs for information resources. The importance of recognizing the role of information resources in the paradigm which has served so well as the framework for analysis was emphasized.

Also discussed was the generic means for management of information resources, represented by the university library and specialized information centers, and two specific approaches to meeting information needs were presented: development of an intervention research Information Center and the use of personal computer-based support tools for the individual. Finally, examples of available tools for access to information resources were discussed.

REFERENCES

Bond, G. 1990. "Strictly for personal information." *Byte*, 15(9): 196ff.

> Provides a review of some of the available personal information managers.

Bowker, R. R. 1987. *North American Online Directory*. New York: R.R. Bowker.

> Provides an inventory of available online databases; serves as one source for the listing of data bases in this chapter.

Carroll, Bonnie, and Betty Maskewitz. 1980. "Information analysis centers," in *Annual Review of Information Science and Technology*, volume 15. White Plains, NY: Knowledge Industry Publications, Inc., 151.

> Provides a review of the literature relating to the role, operation, and management of information analysis centers.

COSATI (Committee on Scientific and Technical Information). 1969. *SATCOM Report: Scientific and Technical Communication, a Pressing National Problem and Recommendations for Its Solution*. Washington: National Academy of Sciences.

Serves as the definitive description of the needs for information in support of research and development and evaluates the alternative means for meeting them.

Cuadra, Carlos. 1989. *Online Database Selection: A User's Guide to the Directory of Online Databases*. New York: Cuadra/Elsevier.

Provides an inventory of available online data bases; serves as one source for the listing of data bases in this chapter.

Directory of Periodicals Online. 1985. Washington, DC: Federal Document Retrieval Inc.

Provides an inventory of available online data bases; serves as one source for the listing of data bases in this chapter.

Drazan, Joseph Gerald. 1982. *An Annotated Bibliography of Eric Bibliographies, 1966-1980*. Westport, CT.: Greenwood Press.

Provides an overview of the kinds of activities involved in the services of information analysis centers.

Edelhart, Mike. 1985. *Omni Online Database Directory*. New York: Collier Macmillan Publishers.

Provides an inventory of available online data bases; serves as one source for the listing of data bases in this chapter.

ERIC Clearinghouse. 1983. *How to Prepare for a Computer Search of ERIC: A Non-technical Approach*. Syracuse, NY: ERIC Clearinghouse on Information Resources, Syracuse University.

Provides an illustration of the means by which data bases can be searched.

Ferguson, Douglas, Ngal K. Kaske, Gary S. Lawrence, Joseph R. Matthews, and Robert Zich. 1982. "The CLR public online catalog study: an overview," *Information Technology and Libraries*, 1 (2) 84-97.

Provides the definitive review (as of the date) of the status and operations of online public access catalogs.

Gale Research. 1982 *Abstracting and Indexing Services Directory*. Detroit: Gale Research Co.

Provides a basic reference tool from which the array of indexing and abstracting journals was drawn; others may be readily identified from it.

Gale Research. 1984. *Online Database Search Services Directory.* Detroit: Gale Research Co.

> Provides an inventory of available online data bases; serves as one source for the listing of data bases in this chapter.

Glossbrenner, A. 1987. *How to Look it up Online: Get the Information Edge with our Personal Computer.* New York: St. Martin's Press.

> Provides a tutorial introduction to the combined use of microcomputers and online access to data bases.

Greenwood, Peter W. 1972. *Alternative Models for the ERIC Clearinghouse Network.* Santa Monica, CA: Rand.

> Reviews the alternative means for organizing a network of information analysis centers.

Hall James L. 1983. *Online Bibliographic Databases: A Directory and Sourcebook.* Detroit: Gale Research Co.

> Provides an inventory of available online data bases; serves as one source for the listing of data bases in this chapter.

Kemp, D. Alasdair. 1979. *Current Awareness Services.* London: Clive Bingley; New York K. G. Saur.

> Discusses one type of service provided by information analysis centers.

Lambert, Steve, and Suzanne Ropiequet (eds). 1986. *CD-ROM: The New Papyrus.* Redmond, Washington: Microsoft Press.

> Provides a very readable discussion of CD-ROM as means for information distribution and access.

National Referral Center (U.S.) 1979. *Directory of Federally Supported Information Analysis Centers.* Washington: Library of Congress.

> Provides an inventory of information analysis centers.

Seymour, Jim. 1989. "A guide to PIMs." *PC Magazine,* 8(5), March 14, 1989: 77-78 and 8(6): 77-78.

> Discusses the use of PIMs (personal information managers).

Trester Delmer J. 1981. *ERIC–The First Fifteen Years 1964-1979: A History of the Educational Resources Information Center.* Columbus, Ohio: SMEAC Information Reference Center, College of Education, Ohio State University.

> Provides a review for the development and operation of ERIC.

Vigil, Peter J. 1986. "The software interface," in *Annual Review of Information Science and Technology,* volume 21. White Plains, NY: Knowledge Industry Publications, Inc., 65.

Discusses the literature relating to man-machine communication.

Whitehall, Tom (ed). 1986. *Practical Current Awareness Services from Libraries* Brookfield, VT: Gower.

Discusses a specific kind of services available from libraries and information analysis centers.

Chapter 6

Meta-Analysis in Intervention Research– Methods and Implications

Steven R. Forness
Kenneth Kavale

The field of special education is illustrative of the use of meta-analysis in social research to guide decisions about intervention. Perhaps more so than other areas of sociobehavioral research, special education is a field that lends itself to use of this technique because of its recent history of rather discrete intervention procedures that continue to be used despite conflicting scientific evidence regarding their efficacy (Forness and Kavale 1987, 1989). The present chapter briefly describes the methodology of meta-analysis, including its limitations, along with a summary of meta-analytic findings and their implications for special education research and practice. It will conclude with practical suggestions and considerations for using the technique in the generic area of intervention.

OVERVIEW OF META-ANALYTIC METHODS

Meta-analysis is a method of research synthesis that aggregates findings across a particular area of research by converting data in each study to a common metric. Its aim is to use this metric as an inductive synthesis to define the relative effectiveness of a particular procedure across several studies, to clarify the parameters of the phenomena that appear to govern its effectiveness, and even to place this relative effectiveness in the context of other procedures used with similar populations. A growing body of methodological concerns has begun to qualify the use of meta-analysis, and the reader is urged to consult these sources for a more complete understanding of the technique (Glass, McGaw, and Smith 1981; Hedges 1982; Hedges and Olkin 1985; Hunter, Schmidt, and Jackson 1982; Kavale 1984; Orwin 1983; Slavin 1984). Table 1 provides a brief summary of four components of meta-analysis: the effect size statistic; a selected list of related study variables that should be coded when gathering data from each study; the use of inferential statistics in which mean effect sizes $(\overline{ES})$ may be further analyzed in relation to such study variables; and selected issues involving the validity of obtained effect sizes. Not included is the issue of representativeness and sampling of studies to be synthesized, since this topic is covered in other chapters in this volume and applies equally to meta-analysis as well.

As noted in Table 1, effect size (ES) is computed by subtracting the obtained mean of the untreated subjects $(\overline{X}c)$ from the mean of the treated subjects $(\overline{X}e)$ and dividing the difference by a measure of the variance in the sample, the standard deviation of the controls (SDc). An alternative ES for studies using a simple pre-test, post-test design is also depicted. Note that one or several ESs may be obtained from each study depending, for example, on the number of dependent variables employed. $\overline{ES}$s may range from 0 to 1 or greater and may be thought of as a z score or standard deviation unit;

TABLE 1. Components of meta-analysis.

$$\text{Effect Size (ES)} = \frac{\overline{X}e - \overline{X}c}{SD_c} \quad \text{OR} \quad \frac{\overline{X}\ post - \overline{X}\ pre}{SD\ pre\text{-}test}$$

Related Study Data:

1. Age of Ss	5. Type of Outcome Measure
2. Dx of Ss	6. Date of Study
3. Mean IQ	7. No. of Ss Per Study
4. Duration of Tx	8. Quality of Study

Inferential Statistics with $\overline{ES}$ (e.g., Correlations by Age, Anova by Dx Group)

Issues   File-Drawer Hypothesis (Fail Safe N)
          Correlations between $\overline{ES}$ and No. of ESs (Weighted ES Average, Nested Anova)
          Small Sample Size, Estimating True from Observed ES

and negative $\overline{ES}$s are possible, as will be demonstrated below. $\overline{ES}$s can also be converted to other more familiar standard scores or percentile ranks. While a particular $\overline{ES}$ possesses no inherent value, $\overline{ES}$s approaching the range of .40 or greater conventionally tend to be considered important. $\overline{ES}$s in this range are generally sufficient to raise the treated subject from an average percentile rank of 50 to a percentile rank in the mid-60s, or better than nearly two-thirds of the general study population. Caution should be exercised, however, in that each ES cannot be completely removed from the context of comparative values of ESs in each situation.

The collection and coding of related study variables will ultimately depend on research questions generated in previous literature reviews, discussion sections of individual studies, and related sources. These may involve age (i.e., does the procedure work better with younger or older subjects?); diagnosis (i.e., with what type of subjects are best results obtained?); intelligence (i.e., at what level of IQ do subjects seem to respond best?); duration (i. e., for what length of treatment are best results demonstrated or is there a minimum length of treatment associated with highest effect sizes?); outcome measures (i. e., does the procedure seem to demonstrate a better outcome on achievement, teacher ratings, IQ, or some other dependent variable?); date (i. e., do older studies seem to show more optimistic outcomes); number of subjects (i.e., do studies with larger Ns–numbers of subjects–produce more conservative ESs?); and quality of research (i. e., do less carefully controlled studies produce more liberal ESs?). Each of these variables may subsequently serve as dependent or independent variables in statistical analyses designed to determine whether size of individual ESs is associated with particular study characteristics.

Meta-analysis is a deceptively simple technique; and, as noted above, a growing body of statistical procedures is available to guard against misinterpretation of obtained effect sizes. Among these is the problem of the file-drawer hypothesis in which large numbers of studies may remain unpublished, particularly if they demonstrate nonsignificant results. Orwin (1983) has shown how to calculate a "fail-safe" number of studies necessary to rule out the file-drawer problem. Correlations between the mean ES and number of ESs per study may reveal a problem in interdependence of ESs within single studies. Techniques to weight intra-study ESs or use of "nested" analyses of variance may thus be warranted in further interpretation or statistical manipulation. Interpretation of critical methodological or substantive study features may also be compromised in cases where too few ESs are available in a particular area. Resolution of these and other issues is critical in using meta-analysis; and the reader is again cautioned to consult original sources, cited above, for guidance on appropriate statistical procedures and criteria for interpretation.

SUMMARY OF META-ANALYSES IN SPECIAL EDUCATION

Compilation of a dozen recent meta-analytic findings in special education intervention is presented in Table 2. These are arranged in order of their traditional application in the special education process, i.e., children are first "placed" in preschool or other early intervention programs or may be placed in a smaller regular class as a prereferral intervention before being placed in a segregated special class; they are then subject to various instructional programs or teaching methods and may eventually be referred to other professionals for diet or psychopharmacologic interventions. For those not familiar with the instructional or teaching programs depicted, perceptual or psycholinguistic training programs are those which focus on underlying psychologic processes thought to be necessary to academic skills; modality instruction is an aptitude-by-treatment approach in which such psychologic processes are trained differentially depending on the child's profile of strengths or weaknesses in each area; behavior modification stresses use of reinforcement theory in instructional approaches; formative evaluation emphasizes daily recording of data on each child's progress as a means to guide instructional decisions; and direct instruction is a specialized program of highly structured and repetitive drills for basic academic skill development.

Note in Table 2 that each procedure is accompanied by the number of studies available for meta-analysis in that body of literature, the mean overall effect size for each procedure across all studies, and the standard deviation for that effect size, suggesting the range of results obtained across all studies. Further citations for indi-

TABLE 2. Summary of meta-analysis in special education.*

Procedure		Number of Studies	ES	SD
Place:	Early Intervention[1]	74	.68	.43
	Reduced Class Size[2]	77	.31	.70
	Special Class	50	−.12	.65
Teach:	Perceptual Training	180	.08	.27
	Psycholinguistic Training	34	.39	.54
	Modality Instruction	39	.15	.28
	Behavior Modification[3]	41	.93	–
	Formative Evaluation[4]	21	.70	–
	Direct Instruction[5]	25	.84	.64
Refer:	Feingold Diet	23	.12	.42
	Stimulant Drugs	135	.58	.61
	Psychotropic Drugs	70	.30	.75

*Adapted from data available in Kavale and Forness (1985b) with exception: 1. Castro and Mastropieri (1986); 2. Glass et al. (1982); 3. Skiba and Casey (1985); 4. Fuchs and Fuchs (1986); 5. White (1988). Note that an ES of .40 would represent an approximate increase from the 50th to 66th percentile, and an ES of 1.0 to the 84th.

vidual publications of each meta-analysis, including original or subsequent publications of data contained in Kavale and Forness (1985b) are provided in the reference section of this chapter. As depicted, it appears that early intervention along with a cluster of techniques involving behavior modification, formative evaluation, and direct instruction are among the most promising. Also promising is the use of stimulant drugs, such as Ritalin, to enhance classroom performance in hyperactive children. Less impressive but somewhat important are language-based or psycholinguistic training programs. Note that special class placement, perceptual training, modality instruction, and diet modification seem less well advised.

These overall effect sizes are somewhat misleading, at least in a few instances; Table 3 is a depiction of the same effect sizes but with additional focus on particular effect sizes of note in each meta-analysis. These serve to qualify selected overall mean ESs. Note that reducing class size becomes more efficacious when dependent variables of children's attitudes (e.g., self-concept scales, attitude measures, teacher or peer ratings of social adjustment, etc.)

TABLE 3. Selected meta-analytic findings in LD.

Procedure	$\overline{ES}$	$\overline{ES}$ of Note	Dep. or Indep. Variable	Implications
Class Size	.31	.47	Attitudes (Not Achieve)	When Class Size Drops Near 20
Special Class	−.12	.29	LD/BD Children	Small N of Studies with These Groups
Psycholinguistic	.39	.63	Expressive Language	Opportunity for Espression, Especially Younger Children
Behavior Mod.	.93	1.57	Academic (Not Behavior)	Supported also by Single Subject Meta-Analyses Using "PND"
Formative Eval.	.70	1.12	Combined with Behavior Mod.	Higher ESs for Use of Graphs and Systematic Analysis
Stimulant Drugs	.58	.38	Academic Gains	Not Just Behavior But Concentration as Well

are used as measures of effect, as opposed to academic measures. Further analysis suggests that this becomes more pertinent as class size drops near or below 20 pupils per class. Special class placement also moves from a negative to a more positive effect size when diagnostic groups are analyzed separately. Most studies were done on children with mild mental retardation, but few studies performed on children with learning disabilities or behavior disorders suggest a positive outcome for special class placement. It seems clear that the question of special class efficacy for these latter groups may as yet be unresolved. Psycholinguistic training, as well, seems to be more effective in producing gains in expressive language, as opposes to gains in other underlying linguistic processes, thus enhancing children's opportunity for verbal expression.

Behavior modification, often regarded as merely a means of social or behavioral control, seems to produce its more dramatic gains in *academic* skill development. Although caution should be exercised in interpretation here, because only group-design studies were included, a more recent technique of meta-analysis for single-subject studies, i.e., percent of non-overlapping data or "PND" (see Scruggs et al. 1988), demonstrated effect sizes in the same general range. Formative evaluation is often considered, an integral part of behavior modification, but this is not necessarily so; and, in those studies where both were combined, effect sizes were much larger. Use of graphic displays of daily data and of systematic rules to analyze daily trends also added to the power of this technique. Finally, although stimulant drugs have their greatest impact on classroom behavior, a not insubstantial effect is also evident when academic achievement is used as a dependent measure of outcome in stimulant medication. All of these findings can then be taken in the aggregate, thus allowing practitioners to sift and weigh the various interventions in a comparative fashion.

Although this introduction to the topic of meta-analysis is quite brief, Tables 2 and 3 demonstrate how overall effect sizes can begin to suggest not only the relative efficacy of various intervention strategies but also specific child or outcome measures that are likely to be differentially affected or at least deserving of further examination. Meta-analysis is, however, only one technique in the overall process of determining choice of intervention. While it provides a quantitative measure of efficacy, such a metric can indeed be misleading, as demonstrated in Table 3. Its advantage, however, is that such a metric becomes a starting point for further analysis and discussion in a much more systematic fashion than traditional narrative reviews.

PRACTICAL CONSIDERATIONS AND IMPLICATIONS

There are a number of considerations in the development and use of meta-analysis that may enhance or limit the use of obtained effect sizes and their interpretation in decision making in the area of intervention. Having introduced the reader to basic considerations in meta-analysis and illustrative uses in the area of special education, it seems essential that more practical considerations be discussed now that a common ground for such a discussion has been established. The following sections, therefore, will detail some practical suggestions in each of the five major steps involved in conceiving, executing, and using meta-analysis in intervention research: (1) setting goals or objectives for the meta-analysis, i.e., determining its purpose and scope; (2) searching available literature for relevant studies or sources of data, i.e., determining when a literature base is adequate and representative; (3) collecting data for entry into meta-analytic calculations, i.e., determining what information needs to be coded and entered into the database; (4) analyzing the data according to appropriate procedures, i.e., determining which statistical analyses are essential for a sound interpretation of obtained effect sizes; and (5) interpreting the findings, i.e., determining whether or not results are strong enough and sufficiently unbiased to be able to draw conclusions in a specific area of research, policy, or clinical intervention.

Purpose of the Meta-Analysis

In any individual research study, literature review, technical report, or related document, there are a number of possible levels of interpretation, of which the writer or researcher who is the author of the document may not always be conscious. Current examples abound in special education wherein proponents for mainstreaming children with handicaps into regular classes have seized upon some aspects of formative evaluation, described above, and turned otherwise obscure studies on continuous monitoring of classroom performance into such a *cause célèbre* that authors of these studies have suddenly found themselves propelled into the limelight of the debate on mainstreaming. Their data, for example, on number of words read by children with and without learning disorders, which was originally intended to serve as a measure of efficacy of a new technique, is now being used in formal or informal debate as an indication of how close (or how far) children with handicaps are from functional readiness for regular classroom integration. Another example involves meta-analysis on early intervention (Castro and Mastropieri 1986), which was intended to highlight gaps in research knowledge but was actually used by a state department of education to support its lack of involvement in early intervention because certain practices were not supported in the research data base.

Meta-analysis indeed has even more potential for such unintended uses, and the scholar attempting to do such an analysis needs to be clear at the outset what purposes are to be served. This is not to say that determination of research needs, policy development at the macro-level, and intervention decisions at a micro-level are not all possible in a single meta-analytic study; but it is to say that certain decisions for subsequent steps of a meta-analysis may indeed be driven by its initial goals.

In a meta-analytic study to determine future *research* needs in an area of intervention that may be controversial, for example, it might be quite advisable to include as many studies as possible, even those which may not meet rigorous research design criteria. In such an analysis, possible clues to promising research variables may indeed emerge even from poorly designed studies. In a meta-analytic study of the same topic to determine best *clinical* practice, on the other hand, one may indeed wish to include only studies of a certain level of scientific rigor. The potential harm in deciding to do research on a specific aspect of intervention, it could be argued, is considerably less than that involved in deciding to choose a particular intervention for a given client or pupil. In deciding to serve both purposes, furthermore, it is quite possible that choosing to include both well- and poorly designed studies is acceptable, providing that one pays particular attention in data collection to evaluation of research integrity, for example, ratings by judges of validity or reliability of dependent measures, sample selection, subject matching, and the like. Thus, scholars are advised to plan subsequent steps in accordance with carefully selected goals, since the potential for an incomplete or ill-conceived database is one that should not be discovered after all studies are coded and all judges have submitted their ratings of scientific integrity.

Selection of Literature for Data Base

This step is among the most crucial in conducting any meta-analysis and is the one perhaps most likely to invalidate results. While computer searches of available literature appear *de rigueur* in any comprehensive literature survey, including meta-analyses, they often prove to be markedly insufficient as the only source of literature citations. Inappropriateness of key words, lack of collaborative publication in common journals on interventions that are likely to be interdisciplinary, and representativeness of journals or other sources surveyed in a particular computer service all continue to be problematic, despite recent gains in computer networking. At a minimum, careful reading of each document and crosschecking of secondary references cited in each obtained source is essential. Scholars conducting a meta-analysis must therefore be quite familiar not only with the special intervention under study but with its specific context within a more general area of inquiry, for example social skills training within the general area of social adjustment, cognitive behavioral techniques within the general area of behavioral analysis, or stimulant medication within the general area of child psychopharmacology. Not to be thus grounded may lead to a number of problems in deciding how to define the particular technique under study, how to determine the parameters that will serve to operationalize that definition, and how to best include studies that may involve more than one treatment approach.

It is often helpful to have other consultants, experts in the specific area of inquiry, to review the proposed list of studies to be meta-analyzed in the context of the specific questions to be addressed. Those who are actively engaged in research, teaching, program development, or related areas are more likely to be able to spot omissions or inappropriate sources because of their long-standing familiarity with the data base of relevant literature. This may be particularly true in regard to sources less apt to be immediately accessible, for example, technical reports, papers presented at scientific meetings, dissertations, etc. Such prior review of a potential data base can often be combined with judgments or ratings on scientific rigor of individual studies though there are occasions when separate panels of raters or judges for each purpose might be needed to ensure a less biased assessment.

Data Collection

There are a great many decisions involved in this particular step; and these become much more critical in relatively large data bases with potential for inferential statistics among ESs and related study variables. As outlined in Table 1 and discussed earlier in this chapter, the mean of the experimental subjects, the mean of the controls, and the standard deviation of the controls are the basic data to be entered into the ES equation. Even these simple metrics may be difficult to obtain. Frequently, for example, one of these may be omitted from both text and tables of even well-regarded studies. It is often necessary to contact the author directly for such data or to work backward from F ratios, p values, and the like in order to calculate means or standard deviations or even to obtain numerical values of related study variables. A related problem involves inter-dependence of studies, in that one or several related interventions or assessments may have been performed on the same sample of subjects or a single study may have been reported on two separate occasions with only moderately different emphases. All of these considerations were indeed a factor in a recent meta-analysis of presumably classic symptoms of brain-injured and non-brain-injured children drawn from prototype studies in this area (Kavale and Forness 1985a).

Outlined in Table 1 are examples of fundamental pieces of information that may be critical in interpretation of obtained ESs. Depending on the particular helping profession involved, data on age, diagnostic category of client, intelligence, socioeconomic class, ethnicity, family status, living arrangements, or a wide variety of other predictor variables may be necessary in interpreting which treatments appear to be most appropriate for which clients. The selection of these data for inclusion on data collection forms is often driven by conclusions from previous narrative literature reviews or representative individual studies. Dependent variables, such as choice of measurement instrument, may need to be entered and coded using rather general categories, though in larger databases it is sometimes possible to obtain sufficient data to examine the outcome of a specific test. In the meta-analysis in Table 2 on stimulant drugs, for example, it was possible not only to assess the impact of stimulants on scores of standardized academic achievement tests but also to determine their differential impact on three specific achievement tests in common use (Kavale 1982). The advantage, in this instance, was that each of the three tests had very different structural and psychometric properties. These differences and the fact that ESs on the three tests were .322, .424, and .628, respectively, allowed inferences about the specific impact of stimulant drugs that may have gone unnoticed without such a level of specificity in data collection.

Even study variables that may not ordinarily be considered in traditional literature reviews can become quite informative in meta-analyses. Date of study, funding source, and author affiliation with a particular research group are all examples of variables that may pinpoint previously unconsidered sources of research bias, when subsequently analyzed for overall magnitude of ES in each instance.

Data Analysis

Although the calculation of effect size as depicted in Table 1 is remarkably simple, the interpretation of effect size is not. As indicated previously, the magnitude of a particular effect size is often considered to be significant in some circumstances but not in others. This magnitude might further need to be determined across the full spectrum of measures of central tendency, for example, mean, range, standard deviation, median, and percent of ESs below .40, above .80, or at other cut-off points. As also indicated above, the independence of obtained ESs is also a factor here, in that a single study may readily produce more than a dozen ESs, for example two different diagnostic groups with outcome measures on four independent variables at two different points in time. Considerations for controlling such artifacts through statistical manipulation are beyond the scope of this chapter, but various basic references on this topic were cited in the previous section.

It should be clear, however, that once the question of intrastudy interdependence of ESs is satisfactorily resolved, each ES becomes in effect the equivalent of an individual subject in a single research study. Inferential statistics can then clarify interpretation of the overall mean ES across all studies or of groups of ESs across certain study variables. Use of t or F tests to examine ES differences between or among groups of subjects is not a methodologically pure technique, however, particularly if the question of independence of observations has not been fully established. These and similar analyses may be impossible to perform reliably in one large factorial analysis because of insufficient data points in a given area. Performing a series of separate but nonindependent inferential tests may also produce spurious significance levels.

Correlational analyses between the mean ES and other study

variables can be quite revealing or, on occasion, also potentially misleading. Magnitude of *r* between the mean ES across all studies (or a specific mean ES across one form of intervention) and a variable such as age of subjects can suggest, for example, that an intervention is more effective only for older subjects. Constructing intervals of ages for children according to recognized developmental periods and computing mean ESs for subjects at each interval is yet another way of examining critical-period hypotheses in regard to specific interventions. Lack of sufficient data points, however, must be taken into account as well as the potential interdependence of ESs, as mentioned above. Correlation with IQ or with mean length of treatment may likewise serve to pinpoint efficacy of certain interventions, although analyses of covariance to control for such variables is also possible in large data bases. The reader is cautioned, however, that use of inferential statistics is at least subject to the same assumptions that characterize their use with groups of individual subjects, if not more so, and that the potential hazards of misinterpretation are indeed magnified proportionately in meta-analysis.

Interpretation of Findings

As indicated in Tables 2 and 3, there are a number of potential levels of interpretation of a given ES as well as a number of different purposes of interpretation. Table 2 provides an example wherein an overall ES across a given area of inquiry is compared with the magnitude of ESs across other largely unrelated interventions in a given field. Table 3 exemplifies the process whereby the efficacy of a given technique is pinpointed for certain salient independent or dependent variables related to that technique. The ESs obtained in either of these processes can further be interpreted in regard to (1) needed research, for example, very few studies of special class placement have apparently been performed on children with learning or behavior disorders but special placement indeed seems more promising for this group; (2) policy development, for example, training of teachers in methods of direct instruction, including reinforcement theory and formative evaluation as associated components, seems better advised than training them in process training; or (3) clinical intervention, for example, use of diet intervention to control behavior generally seems not to be an effective treatment, all other things being equal, though a few children apparently respond in given instances.

There is undoubtedly apt to be controversy at all levels of interpretation, especially when cherished approaches are not supported by $\overline{ES}$s of sufficiently significant magnitude (see, for example, Forness, Kavale, and Nihira 1987). In reporting meta-analytic results, it is incumbent on professionals and scholars to be quite clear in their interpretations and to distinguish among interventions that are not supported in spite of extensive and well-controlled research, interventions that are not yet supported because of insufficient or ill-conceived research, and interventions that are unsupported only under certain conditions or only for certain types of clients. Likewise, meta-analytic support for new or promising interventions must be tempered by consideration of the same parameters, for example, relative strength of this support across selected conditions or subjects. As mentioned above, drawing inferences from meta-analysis is governed by the same conventions which govern research reporting in individual research studies, only more so.

CONCLUSION

There is no question that meta-analysis has advanced both the cause and conduct of intervention research and raised the level of discourse regarding intervention to a different level, one that is arguably more objective than narrative reviews or quantitative assessments. The pitfalls in interpretation of meta-analytic findings are not unlike those which characterize interpretation of any research study, although the stakes are decidedly larger. Meta-analysis has, however, established itself in the increasing array of techniques used by clinicians, policymakers, and researchers to guide their respective endeavors.

REFERENCES

Castro, G. and M. Mastropieri. 1986. The efficacy of early intervention programs: A meta-analysis. *Exceptional Children*. 52, 417-424.

Forness, S. and K. Kavale. 1987. Holistic inquiry and the scientific challenge in special education: A reply in Iano. *Remedial and Special Education*, 8(1), 47-51.

Forness, S. and K. Kavale. 1989. Identification and diagnostic issues in special education: A status report for child psychiatrists. *Child Psychiatry and Human Development, 19,* 279-301.

Forness, S., K. Kavale, and K. Nihira. 1987. Micro-interpretation of a meta-analysis: A reply to Lawson and Inglis. *Learning Disability Quarterly, 10,* 249-252.

Fuchs, L. S. and D. Fuchs. 1986. Effects of systematic formative evaluation: A meta-analysis. *Exceptional Children, 53,* 199-208.

Glass, G. V., L. S. Cahen, M. L. Smith, and N. N. Filby. 1982. *School Class Size: Research and Policy.* Beverly Hills, CA: Sage.

Glass, G., B. McGaw, and M. A. Smith. 1981. *Meta-Analysis in Social Research.* Beverly Hills: Sage.

Hedges, L. V. 1982. Fitting categorical models to effect sizes from a series of experiments. *Journal of Education Statistics, 7,*119-137.

Hedges, L. V. and I. Olkin. 1985. *Statistical Methods for Meta-Analysis.* New York: Academic Press.

Hunter, J. E., F. Schmidt, and G. Jackson. 1982. *Meta-Analysis: Cumulating Research Findings Across Studies.* Beverly Hills, CA: Sage.

Kavale, K. A. 1982. The efficacy of stimulant drug treatment for hyperactivity: A meta-analysis. *Journal of Learning Disabilities, 15,* 280-289.

Kavale, K. A. 1984. Potential advantages of the meta-analysis technique for research in special education. *Journal of Special Education, 18,* 61-72.

Kavale, K. A. and S. R. Forness. 1985a. Historical foundation of learning disabilities: A meta-analysis assessing the validity of the Strauss and Werner exogeneous versus endogeneous distinction. *Remedial and Special Education, 6,* 44-52.

Kavale, K. A. and S. R. Forness. 1985b. *The Science of Learning Disabilities.* San Diego: College-Hill Press.

Orwin, R. G. 1983. A fail-safe N for effect size in meta-analysis. *Journal of Educational Statistics, 8,* 157-159.

Scruggs, T., M. Mastropieri, S. Forness, and K. Kavale. 1988. Early language intervention: A quantitative synthesis of single-subject research. *Journal of Special Education, 22,* 259-283.

Skiba, R. and A. Casey. 1985. Interventions for behavior disordered students: A quantitative review and methodological critique. *Behavioral Disorders, 10,* 239-252.

Slavin, R. 1984. Meta-analysis in education: How has it been used? *Educational Researcher, 13,*(8), 6-15.

White, W. A. T. 1988. A meta-analysis of effects of direct instruction in special education. *Education and Treatment of Children, 11,* 364-374.

Chapter 7

Systematic Research Synthesis–
Conceptual Integration Methods
of Meta-Analysis

Jack Rothman
JoAnn Damron-Rodriguez
Edmond Shenassa

THE GROWTH OF SOCIAL SCIENCE KNOWLEDGE

The social sciences are in the midst of a vast knowledge explosion. A burgeoning number of scholars are projecting a complex collage of ideas and findings in an ever-increasing number of written forms. These developments have been propelled by an expanded cadre of social scientists together with substantial governmental support for social research. There has been vastly increased acceptance of social science knowledge by officials and the public since World War II. Developments also have been aided by improved research methodology and leaps in computer technology.

Rogers' (1983) account conveys the dizzying rate at which new information is compiled in the social sciences. In 1962 he located 405 articles on "diffusion of innovations" for a book with the same name. Nine years later the number of articles relating to this topic had almost quadrupled to approximately 1,500, and by 1983 had doubled once again to 3,085. Wurman (1989) indicates that this knowledge overload has led to a contemporary ailment that he designates "information anxiety." This condition has been fueled, he states, by the fact that the last 30 years has produced more knowledge than the previous 5000, and that the sum of printed information doubles every eight years. It is, at best, difficult for the serious scholar to keep abreast of this outpouring of new knowledge.

Voices from disparate fields of the social sciences and social professions have asserted that the effort to accumulate new knowledge should be accompanied by a concerted effort to also organize existing knowledge. Guetzkow (1978), a noted political scientist, states the point in this way:

> It's time for consolidation. . . . Our next task . . . is to utilize the important advances being made in the processing of information with the aid of computers in order to benefit from the fruits of the labors of others. . . . I hope that . . . scholars will build more cumulatively, so that their researches are less fragmented and ephemeral. (vii, ix)

Glass, McGaw, and Smith (1981), who are based in the field of educational psychology, ask whether one needs "to flounder in the riches of empirical inquiry and sink to confusion [or if] the rubble ought to be sifted and culled for whatever consistency there is in it" (11). They contend that such activity is a "genuinely important scholarly endeavor" (12). Glass and his associates have sought to advance the methodology of meta-analysis as a way to achieve that goal.

Meta-analysis and traditional literature reviews have become two poles representing available methods for integrating research knowledge. What is not sufficiently recognized is that there is an alternative that combines features of both. In the discussion that follows we will examine techniques of research consolidation and delineate a method of conceptual integration of research findings as an option.

TRADITIONAL REVIEWS AND META-ANALYSIS

The traditional literature review has a long history and a central role in scientific advancement (Cook and Leviton 1980). One form consists of a brief overview of previous work presented at the beginning of a research paper. The other is a full analytic article that may appear in a journal or annual review series. The preliminary platform piece presents a concise summary of several previous studies in a few pages, often as preface to a research report. It often appears that the authors of such reviews have cited a number of studies with which they were familiar and which they used in ongoing work, supplemented sometimes by a day or two in the library. The impression in many cases is of a fragmentary, convenient, and sometimes self-serving dip into the literature. These reviews frequently lend support to an author's current study by: (1) justifying the research by showing how little empirical work has been completed on the subject, or how existing research is contradictory and inconclusive; or (2) demonstrating that available research is consistent with the hypothesis or line of inquiry that the author is pursuing. Of course, such reviews can also be more substantive and balanced.

The "review article" is an extension of the traditional approach and is broader, often more detached, and self-contained. It frequently has an amorphous quality, however. Often it treats studies one at a time rather than providing a tightly integrated aggregation or a sense of direction. Both types of reviews have been subjected to criticism for lacking rigor and specificity (Light and Pillemer 1982; Jackson 1978; Cooper and Rosenthal 1980). The basic concern is the absence of a systematic methodology, which leads to researchers overlooking the magnitude and direction of experimental relationships and to bias or gaps in the sample of studies that are reviewed. Also, a precise delineation of sources that were employed for retrieving information ordinarily is not indicated, and the procedures and parameters of the search are vague—making it impossible to evaluate conclusions or to replicate the investigation independently.

Counterpoised to the qualitative or narrative review is the quantitative approach of meta-analysis. It seeks to arrive at a common metric that incorporates multiple studies into a single statistic. Meta-analysis estimates "average effect size" or a similar summary statistic signifying the influence of a causal variable (or intervention) on an outcome or dependent variable. It attempts to make clear its sources of primary studies, the parameters of the search, means of evaluating studies for inclusion, etc. The purpose is to produce objective knowledge about a theory or issue by compacting existing knowledge in cumulative, uncontested form. The process is painstaking, lengthy, and self-conscious. Meta-analysis is described amply by Forness and Kavale in Chapter 6, but a succinct presentation of a few key points will aid this analysis.

A number of different approaches to meta-analysis have developed since the 1970s. Fischer (1990) identifies five different variants of meta-analysis: (1) effect size (Glass 1976); (2) study effect meta-analysis–SEM (Bangert-Drowns 1986); (3) combined probability (Rosenthal 1984); (4) data pooling with tests of homogeneity (Hedges 1982); and (5) data pooling with sampling error correction (Hunter, Schmidt, and Jackson 1982). These methods, all of which aggregate findings across studies, may be divided into two general categories. One is the original approach introduced by Glass (1976), which combines significance levels of differences in mean scores between experimental and control groups, determining whether a specific effect is significant over a number of studies. The second type aggregates effect sizes for an examination of the strength of association. The latter approach is more rigorous in that it controls for nonindependence of data and avoids bias from studies which purport multiple significant results. It is also highly selective regarding the quality of research it uses, whereas the "Glassian" approach typically incorporates all available studies having the requisite statistical structure.

In its short history, meta-analysis has evolved into a widely used tool encompassing large numbers of studies in divergent fields of the social sciences and social professions. For example, Glass notes 36 different fields which employ meta-analytic techniques. The utilization of these methods are applicable to areas of research where a large number of quantitative studies have been completed. Examples are Johnson et al.'s (1981) analysis of 122 studies of cooperative and competitive behavior; Glass and Smith's (1979) synthesis of 300 studies of the effect of class size on achievement; and Smith, Glass, and Miller's (1980) comparison of 475 studies of the effects of psychotherapy. By reducing data to a single embracing metric, meta-analysis avoids the cognitive overload and uncertainty that frequently occurs in qualitative reviews of large numbers of studies.

LIMITATIONS OF META-ANALYSIS

Despite its early promise, meta-analysis has a down side. It conveys an aura of scientism, but is replete with judgments and compromises (Cook and Leviton, 1980; Nurius and Yeaton 1987)–defects of the traditional review that this method was devised to circumvent. The major criticisms have been grouped into four broad categories by Glass, McGaw, and Smith (1981): (1) the "apples and oranges" problem (grouping different types of studies together); (2) use of data from inadequate primary studies; (3) bias in sampling from the literature; and (4) nonindependent data used in different reports from the same data set.

An additional problem is what Fischer (1990) describes as a "positive bias." The frequent reiteration of a statistical relationship produces, in the words of Cook and Leviton (1980), an "unwarranted psychological sense of security" (450), leading to undue lessening of caution and skepticism.

As these criticisms imply, the statistical aggregation of data– which is the hallmark of meta-analysis–does not automatically guarantee an objective or scientifically-sound procedure or conclusion. There also exists the controversial and more technical question of what precise statistical techniques and formulae to employ for various types of analysis. A frequent fault in assessing alternative knowledge synthesis methods is that scholars a priori compare a "bad" qualitative literature review with a "good" meta-analysis, in proverbial strawman fashion. The challenge, rather, is to seek increasingly valid and useful methods applying a variety of approaches.

SYSTEMATIC RESEARCH SYNTHESIS: ANOTHER OPTION

Systematic Research Synthesis (SRS) is a procedural amalgam that uses structured protocols reflected in meta-analysis together with the flexible integrative qualities of the traditional review. It is procedurally rigorous, without seeking statistically summative means of representing conclusions. This procedure applies the virtues of both discipline and creativity to the process of "making sense" of massive and disorderly research evidence. If meta-analysis is defined as working at a higher level, or beyond reliance on findings of a single study, SRS fits well under the rubric.

SRS has four basic features. First, it entails a *planful structuring* of explicit steps and operations in the synthesis. This is consistent with Cooper's (1984) description of research review as parallel to scientific inquiry itself.

A second feature of SRS is that it *provides conceptual rather than statistical data integration.* SRS creates a conceptual synthesis of findings that present a consensus of research in a given area. It is an approximating rather than a determinant integration. The synthesis process entails a degree of invention that makes a new integrated whole from the parts of a body of research findings. Though this provides for unity, the result is less exacting than meta-analysis in stating the strength and direction of findings. Conceptual integration requires qualitative judgments that are subject to reliability questions.

There is a dilemma here. Light and Pillemer (1984) state that "statistical precision" is not a substitute for "conceptual clarity" in knowledge building. The reverse, of course, also holds: conceptual clarity cannot substitute for statistical precision. Each emphasis contributes differently to knowledge aggregation and advancement.

Third, SRS permits a *very broad range of evidence* on any given issue. Meta-analysis must be constrained by statistical strictures in selecting studies from the existing research pool. The conceptual integration of findings allows for more comprehensive coverage, including quantitative studies (of varied types) and qualitative findings. The interdisciplinary and diverse nature of social research suggests use of integrative methods that do not bias results by excluding research from particular disciplines or methodologies, for example, ethnographic studies by anthropologists.

Fourth, the goal of systematic research synthesis as employed by the authors in intervention research differs from other data synthesis: it seeks to *aid in practice and policy development* as well as to accumulate new knowledge. This purpose differs from both traditional reviews and meta-analysis in terms of its audience. The aggregation of findings in SRS, as applied by the authors, is meant to provide an instrumental information set on the basis of which to design action or professional intervention. The result is one or more hypotheses or promising "hunches" about means to solve a given behavioral or social problem and supposes further pilot-testing and intervention development. Since the prescriptive conclusions of SRS assume a next step of empirical pilot-testing, the "approximation" limitation is mitigated. Either the conclusion stands up to experimental evaluation during trial implementation, or it is found to lack foundation operationally.

THE CREATIVE ELEMENT IN SYSTEMATIC RESEARCH SYNTHESIS

We view as an advantage a criticism of the intellectually discretionary character of conceptual (or qualitative) summaries of data. Advocates of traditional meta-analysis believe that the control inherent in their highly structured methodology serves well the aim of finding the truth. These rigid strictures, however, can also narrow, and even distort, the search for new knowledge and increased understanding. Jackson (1978) writes of the need for "creativity in integrative reviews," viewing openness as a "resource" that facilitates bringing conceptual order out of inchoate data.

In his survey of writings on synthesis, Jackson found no references among social scientists to application of creativity to the task. However, in the "hard" sciences this factor was acknowledged and valued by scholars. A highly regarded member of the Committee on Scientific and Technical Communications of Sciences and Engineering wrote to Jackson in a personal communication:

> Those publications [integrative reviews] can do the task adequately only if their authors invest a great deal of thought–and really *creative* thought–in their preparation. There is a great deal of intellectual challenge in this kind of activity (emphasis in the original). (50)

Jackson hypothesizes that the total absence of such views among social science scholars was because "they judged creativity to be too ephemeral or metaphysical to be of use to a scientific task" (50). This may be influenced by the previously noted posture of scientism which includes, perhaps, a striving to raise the status of the field to the level of the older physical and natural sciences through means perceived to accomplish this legitimation.

The importance of intellectual creativity in synthesis is discussed by Gibson, an engineering scholar (1964). He conceives of the synthesis task as follows:

> To arrange the new facts and the old knowledge in consistent and satisfying patterns. . . . Its outputs are . . . increased understanding that comes when the new and strange are logically related to the old and familiar . . . [it is] the power of producing new facts by extrapolation from well-established knowledge. (37-38)

Rothman (1980) states the notion in this way:

> The task is on the one hand extremely tedious and on the other, highly imaginative. It may be necessary to sift through sometimes hundreds of studies in order to group similar elements, and visualize connections among distinct languages, concepts, and findings from diverse disciplines and contexts. Clusters of data comprising a consensus of findings must be constructed, and appropriate statements constituting generalizations must be composed. (74)

Some social scientists, such as Posner and Strike (1982), acknowledge this aspect of synthesis with terms such as conceptual innovation and inductive interpretation. In this way one can seek the "essence" of the study–what did the author really mean and what do the data say cumulatively, in context, and in light of the cognitive history of the topic. Also, peripheral data that are not central to the original researcher's purpose but vital to another purpose can be extracted and exploited.

Jackson reminds us, in keeping with SRS, that creativity should not be read to mean "mindless eclecticism," and that "creative insights should be as rigorously verified as is possible" (51). It is indeed necessary for conceptual synthesis to be scientifically responsible. But there may not be as wide a methodological gap here as would appear. Nurius and Yeaton (1987) point to multiple "hidden judgements" that beset typical meta-analysis, and Fischer (1990) contends that substantive reviews optimally should process information both qualitatively and quantitatively. Also, SRS often presupposes the further careful field testing of its action inferences in real-world settings as a check on the results of conceptual integration–a step that is typically omitted in meta-analysis.

THE PROCEDURES OF SYSTEMATIC RESEARCH SYNTHESIS

In this section we delineate a set of steps for SRS. In order to anchor the discussion, we present an example in which the process was applied in a study of case management intervention in the human services field. This project was conducted through the Center for Child and Family Policy Studies at UCLA, in collaboration with the Los Angeles County Department of Mental Health. Because of the varied definitions of case management and numerous forms of practice, the Department requested aid to design more coherent case management practices. The project was performed in an intervention research framework and the results are reported elsewhere (Rothman 1992). This discussion is an expansion of that description of the methodology. The steps are identical with standard meta-analysis procedures, except for steps 5 and 6:

1. Defining the problem/goal
2. Identifying general knowledge areas relevant to the problem/ goal
3. Identifying specific data sources
4. Determining appropriate descriptors for the search
5. Establishing procedures for codifying, assessing, and managing information
6. Establishing procedures for developing consensus findings and intervention guidelines

Defining the Problem/Goal

In the normal procedure, a bounded practical problem or goal is designated at the outset. Problem and goal are ordinarily opposite sides of the same coin, stated one way or the other for reasons of preference or convenience. In the human services context, a problem may be stated as client reluctance to use a given agency service, and the goal may be to develop a method for stimulating a greater degree of service utilization. In this illustration, the problem was lack of empirically-based intervention principles for conducting case management. The goal was to construct a set of such intervention modalities by identifying relevant research in the literature and designing appropriate applications.

Nurius and Yeaton (1987) note the need, as in standard research procedures, to make any theoretical filters explicit at this stage because they will influence the structure of the review. By specifically selecting the questions for inquiry, the researcher distinguishes relevant from irrelevant material. The most fertile research areas for synthesis are those that have generated an appreciable interest (and empirical evidence to draw upon) within the field (Cooper 1984). For example, concern about psychosocial support of families with HIV positive infants might not be well served at this time by compiling available research studies. The problem is too new to have a solid base of empirical data at hand. In that instance, it would be more useful to focus energy on conducting original research. Further SRS, typically focuses on creating a procedure, technique, or strategy that will aid in fulfilling human service professionals' goals. This directs the researcher's attention to data having such applied potential, and to an assessment of whether available research can contribute to that purpose.

Identifying General Knowledge Areas Relevant to the Problem/Goal

At first blush the identification of knowledge areas pertinent to a given development undertaking may seem simple and obvious. Experience shows that this is not the case, however. For example, with regard to the problem of reducing dependency of elderly clients, the multiple knowledge sources might include the fields of medicine, gerontology, psychology, social work, nursing, rehabilitation and several others. For particular problems, the potential number of knowledge areas may be so numerous as to prohibit exploitation of them all. Judgment must ordinarily be exerted to allow a sweep which covers enough knowledge areas to make the search productive and meaningful, without being so broad as to rule out the feasibility of managing the data that is collected. This type of judgment requires delineating the most pertinent knowledge areas, as well as their appropriate number and blend, relative to the task at hand. The issue goes to the design of an inquiry and involves the same questions of scope and relevancy that pertain to planning research generally.

A comprehensive search methodology that cuts across knowledge fields is strongly recommended by many scholars (Glass, McGaw, and Smith 1981; Light and Pillemer 1984). In social science research, the interdisciplinary nature of human behavior calls for incorporating multiple bodies of both basic and applied knowledge. Disciplinary bias may substantially skew findings as different paradigms are utilized to investigate similar social phenomena. These disciplinary differences make knowledge integration difficult, compounded, as well, by respective language differences. Thomas (1967) has outlined areas in sociology relevant to social work: examples related to the client population were social stratification, race and ethnic relations, personality and social structure, disorganization and deviant behavior, and the sociology of mental illness and criminology. In the search of general knowledge areas for research synthesis, a similar translation between disciplines and from basic to applied practice areas must be made.

In regard to the subject of case management and the resource base of the illustrative project, the project staff delineated five knowledge areas: psychology, sociology, social work, health, and mental health. It was recognized that the ends being sought are practical in nature, therefore it is important to have a mix of basic and applied research sources. It is neither necessary nor desirable to confine the search to pure science fields, as the clinical or professional fields may offer especially pertinent intervention data and hunches to inform the direction of application.

Identifying Specific Data Sources

The delineation of knowledge areas to be explored is a necessary but not sufficient step in the conduct of a retrieval program. Knowledge is reported and stored in a variety of different forms and sources. Among these are:

Computerized Data Bases–Educational Resources Information Center (ERIC), Smithsonian Science Information Exchange, Enviroline, Health Planning and Administration, etc. Cooper (1984) emphasizes the importance of computer searches as efficient means to conveniently scan an enormous amount of material with phenomenal speed. However, this does not preclude the use of manual methods and has its peculiar problems: the difficulty in finding encompassing yet delimiting key words; sorting out an indicative rather than an informative search yield; and filtering the "catch" from the broad-net computer yield.

Hard Copy Sources (*Indexes, etc.*)–*Psychological Abstracts, Sociological Abstracts, Social Science Citation Index, Social Sciences and Humanities Index*, etc. Reviews and synthesized works can also be valuable–Annual Review of Sociology, Annual Review of Psychology, Schizophrenia Bulletin, Smoking and Health Bulletin, relevant books and monographs containing reviews, etc. These methods allow for substantiating the results of the computer search as well as complementing it. Most recent articles may not be found through computerized searches. Classic articles which are theoretically relevant may be found only through the review of nonempirical articles. Scanning books on library shelves with similar call numbers may be helpful. Relevant topical encyclopedias such as the *Encyclopedia of Social Work* or the *Encyclopedia of Aging* in the Social Sciences may prove productive.

Unpublished Sources–Dissertations, conference papers, government reports, and correspondence. Cooper (1984) describes a bias toward publishing positive findings and a tendency to look less favorably at findings that are counterintuitive. Unpublished work can assist in balancing this, but unpublished material may also be accused of insufficiently rigorous scientific methodology. Unpublished materials may be particularly relevant to applied work as they often report program evaluation findings.

For purposes of the illustrated project, researchers used computerized data bases systematically as the core source. They used the other sources in a supplementary and informal fashion. Four computerized data bases identified as fundamental for this study were scrutinized from the point in time of the search at the end of the 1980s back to the earliest time for which data is kept in the data base. The data bases included:

Psychlit (for psychology) (from 1967)
Mental Health Abstracts (from 1969)
Social Work Research and Abstracts (from 1977)
Sociofile (for sociology and related information) (from 1963)
Medline (for public health, nursing, psychiatry) (This base was used for the most recent three year period, in supplementary fashion.)

These data bases were purposely selected to search the several knowledge fields identified earlier.

Determining Appropriate Descriptors for the Search

Cook and Leviton (1980) call descriptors the nomological net. Descriptors are a kind of shopping list with which one enters the warehouse of knowledge. This is complicated, as noted previously, by the absence of a shared language in relevant disciplines and professions. Identical variables may be described in terms of different concepts within each discipline. In the UCLA study, in addition to case management and chronically mentally ill descriptor categories, aspects of the case management process were identified separately, such as advocacy, case coordination, and case planning. Related concepts were also included: community support, service integration, and deinstitutionalization.

An intermediate level of subject matter conceptualization is desirable for intervention research purposes. Broad, amorphous, diffuse theoretical concepts and terms, such as *id, anomie, social sys-*

tem, collective unconscious, and *historical determinism,* are of little practical use. The level of abstraction aimed for is "middle-range." The more finely tuned the descriptors for a given knowledge source, the easier and more effective is the search.

By means of a preliminary review of the literature and piloting of the databases, a set of key words and descriptors was delineated for guiding the search:

advocacy	compliance	relations
case conference	continuing care	multidisciplinary teams
case coordination	continuum of care	psychosocial
case management	deinstitutionalization	rehabilitation
case planning	homelessness	referral
channeling	interdisciplinary team	resource integration
chronically mentally ill	interagency relations	resource mobilization
client advocacy	interorganizational	service coordination
community-based care	analysis	service integration
community support	interorganizational	social support

Establishing Procedures for Codifying, Assessing, and Managing Information

A comprehensive search can yield an unwieldy morass of raw information, including what computer buffs typically refer to as "garbage." Defined procedures are required for dissecting and handling the information that is gathered. The following are key areas to record in systematic fashion:

a. Basic identification–study or document title, author, original source, subject matter, or main themes addressed;
b. Research study characteristics–variables, social context, types of subjects, study design and methodology, instruments used;
c. Abstract or summary–theoretical perspective and conceptual framework, problem context, hypothesis, further description of methodology, and findings;
d. Substantive subcategories of the synthesis investigation–relevant variables or search descriptors;
e. Quality and relevance of the information–evaluation of study methods, limitations, relationship to other studies, utility for the project purpose.

Reviewers are advised to "stay close to the data" in recording findings. The retrieval should report what the specific findings are rather than the implications, conclusions or elaborations by the author.

Through the methods described in the case management project, 783 published items (journal articles, research reports, monographs) we initially retrieved. The majority of these found to be nonempirical. Also, there was considerable duplication across different data bases. We added to this pool other pertinent reports, books, and monographs that came to the attention of the staff informally. The staff reviewed each item and identified empirical studies assessed to be suitable by content for inclusion in the data pool. Articles that were found to have obvious methodological defects, such as an inadequate number of subjects, an unrepresentative sample, loose procedures, or logical inconsistencies, were omitted. The staff then coded items into 29 subject-matter categories.

Assessing a study for purposes of inclusion in the synthesis information pool may involve a larger or smaller set of criteria. These may be from among the following: validity, reliability, representativeness of the sample, logic of the design, comparability of the comparison groups, and match between the form of data and the statistical techniques.

Cooper (1984) warns that the predisposition of the reviewer affects the outcome of the review assessment and cites evidence that reviewers judge counter-attitudinal studies to have poorer research designs. He found that even disinterested judges could not agree on what constitutes a high quality study.

An issue may be what Rothman (1974) describes as "elegance versus bulk." Some argue for "elegance": i.e., Slavin (1986) in his methodology for Best Evidence Synthesis (BES) and Eysenck (1978) in describing lenient inclusion criteria as an "abandonment of scholarship." Glass, who is probably the leading scholar in developing formal meta-analysis methodology, places himself squarely on the side of an inclusionary approach. While strongly championing high quality research, he comments: "It hardly follows that after a less-than-perfect study has been done, its findings should not be considered" (Glass 1978, p. 355). He argues for aggregating as much information as can reasonably be integrated, and against the "profligate" discarding of hundreds of findings. Even imperfect studies can help "converge on true conclusions" (p. 355). This embracing perspective is joined by other investigators, including Cooper, 1984; Jackson, 1978; and U.S. General Accounting Office, 1983. The wisest perspective is suggested by Forness and Kavale (Chapter 6) in their observation that choice in this matter needs to be based on the purpose and context of the study.

In the UCLA study, there occurred a lapse of three years between the time the information retrieval search was conducted, a basic synthesis was completed, and a manuscript was accepted for publication. To make the information pool used in the synthesis current, a subsequent retrieval procedure was performed for the years 1988, 1989, and 1990. This update was less comprehensive, drawing on two of the original data bases–Sociofile and Psychlit, and included another, Medline, to add breadth. These treatments yielded some 70 additional empirical study reports, which were integrated into the previous synthesis of 132 studies.

The code sheet for treating information contained the following categories:

General Areas

1. *Target Populations:* chronically mentally ill, elderly, children, developmentally disabled, handicapped, etc.
2. *Community Context:* special community situations, rural, Black, Hispanic, Asian American, Native American, etc.
3. *Models of Case Management:* different approaches such as use of paraprofessionals, special team arrangements, etc.
4. *Interorganizational Relationships:* patterns of linkage with supportive resources
5. *Funding and Financial Arrangements:* use of financial arrangements such as purchase of service, joint funding, pooled funding, etc.
6. *Social Supports (formal and informal):* use of social supports of both a formal nature (agencies) and informal (families, friends, self-help groups, etc.)
7. *Staffing:* type and level of staff employed, professional, paraprofessional, volunteers, etc.

8. *Training and Supervision:* type and amount of training and supervision
9. *Planning of Services:* aspects of the planning process in designing and establishing services
10. *Information Systems:* information systems for tracking clients, accounting for materials, and planning
11. *Legal Issues and Clients' Rights:* preserving clients' rights and assuring their legal position
12. *Organizational Evaluation:* evaluation of issues and experiences on the organizational level
13. *General Case Management:* general support for case management, comparing case management with other approaches
14. *Other General Variables:* (specify)

The Case Management Treatment Process

15. *Client Identification and Outreach:* delineation of the target population, and methods of identifying individual clients within that population. This includes outreach and marketing to find clients unaware of existing services or unable to use them.
16. *Intake:* interview procedures, determinations of eligibility, and initial involvement of clients in the service.
17. *Individual Assessment or Diagnosis:* establishment of helping relationship with client and collection of basic information for service planning: current and potential level of functioning, social supports, service needs, and client attitudes concerning the service situation
18. *Goal Setting:* establishment of expectations reflecting the capacities of the program and the preferences of the client.
19. *Resource Identification and Inventory:* identification of formal and informal resources for supporting client
20. *Getting General Agreement by Community Agencies:* arrangements for collaboration among different agencies. Entails developing policies and procedures that facilitate referrals, including transfer of funds for service provision. Many of these arrangements must be made initially at the policy and administrative level, but implemented at the clinical level.
21. *Service Planning:* specification of short- and long-term ob-

jectives, actions, time frames, other agencies to be relied on, and potential barriers to successful service provision

22. *Linking Clients to Needed Services and Supports:* connecting clients to formal services and informal social supports. This subject is distinguished from referral in entailing assertive implementation such as providing transportation and assisting with intake in another agency. It includes materials on case manager skills in negotiation, communication, and interprofessional relationships.

23. *Monitoring Service Delivery:* tracking the service plan after initiation to verify that the client's external supports and service agency are engaged in the manner designated

24. *Reassessment:* provisions for modifying plans as new support opportunities arise or old ones change

25. *Advocacy:* role of case manager in appealing denial of service benefits and seeking to achieve fair access. This subject includes both policy and legislative approaches to changing service patterns in delivery systems.

26. *Evaluation (individual level):* determination of effectiveness of service for individual clients and prognosis for future service requirements for particular individuals

27. *Monitoring Relationships:* monitoring former clients in order to remain accessible if similar or new services should be required at a future time

28. *General:* general discussion of the treatment process

29. *Other Treatment Process:* specific topics not covered above

Each article was coded into as many categories as applied. Key concepts in each study report were delineated through a content analysis. A separate folder was prepared for each category, containing information on all studies dealing with that category or variable. These, then, became the raw material for further analysis.

Given the large number of relevant studies available, we worked primarily with the abstracts that had been yielded through the computerized data systems. When a particular study seemed important, or if too little information was provided, the entire article was obtained and reviewed.

In previous research synthesis projects, the senior author has used alternatively as the basis for analysis both complete articles (Rothman 1974; Rothman and Hugentobler 1986) or data base abstracts (Rothman 1991; Rothman, Gant, and Hnat 1985). Articles provide fuller information and allow for a firmer assessment of methodology and wider extraction of findings. Abstracts contain constricted information about the study, but permit integration of the most salient conclusions from a much greater volume of reports. There is a trade-off between depth and breadth.

There is an interesting methodological issue here that merits discussion. The benefits of full reports are often less than ideal. Those who have conducted meta-analysis projects are aware that complete articles often have insufficient detail concerning methodological and substantive matters. This is because they may be part of a larger published or unpublished work, or are one of a series of articles originating from a single study, with important background information scattered among them. Also, sadly, written presentation skills of many of those in the behavioral and social sciences are often wanting, resulting in gaps and distortions in information.

Allowing that abstracts limit the amount of information available from each study, the advantage gained from being able to aggregate a considerably larger pool of studies may be substantial. There is a natural tendency to favor fuller information and to eschew summarizations. The senior author began in this area of work with that predisposition, but computerized information systems were found to represent a technological advance that demanded exploitation on its own terms. New technology often necessitates changes in established outlooks and procedures. For example, use of the telephone for research interviewing was initially rejected because it eliminated face-to-face interaction. Over time, the telephone, despite its limitations, became a recognized means of conducting survey interviews, especially for specific purposes and circumstances. The same kind of considerations may be necessary in this instance. Notwithstanding, SRS does not assume or require a more or less expansive or exacting retrieval strategy. Developers are free to select from these approaches within the SRS methodological framework.

The purpose and the context of a given project has a bearing on the specific procedures employed. In this instance, the study was sponsored by a service agency and funded by that organization. The agency was addressing a pressing immediate problem and desired to have solution tools quickly. Approximately six months were available for active data gathering. In a university-controlled project, the emphasis is squarely on knowledge acquisition and the time frame is longer. To the degree that intervention research is collaborative with community-based agencies and engages critical real world problems, the usual academic time line is contracted. The issue, then, becomes selecting procedures that optimize the practical objectives of intervention research within the given time limits while simultaneously attaining reasonable academic outcomes.

Establishing Procedures for Developing Consensus Findings and Intervention Guidelines

The next step is both routine and imaginative. This is where the systematic and creative aspects of the synthesis are joined. It may be necessary to sift through several hundred studies in order to group similar elements and to visualize connections among distinct languages, concepts, and findings among diverse disciplines and contexts. Uniformities and tendencies in the data are discerned, clusters of data comprising a consensus of findings are identified, and appropriate statements constituting generalizations are composed.

This process is a form of meta-analysis that has been described as conceptual integration (Posner and Strike 1982). It allows for combining in the analysis both quantitative and qualitative studies, as well as a large amount of quantitative data that does not lend itself to treatment through the usual meta-analytical techniques. Gibson (1964) refers to it as "theoretical research," entailing the "ordering of knowledge." He describes it as follows:

> The input to this [theoretical research] block is new and old knowledge, and the function of this block is to arrange the new facts and the old knowledge in consistent and satisfying patterns which we call theories. Its outputs are new or extended consistent patterns of knowledge–increased understanding that comes when the new and strange are logically related to the old and familiar and the power of predicting new facts by

extrapolation from well-established theories. In other words, the primary function of this block is to reduce the myriad facts emerging from experimental research to systematic and manageable form. (37-38)

The approach employs a set of techniques typically utilized in qualitative research analysis, including clustering, splitting variables, factoring, finding intervening variables, building chains of evidence, and subsuming particulars into the general (Miles and Huberman 1984). Jackson (1978) adds to this the use of analogies and metaphors, employing abstractions, and applying principles of parsimony.

Paisley (1991) discusses computer techniques for dealing with "full-text data bases" in a way that also describes qualitative meta-analysis. MESH indexing involves looking for markers that comprise different wordings for the same term. This is referred to as disambiguating terms. Hypertext links involve making connections between similar sections of text, both within articles and across articles. Paisley also speaks to the importance of reducing findings and conclusions to intervention relevant propositions.

The synthesis process also often includes finding an intervening variable that explains and reconciles different conclusions. Consensus findings can be generated by raising or lowering the level of abstraction of a conceptual category as illustrated in Glaser and Strauss (1967): "Instead of writing about how doctors and nurses give medical attention to dying patients according to patient's social value, the analyst can talk of how professional services are distributed according to the social value of clients" (243).

Findings from different studies may be synthesized to minimize or maximize congruencies, i.e., a consensus finding may state the relationship of variables as they are supported and also include subgeneralizations showing inconsistencies among findings as they relate to different circumstances or groups (only white, middle-class women, etc.). Synthesis can entail the creation of new concepts, or the modification, transformation, or reorganization of current ones.

In the case management project, all the studies within a category (such as informal helping networks) were analyzed accordingly.

Studies treating an identical subarea (such as family support or self-help groups) were grouped together. Generalizations were formulated from a consensus in findings among different researchers studying different subjects in different settings.

In most instances, findings converged in a particular direction. This may be related to a rather high level of abstraction in the shaping of generalizations. When there was no consensus among findings, no generalization was drawn. In some instances, such as in evaluating the effectiveness of case management, a strong positive trend was reported, but a smaller negative tendency was also indicated. In cost consequences of case management, no common direction of fundings was found and this was noted. Generalizations represented those specific areas in which near uniform consensus was discerned in the literature.

In the case management study, action guidelines (policy, program, or practice implications) were extrapolated from each generalization. These were formulated in a tightly controlled fashion and closely adhered to the essence of the data. They were clear, bounded, logical applications of the knowledge generalizations. It might be said that a disciplined but creative inferential leap was made from data in descriptive form to its derived prescriptive form. This process of design has been treated elsewhere in the literature and will not be explicated here (Thomas 1984; Mullen 1978; Rothman 1978).

RESULTS AND SUBSEQUENT STEPS IN SRS PROCEDURES

The research synthesis lent itself to clustering in five broad categories. These included: practice roles in case management; linking clients to informal helping networks; linking clients to service agencies; staffing and training for case management; and evaluation of case management services. The presentation format is illustrated below.

Generalization 1: Social supports have been found to aid highly dependent clients with their adjustment problems and to facilitate their sustained functioning in natural settings (Beels et al. 1984; Brown and Harris 1978; Caton et al. 1981; Field and Yegge 1982; Greenblatt, Becerra, and Serafetinides 1982; Grusky et al. 1985;

Hammaker 1983; Henderson, Byrne, and Duncan-Jones 1981; Leff et al. 1982; Steefanik-Campisi and Carol 1988; Syrotvik and D'Arcy 1984; Wan and Weissert 1981).

1a: Case managers have been found to be able to enlist family members as helping partners in case management functions and to train them for this role (Caires and Weil 1985; Downing 1985; McGill et al. 1983; Seltzer et al. 1984; Stoller 1989; Thompson and Barnsley 1981; Weil 1981).

1b: Contact with family members may be differentially beneficial to clients (Brown, Birley, and Wing 1972; Grusky et al. 1985; Hooley 1985; Memmott and Brennan 1988; Vaughn and Leff 1976).

1c: Long-term impaired clients may place severe emotional, material, and social strains on their families. Families may thus experience a great deal of difficulty in supporting their dependent relative in a natural setting (Brown, Birley, and Wing 1972; Deimling and Bass 1984; Doll 1976; Grella and Grusky 1989; Keating 1981; Noelker 1983; Seccombe, Ryan, and Austin 1987)

Action guidelines parallel the consensus findings. Their construction draws on the particulars of the studies upon which they are based.

Action Guideline 1: Informal social networks are a potential source of support and sustenance for long-term impaired clients that should be vigorously utilized by case managers. This might include instrumental aid, emotional assistance, and social companionship.

1a: To facilitate case management, family members may be enlisted as collaborators in providing case management for their impaired relative. Although such assistance is often elicited on an informal basis, family members may be trained for the role formally or informally. If a family involvement format is adopted, case managers may also need to receive special training in how to effectively collaborate with the family members.

1b: Case managers should not automatically assume that contact with family members will be beneficial to the client. They should carefully assess the nature of the relationship of the client with family members prior to accenting family involvement in the life of the client. If the case manager does not have the knowledge or skills to assess dynamics, such as expressed emotion in the family, he or she should: (a) learn the necessary assessment procedures, (b) attempt to gain this information by contacting knowledgeable therapists, or (c) attempt to bring in an expert for an assessment of maladaptive interaction patterns in the family. Standardized forms may be utilized to allow routine, simplified family assessment by case managers.

1c: Dependent clients can place severe strains on the family, causing it to deteriorate. Several factors may be important to facilitate successful functioning of clients in their families, and thereby avoid liabilities and expenses incurred with institutional care. First, assure that the patient's relatives are able to help or will receive adequate assistance to carry out their support role. In cases where the client can be released to stay with relatives, the client's adjustment to the community and general functioning should be monitored by case managers or other appropriate personnel. Help that might be provided to less solid families might include education, consultation, emotional support, temporary respite care, and personal encouragement.

In an intervention research framework, these action concepts are viewed as tentative and suggestive. They constitute early intervention design constructs that must be field-tested to refine and operationalize them and to confirm or disavow their utility as reliable practice tools. Systematic research synthesis provides a means to generate intervention tools that hold promise along these lines because they emerge from accumulated research knowledge.

REFERENCES

Bangert-Drowns, R. L. 1986. Review of developments in meta-analytic method. *Psychological Bulletin, 99*(3), 388-399.

Beels, C., L. Gutwirth, J. Berkeley, and E. Struening. 1984. Measurements of social support in schizophrenia. *Schizophrenia Bulletin, 10*, 399-411.

Brown, G. and T. Harris. 1978. *Social Origins of Depression: A Sudy of Psychiatric Disorder in Women*. London: Tavistock.

Brown, G., J. Birley, and J. Wing. 1972. Influence of family life on the course of schizophrenic disorders: A replication. *British Journal of Psychiatry*, 121, 241-258.

Caires, K. and M. Weil. 1985. Developmentally disabled persons and their families. In *Case Management in Human Service Practice*, edited by M. Weil and J. M. Karls. San Francisco: Jossey-Bass, 233-275.

Caton, C., J. Fleiss, S. Barrow, and J. Goldstein. 1981. *Rehospitalization in Chronic Schizophrenia, I: Predictors of Survivorship in the Community*. New York: New York State Psychiatric Institute.

Cook, T. D. and L. C. Leviton. 1980. Reviewing the literature: A comparison of traditional methods with meta-analysis. *Journal of Personality*, 48, 449-472.

Cooper, H. M. 1984. *The Integrative Research Review: A Systematic Approach*. Beverly Hills, CA: Sage.

Cooper, H. and R. Rosenthal. 1980. Statistical versus traditional procedures for summarizing research findings. *Psychological Bulletin*, 87, 442-449.

Deimling, G. T. and D. M. Bass. 1984, November. Mental status among the aged: Effects on spouse and adult-child caregivers. Paper presented at the annual meeting of the Gerontological Society of America, San Antonio, TX.

Doll, W. 1976. Family coping with the mentally ill: An unanticipated problem of deinstitutionalization. *Hospital and Community Psychiatry*, 27, 183-185.

Downing, R. 1985. The elderly and their families. In *Case Management in Human Service Practice*, edited by M. Weil and J. M. Karls. San Francisco: Jossey-Bass, 145-169.

Eysenck, H. 1978. An exercise in mega-silliness. *American Psychologist*, 33, 517.

Field, G. and L. Yegge. 1982. A client outcome study of a community support demonstration project. *Psychosocial-Rehabilitation Journal*, 6(2), 15-22.

Fischer, J. 1990. Problems and issues in meta-analysis. In *Advances in Clinical Social Work*, R. E. *Research*, edited by Lynn Videka-Sherman and William J. Reid. Silver Spring, MD: NASW Press, 297-325.

Gibson, R. E. 1964. A systems approach to research management. In *Technological Innovation: An Introduction*, edited by James R. Bright. Homewood, IL: Richard D. Irwin, Inc., 34-57.

Glaser, B. and A. L. Strauss, 1967. *The discovery of Grounded Theory: Strategies for Qualitative Research*. Chicago: Aldine Publishing Company.

Glass, G. V. 1976. Primary, secondary and meta-analysis of research. *Educational Researcher*, 5, 3-8.

Glass, G. V. 1978. Integrating findings: The meta-analysis of research. *Review of Research in Education*, 5, 351-379.

Glass, G. V. and M. L. Smith. 1979. Meta-analysis of research on class size and achievement. *Education Evaluation and Policy Analysis*, 1, 2-16.

Glass, G. V., B. McGaw, and M. L. Smith. 1981. *Meta-Analysis in Social Research*. Beverly Hills, CA: Sage.

Greenblatt, M., R. Becerra, and E. Serafetinides. 1982. Social networks and mental health: An overview. *American Journal of Psychiatry*, 139, 977-984.

Grella, C. E. and O. Grusky. 1989. Families of the seriously mentally ill and their satisfaction with services. *Hospital and Community Psychiatry*, 40, 831-835.

Grusky, O. et al. 1986. Models of local mental health delivery systems. In *The organization of mental health services*, edited by W. Richard Scott and Bruce L. Black. Beverly Hills, CA: Sage Publications, Inc., 159-196.

Grusky, O., K. Tierney, R. Mandersheid, and D. Grusky. 1985. Social bonding and community adjustment of chronically mentally ill adults. *Journal of Health and Social Behavior*, 26(1), 49-63.

Guetzkow, H. 1978. Forword. In *Organizational Effectiveness: An Inventory of Propositions*, edited by James L. Price. Homewood, IL: Richard D. Irwin Inc.

Hammaker, R. 1983. A client outcome evaluation of the statewide implementation of community support services. *Psychosocial-Rehabilitation Journal*, 7(1), 2-10.

Hedges, W. D. 1982. Fitting categorical models to effect sizes from a series of experiments. *Journal of Educational Statistics*, 7, 119-137.

Henderson, S., D. Byrne, and P. Duncan-Jones. 1981. *Neurosis and the Social Environment*. Sydney: Academic Press.

Hooley, J. 1985. Expressed emotion: A review of the critical literature. *Clinical Psychology Review*, 5, 119-135.

Hunter, J. E., F. L. Schmidt and G. B. Jackson. 1982. *Meta-Analysis: Cumulating Research Findings Across Studies*. Beverly Hills, CA: Sage.

Jackson, G. B. 1978. *Methods for Reviewing and Integrating Research in the Social Sciences*. (Final technical report to National Science Foundation). Washington, DC: The George Washington University.

Johnson, D. W., G. Maruyama, R. Johnson, D. Nelson, and L. Skon. 1981. Effects of cooperative, competitive, and individualistic goal structures on achievement: A meta-analysis. *Psychological Bulletin*, 89, 47-67.

Keating, D. 1981. Deinstitutionalization of the mentally retarded as seen by parents of institutionalized individuals (Doctoral dissertation, Temple University). *Dissertation Abstracts International*, 42(6), 2505B.

Leff, J., L. Kuipers, R. Berkowitz, R. Eberlein-Vries, and D. Sturgeon. 1982. A controlled trial of social intervention in the families of schizophrenic patients. *British Journal of Psychiatry*, 141, 121-134.

Light, R. J. and D. B. Pillemer. 1982. Numbers and narrative: Combining their strengths in research review. *Harvard Educational Review*, 52, 1-26.

Light, R. J. and D. B. Pillemer. 1984. *Summing Up: The Science of Reviewing Research*. Cambridge, MA: Harvard University Press.

McGill, C., I. Falloon, J. Boyd, and C. Wood-Silverio. 1983. Family educational intervention in the treatment of schizophrenia. *Hospital and Community Psychiatry*, 34, 934-938.

Memmott, J. and E. M. Brennan. 1988. Helping orientation and strategies of natural helpers and social workers in rural settings. *Social Work Research and Abstracts*, 24(2), 15-20.

Miles, M. B. and A. M. Huberman. 1984. *Qualitative Data Analysis: A Source Book of New Methods*, Beverly Hills: Sage Publications, 1984.

Mullen, E. J. 1978. The construction of personal models for effective practice: A method for utilizing research findings to guide social interventions. *Journal of Social Service Research*, 2, 1, 45-63.

Noelker, L. S. 1983, November. Incontinence in elderly cared for by family. Paper presented at the annual meeting of the Gerontological Society of America, San Francisco, CA.

Nurius, P. S. and W. H. Yeaton. 1987. Research synthesis reviews: An illustrated critique of 'hidden' judgements, choices and compromises. *Clinical Psychology Review, 7*, 695-714.

Paisley, W. 1991. New media and methods of health communication. Prepared for the conference on Effective Dissemination of Clinical and Health Information. University of Arizona and Agency of Health Care Policy and Research, Tucson, Arizona.

Posner, G. J. and K. A. Strike. 1982. Accommodation of a Scientific Conception–Toward a Theory of Conceptual Change. *Science Education* 66, 211-227.

Rogers, E. 1983. *Diffusion of Innovations*. New York: The Free Press.

Rosenthal, R. 1984. *Meta-Analytic Procedures for Social Research*. Beverly Hills, CA: Sage.

Rothman, J. 1974. *Planning and Organizing for Social Change*. New York: Columbia University Press.

Rothman, J. 1978. Conversion and design in the research utilization process. *Journal of Social Service Research*, 2(1), 117-131.

Rothman, J. 1980. *Social R&D: Research Development in the Human Services*. Englewood Cliffs, NJ: Prentice-Hall.

Rothman, J. 1991. *Runaway and Homeless Youth: Strengthening Services to Families and Children*. New York: Longman.

Rothman, J. 1992. *Guidelines for Case Management: Putting Research to Professional Use*. Itasca, IL: F. E. Peacock Publishers.

Rothman, J., M. Hugentobler. 1986. Planning theory in social work community practice. In *Theory and Practice of Community Social Work*, edited by Samuel H. Taylor and Robert W. Roberts. New York: Columbia University Press, 125-153.

Rothman, J., L. M. Gant, and S. A. Hnat. 1985. Mexican-American family culture. *Social Service Review, 59*(2), 197-215.

Seccombe, K., R. Ryan, and C. D. Austin. 1987. Care planning: Case managers' assessment of elders' welfare and caregivers' capacity. *Family Relations*, 36, 171-175.

Seltzer, M., K. Simmons, J. Ivry, and L. Litchfield. 1984. Agency-Family partnerships: Case management of services for the elderly. *Journal of Gerontological Social Work*, 7(4), 57-73.

Slavin, R. E. 1986. Best-evidence synthesis: An alternative to meta-analytic and traditional reviews. *Educational Researcher, 15*, 5-11.

Smith, M. L., G. V. Glass, and T. I. Miller. 1980. *Benefits of Psychotherapy*. Baltimore: Johns Hopkins University Press.

Stefanik-Campisi, C. and T. R. Carol. 1988. Case management and follow-up of a chemically impaired nurse. *Perspectives in Psychiatric Care*, 24, 114-119.

Stoller, E. P. 1989. Formal services and informal helping: The myth of service substitution. *Journal of Applied Gerontology*, 8(1), 37-52.

Syrotvik, J. and C. D'Arcy. 1984. Social support and mental health: Direct, protective and compensatory effects. *Social Science and Medicine*, 18, 229-236.

Thomas, Edwin J. 1967. Types of contributions behavioral science makes to social work. In *Behavioral Science for Social Workers*, edited by Edwin J. Thomas. New York: Free Press, 3-13.

Thomas, E. J. 1984. *Designing Interventions for the Helping Professions*. Beverly Hill, CA: Sage.

Thompson, A. and R. Barnsley. 1981. Person crisis: A report from the people. *Canada's Mental Health*, 29(3), 21-27.

U.S. General Accounting Office. 1983. *The Evaluation Synthesis*. Institute for Program Evaluation: Methods, Paper 1, Washington, DC.

Vaughn, C. and J. Leff. 1976. The influence of family and social factors on the course of psychiatric illness. *British Journal of Psychiatry*, 129, 125-137.

Wan, T. T. and W. G. Weissert. 1981. Social support networks, patient status, and institutionalization. *Research on Aging*, 3, 240-256.

Weil, M. 1981. Report on Fiesta Educativa. Unpublished manuscript, University of Southern California, School of Social Work, Los Angeles.

Wurman, R. S. 1989. Information overload. *Los Angeles Times Magazine*, 5(4), 8-12.

DESIGN

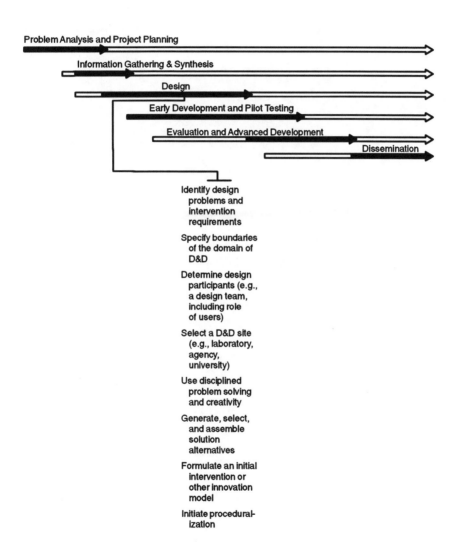

Problem Analysis and Project Planning

Information Gathering & Synthesis

Design

Early Development and Pilot Testing

Evaluation and Advanced Development

Dissemination

Identify design
  problems and
  intervention
  requirements

Specify boundaries
  of the domain of
  D&D

Determine design
  participants (e.g.,
  a design team,
  including role
  of users)

Select a D&D site
  (e.g., laboratory,
  agency,
  university)

Use disciplined
  problem solving
  and creativity

Generate, select,
  and assemble
  solution
  alternatives

Formulate an initial
  intervention or
  other innovation
  model

Initiate procedural-
  ization

Chapter 8

Design of Social Intervention

Edward J. Mullen

This chapter discusses methods and issues in the design of social intervention, the third phase of Intervention Design and Development. The methodology of intervention research is not well developed, and design is the least developed aspect. In social work, research has usually not been a significant source for program design. While research findings are often referenced, it is generally not the case that such findings in a systematic way form the basis for social work interventions. And, for those approaching the topic from a "pure" social science research background, the world of design will be especially problematic.

Social scientists have typically engaged in research activities which either describe an existing phenomenon or test the implications of a phenomenon. For social scientists, design most typically means the structuring of a research study, but in the context of intervention research it means the formulation of intervention constructs. Not only will the typical social scientist be unaccustomed to this process, but more than likely will quickly conclude that he or she has not been trained for such tasks. This is a strange state of affairs, since social scientists expect that the findings of their research will be beneficial to society, and hope that their findings will be used, but when they refer to the use of research findings, they mean only that someone will become aware of the findings. Somehow, this awareness is thought to influence people in their decisions, but researchers generally do not expect that their findings will be converted systematically into practice applications.

In contrast, the Intervention Design and Development framework used in this book is based on the assumption that research findings can be converted systematically into social interventions. This chapter examines the nature of this conversion and design process, discussing methods and issues. It draws from the work of Rothman (1980) and Thomas (1984, 1985), as well as from Mullen's (1978, 1981, 1983, 1988) and Mullen and Schuerman's (1990) work in the area of personal intervention modeling and expert system development.

Design is a stage of purposive planned change, one of several alternative processes leading to the development of social interventions (Glaser, Abelson, and Garrison 1983; Zaltman 1979). New interventions come about through a variety of means in addition to disciplined design and development. Costello (1968), reflecting on his experiences in New York City, describes such other routes to change including the confluence of forces, event-dominated change, accidental innovation, and external intervention. Indeed, in the human services it is probable that these other routes to change are most typical, and that planned change is the exception. Even within a planned change framework, intervention designs contain other elements and "emerge from a complex mixture of political considerations, the personal influence of key stakeholders, economic constraints, and the availability of necessary program staff and technology" (Rossi and Freeman 1985: 61).

Design methods also differ depending on the particular model of planned change dominating the social intervention research. Glaser, Abelson, and Garrison (1983) identify a wide range of perspectives and models applicable to planned change. They suggest that a general problem-solving paradigm has become the most popular for depicting the stages of planned change. In social work and other human service fields, the problem-solving model is a dominant paradigm used by professionals to describe both the process of intervention as well as the process of research. Glaser, Abelson, and Garrison also find that those who subscribe to the problem-solving framework generally propose similar stages including some pressure for action (problem, need, discrepancy); clarification of pressure source (diagnosis, analysis, assessment); search for knowledge (existing or development of new knowledge); specification of alternatives; implementation; and evaluation (Glaser, Abelson, and Garrison 1983: 155). However, practice rarely proceeds in such an orderly fashion. Social intervention research may begin at any of these stages, and there is usually backtracking.

Design is the ground on which this analysis stands. From that vantage point, however, it will look back on relevant steps leading to the design function, and forward to certain follow-up requirements.

Social intervention research has been enriched by concepts and methods emerging from evaluation research and policy analysis, and this chapter draws on these contributions. However, the primary focus is on social intervention research as viewed through the social research and development framework and the developmental research paradigm. Although it is instructive to consider design by contrasting its place within the various design and development approaches, as noted in the introductory chapter, these various approaches have been joined in this book under the general term "Intervention Design and Development" (IDD) which is in turn within the broader area of intervention research. The integrated IDD model as presented in Chapter 1 brings together important common features in social research and development, developmental research, and related approaches. Accordingly, the focus of this chapter–design–is conceptualized as the third phase in IDD. However, because interesting issues are identified by contrasting alternative approaches, such contrasts will be made in this chapter. In social intervention research, whether the perspective is developmental research (Thomas 1984, 1985), social research and development (Rothman 1980), or one of the other major approaches, design is seen as following a phase of problem-focused analysis and information retrieval.

ANALYSIS AND SOCIAL PROBLEM SPECIFICATION

Design activities are preceded by a phase of analysis which identifies a social problem requiring a fresh intervention. That is, during the analysis phase it should be determined that a social problem or need exists for which a suitable intervention does not yet exist. In addition, it should also be established prior to engaging in design activities that a suitable intervention can probably be designed, implemented, and evaluated. Design problems should be formulated only after it has been determined that a social problem exists for which a new intervention is required and that development of the intervention is determined to be feasible.

The importance of this prior analytic work is emphasized in most social intervention research approaches. For example, the social R&D framework starts with identification of a social problem or goal which is of concern to some group or organization. A first step in the research and development process is retrieving information of relevance to the problem or goal from the existing body of social science empirical knowledge (Rothman 1980). Alternatively, in developmental research the first step is problem selection and consists of retrieval of information which can help to specify the nature of the problem needing attention.

A variety of procedures are available for specification of social problems. For example, need assessments can be conducted using a variety of procedures. Typically, these include examination of published reports; systematic surveys of key constituencies; community forums; and analysis of social indicator data describing incidence and prevalence trends and populations involved. It is probably true that, in the area of social intervention, problems are most often identified through less formal mechanisms. Nevertheless, proper identification of a social problem or need provides the foundation for design activities.

Thomas (1984) suggests use of state-of-the-art reviews to establish whether interventions have already been designed which apply to the particular social problem. Rossi and Freeman (1985) also suggest the use of meta-analysis as a source for assessing the existence of effective intervention models. The outcome of these literature reviews indicates whether intervention design is needed.

In addition, prior to design work, it should be established that the proposed intervention is feasible. Thomas (1985) identifies factors requiring consideration in the feasibility assessment, including technical, organizational, economic, financial, political, and use feasibility.

Design initiation assumes that the requirements of this prior analysis phase have been met and design activities are indicated. Having concluded that a social problem exists for which an appropriate intervention does not, and that developmental work is feasible, design problems can be specified.

Two different types of problems are addressed in this chapter, one is a social problem and the other a design problem. As already noted, a social problem is usually the condition requiring the social intervention. A design problem is quite different, referring to the issues requiring attention in the design work. Design problems are illustrated later.

Social Problem Examples

The following two examples illustrate what an initial social problem statement might look like. (1) A group of clinicians or an individual clinician might conclude that a method needs to be found to provide more effective counseling to individuals experiencing depression. (2) A child protective service agency might find that the number of allegations of child abuse and neglect surpasses the capacity of available experts to assess the risk of harm for every case.

FRAMING OBJECTIVE

Closely linked with conceptualization of the problem requiring attention is framing the design objective. It is useful to distinguish between design objectives and intervention objectives. An intervention objective is a statement of a desired change in a social problem or in some condition related to a social problem. A design objective refers to a task to be achieved in the design work. In Thomas's (1984) concept of developmental research, determination of the design objective is the first step in the design phase. In the social R&D formulation, specification of the objective precedes design, providing focus to the information retrieval and the design work.

In its broadest sense, the objective of intervention research is development of a social technology to ameliorate a social problem. Social technology is broadly viewed to include all of those artifacts used by service professionals or change agents to achieve their intervention objectives. Egea (1975) contrasts embodied technology (a product–a machine, a software program) and disembodied technology (a concept or process). In engineering as in industry the focus most often may be a tangible technology, while in social intervention the technology often may be of an abstract form. Haeffner (1973) similarly contrasts innovations which are products from those which are ideas. He uses the notion of abstractness to distinguish these innovations. For Haeffner, products are innovations which have been demonstrated in practice, whereas product ideas are innovations only tested in the laboratory. In social work, Thomas (1978) has proposed a classification which identifies a broad range of technologies spanning micro and macro levels of intervention. He identifies categories of technology including physical frameworks, electromechanical devices, information systems, assessment methods, intervention methods, service programs, organizational structures, service systems, and social welfare policy. It may be useful to examine how design methods might differ across levels of innovation or technological abstractness and to explore the extent to which the principles of design which have been developed for tangible technologies fit abstract technologies. These distinctions can guide consideration of design methods.

Objectives Examples

Using the prior social problem examples, design objectives could be as follows. (1) To develop an efficient and effective clinical intervention procedure for use with individuals experiencing depression. (2) To develop a computer program capable of assessing the probability of a child's risk of harm from a caretaker.

These examples illustrate different technology types. The first sets as an objective the development of an abstract technology, an interpersonal strategy which could be used to affect the problem of depression experienced by individuals. The second example sets as an objective the development of a software program, which is a tangible technology. The computer program would be used to deal with the problem of insufficient numbers of available experts to assess a child's risk of harm from abuse and neglect. This is an interesting example since the expert knowledge is abstract, whereas the software program which encodes the knowledge is material.

DESIGN DOMAIN

Even more specific objectives must be formed to focus design activities. Thomas (1984) proposes specifying a domain of design in which some intervention elements are assumed to be fixed and, therefore, do not need to be designed, whereas other elements are singled out for attention. When this can be done it simplifies the design task. Mullen (1978) suggests a systems formulation of social work practice with intervention conceptualized as a set of interacting elements. Accordingly, an intervention system would include the social worker, the client, the agency, as well as the particular techniques used. Such conceptions of intervention and its components can be used in design work to frame the areas for design activity. For example, fixed elements might be agency context variables, whereas elements needing to be designed might be particular techniques to be used by a clinician. In community intervention, aspects of the economic system may be fixed and not subject to modification, but relevant statutes can be changed through advocacy with the state legislature. Rothman (1980) suggests additional factors to guide design including structural, administrative, interpersonal, and ethical factors. Another useful classification has been proposed by Thomas (1984). He identifies a detailed set of helping strategy components which could be selected as design elements such as assessment methods, monitoring methods, termination procedures, and implementation methods.[1]

To illustrate the idea of a design domain with the example pertaining to clinical intervention for depressed individuals, the decision might be to design only two components, intervenor relation-

---

1. Thomas identifies the following as components of helping strategies: change objectives; targets of intervention; participants; roles; contexts of helping; adjuncts and props; assessment methods; method of planning intervention; intervention methods; implementation procedures; maintenance methods; termination procedures; monitoring methods; evaluation methods; follow-up procedure; behavior theory; and intervention theory (Thomas 1984:283).

ship qualities (e.g., skilled use of empathic communication) and intervention techniques (e.g., cognitive procedures). The fixed parameters could be elements in the environment (e.g., client's job), agency characteristics (e.g., fee scale), and client qualities (e.g., ethnicity of clients).

DESIGN REQUIREMENTS

Having specified the design domain, design requirements, the conditions the intervention is to satisfy, should be determined. To illustrate with the computer program example, it could be decided that the computer program to be developed must be capable of: use by relatively untrained protective service investigators; assessing risk of harm indicators which are typical of those factors used by protective service experts; making clear how the conclusions reached by the system had been derived from information provided; and determining how much confidence the user could reasonably have in the conclusion reached. Such requirements focus the design work.

DESIGN PROBLEMS

To focus further the design activities, Thomas (1984) proposes the specification of design problems, that is, identification of unresolved issues regarding the elements of the intervention under development. Continuing with the computer program example, design problems might include: What systematic coding system will be used for representing the knowledge to be included in the computer program? What method of knowledge acquisition should be used–should the program learn by being fed new knowledge propositions or should the program be capable of generating and modifying knowledge propositions in interaction with an expert? Or, should the program be capable of discovering new concepts and relationships? Should the system be capable of reasoning from antecedents to consequences as well as reasoning from a goal or conclusion to determine whether or not the facts exist to support the conclusion? These design problems provide further focus. This statement of design objectives, design requirements, and design problems provides a foundation for subsequent steps in the intervention research process.

INFORMATION RETRIEVAL BY SOURCE AND TYPE

Having settled on a problem and objective, additional analysis and information retrieval proceeds with a decision about the type of information to be retrieved. First, will the information retrieved be limited to empirical research findings or will the search include retrieval of theoretical work or experiential data? Second, will the information search be limited to the literature or will it extend to retrieval of information from additional sources, such as experts in the problem area? Frequently retrieval is limited to information available in the literature, but other sources such as experts should be considered.

In the example of clinical intervention with depressed individuals, the type might be a retrieval program including information derived from both empirical research as well as theoretical formulation. Because both sources of information can be useful, Mullen has described systematic procedures for this type of retrieval (Mullen 1988). In the case of computer system development, the source could be experts who assess a child's risk of harm for abuse and neglect. Experts could be interviewed and their knowledge codified and used in the design of the computer program. Alternatively, case examples involving a risk abuse or neglect assessment could be collected and the program designed to infer knowledge rules from the examples.

Thomas (1978, 1984), Rothman (1980), and Havelock (1969) do propose the use of various sources of information in the analysis and retrieval stage. Rothman's (1980) work in the Community Intervention Project was focused on social science empirical knowledge, and the literature served as the primary data source. Typically, social R&D efforts do focus on empirical research data. Rothman (1989) also reports the use of a survey of community knowledgeables to supplement existing empirical knowledge. Patti (1981) suggests that design should draw from ". . . whatever sources of information appear relevant to the goal or problem at hand" (40).

Thomas (1978, 1984) identifies a variety of possible sources including basic and applied research, scientific technology, allied technology, legal policy, social innovation, indigenous research, and practice experience.

While these are issues needing to be addressed in the first two phases of the IDD process, the effect on design possibilities is obvious. It is apparent from these initial observations that the first three phases of IDD are highly interdependent. This interdependence underscores the fact that, while various formulations of the intervention research process may demarcate boundaries around particular stages and provide an order to various steps, these formulations should not be rigid or reified. In the developmental research formulation, determination of objectives, selection of information sources, and gathering and processing of information are included in the area of design, yet they are assigned to prior stages in the social R&D framework. This illustrates the flexibility of current formulations.

CONVERSION AND INTERVENTION DESIGN

From a developmental research perspective, we are deep into design at this point of the social intervention research process. However, from the social research and development perspective, having acquired the necessary information, retrieval ends and design begins. As Rothman (1980) observes, "having acquired information from the knowledge base, it is now necessary to manipulate that information in some meaningful fashion, to convert it into a form that will yield workable design concepts" (83). He sees these concepts as being formulated through a two-step process of conversion and design. (If the research base is already interventive or action-oriented in form, a conversion phase may not be necessary). The information accessed in the retrieval stage is converted into basic action constructs, and through design processes these basic action constructs are used to formulate more specific situational intervention concepts. These resulting concepts form the conceptual plan for development. The task of design, then, is creation of a conceptual formulation or plan which specifies the general form of an intervention which satisfies the goal requirements. In the conversion step, descriptive generalizations developed during the retrieval stage are used to form prescriptive assertions about how to intervene.

While conversion and design are information-based, these processes require creativity and imagination since intervention plans can not simply be inferred from a body of information. Furthermore, information gleaned from the retrieval stage will not include important contextual information required for the design of a situation-specific intervention. Because of the difficulties of logically moving from information gathered during the retrieval stage to conversion and design concepts, Patti (1981) observes that "in the final analysis. . . the task of conversion is an attenuated, idiosyncratic one largely dependent on the blend of personalities, perspectives, and biases of those involved, the time available, and a host of other factors peculiar to each R&D undertaking. Stated differently, it appears unlikely that two R&D teams operating from the same set of generalizations would arrive at the same application concepts. The ability to replicate the conversion process seems highly problematic" (41). Patti's observation underscores the fact that conversion and design include a heavy dose of creativity and imagination and can not be reduced to pure logical inference. Rothman (1980) notes that design is partially an art, tentative and exploratory.

It has been suggested previously that design activities are not indicated if, during the initial analysis phase, it has been determined that appropriate interventions already exist for the social problem of concern (e.g., such as through a state-of-the-art review or a review of a meta-analysis). However, it is probably more often the case that even when interventions already exist, some design work is required to fit the intervention to the particular context. For example, in Mullen's (1978, 1981, 1983, 1988) work on personal intervention modeling, it has been found that existing technologies need to be embedded into each practitioner's own personalized model, and this requires that each practitioner engage in design work. It is probable that these individualized designs could be grouped or clustered into common design types and, therefore, existing interventions could be adapted for a limited number of cluster "situations." These prototypes could then be made available without much further design work by those choosing to adapt them to their needs.

The nature of design work varies depending on how deep the

particular research is in the development cycle. Munson and Pelz (1980) suggest that the need for design, as well as the design methods, differ by level of technological development. Examining innovation in organizations, they describe a matrix of stages and levels of innovation development. They include in the stages diagnosis, design (an innovative solution is developed, adapted, or adopted, and detailed action guidelines are generated), implementation, and stabilization. Glaser, Abelson, and Garrison (1983) describe Munson and Pelz's levels of development as follows: "(1) Innovating occurs at the level of origination . . . when no solution to a problem is known to operate elsewhere. . . . (2) Innovating occurs at the level of adaptation when a few prototype solutions exist but are not well packaged. . . . (3) Innovating occurs at the level of borrowing when many well-packaged innovations exist" (409). For example, at the origination level design is central, giving shape and form to the innovation, whereas at the borrowing level design is much less significant since the intervention is well developed.

Rossi and Freeman's (1985) differentiation of program stages results in similar conclusions since it distinguishes innovative programs, established programs, and those in between needing "fine-tuning," modification, or refinement (46). Conceptual activity in design and evaluation varies depending on the stage.

Example with Depression

The prior example with depression services to illustrate the process of conversion and intervention design. The discussion of this example is organized into two main parts. First, it illustrates how generalizations are formed based on the information gathered. It then provides an example of how this is done for accurate empathy, and then as an alternative, how it is done for cognitive procedures. Following discussion of formulation of generalizations, the example then shows how practice guidelines can be created from these generalizations.

Forming Generalizations

Information retrieval, conversion, and design with many social intervention problems can be conducted by an individual researcher, although most efforts would be enriched when a group of designers work together. In the clinical example in which the goal was an intervention for use with persons experiencing depression, an individual conducted the process. During the initial stage, for purposes of illustration, the example assumes that a decision had been made to draw from two types of information: intervention research findings and theoretical presentations. The source of the information would be limited to recent published reviews of research findings regarding the effectiveness of various forms of psychosocial intervention for depression, as well as major theoretical publications (e.g., Shelton et al. 1991; Wolman 1990; Hargreaves and Shumway 1989). The design domain, as already noted, is limited to intervenor characteristics and intervention techniques. Summary statements could be formulated which presented broad descriptive summaries of the findings from the research and theoretical work.

In this example, a student-clinician took on this design problem and found that the findings regarding accurate empathy, as well as cognitive interventions, turned out to be particularly interesting and relevant to the problem of depression. Several of the generalizations that were developed by this student-clinician are adapted and used to illustrate. As described below, the student-clinician built on the work of prior student-clinicians who had already done the conversion work regarding accurate empathy and cognitive procedures. This is an example of borrowing from prior design work (Munson and Pelz, 1980). These borrowed generalizations and guidelines were combined with original work done by the student clinician in other areas of conversion. It is important to note that design work frequently combines borrowing, adapting, and originating activities. When applied research is the primary type of information retrieved, then borrowing and adapting technologies may dominate and, therefore, design work may be simplified. This is because applied research is practical, that is, it is usually conducted with the intent that the findings be useful. Practice principles may be apparent or easily identifiable when applied research findings are examined for use in design. In the following example, the student-clinician's broader objective is to develop a general intervention strategy or what Mullen has termed a *personal intervention model*. Included in that model is a preferred strategy for clinical intervention with depressed individuals. The discussion is limited to this particular area of the model.

Accurate Empathy. As already noted, this student-clinician borrowed the work done by a prior student-clinician regarding accurate empathy and, as a result, conversion was simplified. The following describes the original work done by the first student-clinician who followed the steps by Mullen for designing personal intervention models.[2] Intervention guidelines are the products resulting from conversion and design. In this illustration, literature reviews were analyzed and codified. The student-clinician used a recording format which included documentation of the component being examined; the specific intervention variable under study, including its description; the reported efficacy of the intervention; and the limiting conditions. These three steps resulted in identification and recording of what can be thought of as substantive findings. In addition, an assessment of the soundness of the evidence was conducted. Conventional criteria were used to judge the validity of research data. The approach to review of the quality of evidence supporting a substantive generalization includes four tasks: (1) specification of the representativeness under which the intervention was studied; (2) identification of the characteristics of the research designs and threats to validity; (3) specification of the consistency of the findings; and (4) specification of the extent of replication of the findings. In this information retrieval method three conceptual areas are formulated: substantive generalizations detailing the character of the relationships between the intervention and its effects on clients; limiting factors specifying the pertinent environmental, organizational, client, and technical conditions under which the interventions reportedly have an effect; and quality-of-evidence factors specifying the nature of the empirical and theoretical grounding. These are illustrated in Figure 1.

Cognitive Procedures. The generation of alternative intervention potentials from available information is generally recognized to be an important step in design work. In the area of practice it is now

---

2. The process of personal intervention modeling is an adaptation of the social research and development process developed by Rothman (Mullen 1978, 1981, 1983, 1988; Rothman 1974).

FIGURE 1. Generalizations regarding accurate empathy.

1-1: Substantive Generalization Regarding Accurate Empathy.

Substantive Generalization: An intervenor's sensitivity to the moment-to-moment feelings of the client and the intervenor's verbal facility to communicate this understanding in a language attuned to the client's current feelings (as measured by the Accurate Empathy Scale) are positively associated with the client's depth of self-exploration (as measured by the Self-Exploration Scale) and are frequently associated with attitudinal, cognitive, and behavioral improvements in clients. A low level of empathic responses (as defined above) is associated with low levels of client self-exploration and is frequently associated with deterioration in attitudinal, cognitive, and behavioral areas. Although associated with intervention outcome, this quality does not appear to be either a necessary or sufficient condition, nor does it appear to be among a set of necessary and sufficient conditions for successful outcomes. Empathy accounts for a relatively small amount of variance in intervention outcomes, yet this amount is often statistically significant (Mullen, 1978, pp. 56-57).

1-2. Limiting Factors

Limiting Generalization: Since most of the research has been based on interventions using intervenors trained in a client-centered approach, it is not known to what extent the substantive generalization would be valid for other types of intervenors. Since most studies incorporated as techniques nonpossessive warmth and genuineness, it is unknown to what extent the substantive hypothesis would be valid independently of warmth and genuineness. Limiting conditions concerning client characteristics and organizational contexts are of unknown relevance, based on the available information (Mullen, 1978, p. 57).

1-3: Quality of Evidence Generalization

Quality of Evidence Factors: The substantive generalization is based on a relatively small number of uncontrolled field studies involving a relatively small number of investigators. The reliability and validity of the Accurate Empathy Scale is questionable, and the subject of much disagreement. It is unclear to what extent accurate empathy is independent of client qualities and the extent to which the qualities are reciprocal (interactive). It is not clear to what extent the reported association between accurate empathy and intervention effects is a function of the particular scales used to measure empathy and its assumed effects and the interdependence of the scales. Since the research is relatively uncontrolled, little is known about the extent to which empathy and the effects are causatively associated. Although the findings favor the substantive generalization, some inconsistency is evident, especially in more recent years (Mullen, 1978, p. 57).

evident that many social problems can be approached via alternate intervention methods. These alternatives should be specified in design work, and their relative merits for the problem at hand should be assessed. At times, alternatives may already be specified in the design problem statements, as is the case with the computer program example. The alternatives in this example had been identified because of prior familiarity with the literature. In the instance of the clinical example, alternatives were identified in the course of the literature review.

Thomas (1984) provides a comprehensive list of design criteria for the selection among alternatives. He includes such dimensions as relative advantage, engineerability, compatibility with other design components, and anticipated usability. Design criteria for assessing relative merit should include innovation requirements (as described above) as well as more inclusive criteria such as those of effectiveness, efficiency, risk, equity, and distributional consequences (Tanenbaum 1987). Efficiency analysis is at times an appropriate approach to the selection among alternative interventions. Cost-benefit and cost-effectiveness analysis, while complex and at times unsuitable, can help to specify efficient design alternatives. Of course, when these techniques are used in program design, assumptions must be made about expected costs, benefits, and effects. To some extent, these assumptions can be informed by prior studies. Equity and distributional consequences can be examined in the efficiency analysis. In social intervention these criteria are especially important since values are usually at stake. Technical methods for assigning values to benefits may be used in design work. The decision-theoretic approach is one such method (Edwards, Guttentag, and Snapper 1975).

In addition to these general criteria, the specific application invokes additional considerations. In the clinical example, the practitioner's own values, knowledge, and skills filtered the options available. The student-clinician in this example determined that generalizations regarding cognitive procedures also were relevant to the goal of developing an intervention for work with depressed clients. These were considered as an alternative to accurate empathy. Once again, this student-clinician was fortunate in that a prior student-clinician had already retrieved this information and had formulated generalizations. Unlike the example of accurate empathy, the type of information examined in the original retrieval stage included both empirical research findings as well as theoretical formulations and so the generalizations draw from both sets. In the instance of the cognitive technologies, the student-clinician adopted the generalizations formulated by the first student-clinician illustrated in Figure 2. When appraising the quality of evidence, encompassing multiple information sources, it is useful to develop summary generalizations concerning the grounding for each source. As already noted in this illustration, two sources were used, namely theory and research. Using the cognitive learning technologies, examples of these two sources are also illustrated in Figure 2. When assessing the quality of evidence supporting theoretical formulations, it is useful to distinguish criteria by theoretical function. That is, theories can be used in intervention design to serve one of three functions: heuristic, instrumental, or technological. In addition to the formal criteria typically used to assess a theory (e.g., derivability, clarity, logical consistency, simplicity, generalizability, cohesiveness, and verifiability), social intervention criteria can also be applied (e.g., relevance and ethical standards). A quality of evidence generalization regarding theoretical information was developed by the student-clinician (Figure 2). In addition, a quality of evidence generalization based on research information was formed by the student-clinician (Figure 2). Finally, a broad summary statement might be attempted as a conclusion, as illustrated in Figure 2, for cognitive learning technologies.

These generalizations are examples of those that might emerge from the information retrieval stage. What remains is the conversion of these various descriptive generalizations into prescriptive formulations that can give direction to intervention. These prescriptive formulations are practice guidelines.

Illustrated are only two alternative interventions, accurate empathy and cognitive procedures. Comparisons should be made using criteria such as those already mentioned and a design choice should be made among the alternatives. In this example, the choice illustrates a variation in that the student-clinician selected both accurate empathy as well as the cognitive procedures for inclusion in subsequent design work. The selection of both follows from the student-

FIGURE 2. Examining alternatives and forming generalizations.

2-1: Substantive Generalization Regarding Cognitive Procedures

---

Substantive Generalization: The cognitive learning therapies are considered by Mahoney and Arknoff (1978) to be of three general types: cognitive restructuring techniques; coping skills techniques; and problem-solving techniques. Each of these general types are composed of more specific techniques. Cognitive restructuring includes rational-emotive therapy, self-instruction, and cognitive therapy. Coping skills techniques include covert modeling, coping training, anxiety management, and stress inoculation. The problem-solving techniques include behavioral problem solving, problem-solving therapy, and personal science. The general class of cognitive learning therapies is seen by Mahoney and Arknoff (1978) as related to and sharing some similarities with behavioral self-control and covert conditioning.

In general, these techniques share a common goal–to increase social functioning by assessing and modifying maladaptive cognitions by means of teaching new, more realistic patterns of thought, feeling, and/or behavior. These various techniques share a common set of intervention principles, as well as principles specific to each technique. The common principles are that the human organism responds primarily to cognitive representations of its environment, rather than to the environment per se; that the cognitive representations are fundamentally related to processes and parameters of learning; that most human learning is cognitively mediated; and that thoughts, feelings, and behaviors are causally interactive. Derivations include the following. (1) In attempting to predict behavior, phenomenology is a better predictor than external reality, and a weighted prediction based on phenomenology and external variables will often be best. (2) Beliefs, attitudes, and other cognitive representations should be modified by procedures that parallel those of the learning laboratory. (3) There is a causal circularity–an interactive (or reciprocal) an interactive (or reciprocal) determinism between cognitive representations on the one hand and feelings, actions, and consequences on the other hand. Cognitions are both the process and product of learning (Mullen, 1988, p. 526, based on Anderson-Ray, 1980).

2-2: Limiting Factors

Limiting Generalization: Concerning the characteristics of the intervenor relevant to the cognitive learning techniques, it is reported that such techniques can be and have been used by a wide range of professional helpers with no particular limitations specified. Intervenors are generally required to play an active role in structuring and controlling the direction of the session. Teacher and enabler roles are seen as important in helping the client clarify thought patterns and learn new patterns and behaviors. The relationship is of obvious importance and the relationship effects appear central, especially manipulation of expectancy. Relatively little training is required to learn these techniques.

The techniques are proposed for and reportedly have been used with a wide range of clients with diverse problems including depression, obesity, smoking, alcohol abuse, stress, sexual problems, phobias, and avoidance patterns. A client limitation is that the client must be able to distinguish between external reality and internal experiences and be able to test hypotheses and try alternative behavior, accepting them as valid. The organizational contexts appropriate for the use of these techniques have not been specified, nor has their use in social work settings (Mullen, 1988, pp. 526-527, based on Anderson-Ray, 1980).

2-3: Quality of Theoretical Information Factors

Quality of Theoretical Information: Cognitive learning principles are based on a combination of psychodynamic and behavioral theories. A well-developed cognitive learning theory has not been devised. Although each of the subtypes has its own set of principles and propositions, a more general, overarching theory is not evident. Mahoney and Arkoff (1978) have outlined four principles and several derivations, cited earlier, that reflect the foundation of cognitive learning theory at its present state of development. Although the theory in its present state of development is too skeletal to merit high marks on the formal criteria normally used to assess scientific theory, it does appear to be developing favorably in terms of derivability, clarity, logical consistency, simplicity, and generalizability. Its potential cohesiveness or fit with the larger body of theoretical development is less clear. Its verifiability also appears to be somewhat problematic, especially due to the concern with internal, cognitive events. Concerning relevance to personal and professional values and to prescriptive knowledge, the general theory seems highly congruent, to the extent of its development. The theory appears to be based on humanistic assumptions. Of some concern is the idea of restructuring the client's cognitions. Because of this idea, special considerations of client consent and involvement of the client in goal formation seem ethically important. Finally, it does appear that this theoretical base lends itself to a heuristic function in model building (stimulating further development of the theoretical system), as well as an instrumental function (providing guidance to the practitioner and client because of the believability of the ideas included in the theory). However, because of a lack of empirical support, it would be premature to consider it as serving a technological function (being used because of its demonstrated validity) (Mullen, 1988, p. 527, based on Anderson-Ray, 1980).

2-4: Quality of Research Factors

Quality of Research Information: Largely untested, coping skills techniques are without an adequate research base from which to draw meaningful conclusions regarding their effectiveness. Cognitive restructuring and the problem-solving therapies are also not well grounded in research evidence, although the small

FIGURE 2 (continued)

amount reported tends to be favorable. Research in this area has generally failed to control for limiting conditions (qualities of the intervenors clients, relationship factors, or organizational contexts), and the quality of the designs and research methods is poor (Mullen, 1988), pp. 526-527. based on Anderson-Ray, 1980).

2-5: Conclusions Regarding Cognitive Procedures

Concluding Summary. Because interest in cognitive therapy has developed relatively recently, neither cognitive learning principles nor intervention techniques have been fully developed or adequately researched. In spite of this, the principles give the practitioner a new way to understand the client that unites the psychodynamic and behavioral perspectives. In addition, many of the techniques hold potential for increasing the efficiency and effectiveness of interventions. Among the most promising of these are self-monitoring, covert counterconditioning, and the entire set of cognitive learning techniques (Mullen, 1988, p. 528, based on Anderson-Ray, 1980).

---

clinician's observation that the two approaches complement one another. In other instances the summary generalizations might suggest that one intervention is more effective or that, while both are effective, one might be less costly. It may also be found that the alternatives are incompatible. Having made a choice the process continues into the conversion stage.

Develop Practice Guidelines

The conceptual task in the conversion process is to take the set of generalizations formulated in the retrieval stage and to specify intervention prescriptions which do not deviate too much from the original generalizations pertaining to accurate empathy. Figure 3 illustrates examples of intervention or action guidelines that might be developed from the generalizations.

While the guidelines resulting from conversion are general, their application to a specific context such as clinical intervention with depressed clients moves into design-related plans. In design planning and formation of specific practice guidelines, the original social intervention problem and goal become pivotal. It is in this step more than any other in the design process, that creativity has an

FIGURE 3. Intervention guidelines.

3-1: Intervention Guidelines Regarding Accurate Empathy

In practice situations where client self-exploration is desirable, intervenor responses that reflect accurate empathy should be used to facilitate client self-exploration.

Expression of low levels of accurate empathy should be avoided, especially with more fragile and vulnerable clients, to avoid harming clients.

Since expression of accurate empathy appears to a large extent to be reciprocal, intervenors should be aware of how they are emphatically relating to their clients and should exert control over their expression of empathy.

Since accurate empathy at best appears to account for only a small portion of variance in intervention effects, other intervention qualities should be used to enhance effectiveness (Mullen, 1978, p. 58).

3-2: Design Articulations Regarding Accurate Empathy

When providing clinical intervention with depressed clients where client self-exploration is desirable, intevenor responses that reflect accurate empathy should be used to facilitate client self-exploration.

Expression of low levels of accurate empathy should be avoided with more fragile and vulnerable depressed clients since this could worsen the depressive condition.

Since expression of accurate empathy appears to a large extent to be reciprocal, clinicians working with depressed clients should be aware of how they are empathically relating to these clients and should exert control over their expression of empathy.

Since accurate empathy at best appears to account for only a small portion of variance in intervention effects and since these effects are generally associated with enhancing self-exploration rather than symptoms of depression **per se**, an intervention specifically designed for depression should include other intervention elements to enhance effectiveness especially cognitive-behavioral and psychopharmacological treatments.

---

impact. Without a creative, pragmatic element, it would be difficult to develop intervention guidelines from what might appear to be interesting but distant empirical and theoretical generalizations. Figure (3-2) also illustrates guidelines that could result from design considerations. These articulated guidelines are quite similar to those formed in the conversion phase but they differ in that the specific application area is included, in this instance work with depressed clients.

Examples of guidelines which take into account design specifications concerning intervention with depressed clients and the generalizations regarding cognitive learning technologies are illustrated in Figure 4 (Anderson-Ray 1980).

These generalizations and guidelines from the clinical intervention example have been presented in some detail for purposes of illustration. (Other examples are in the chapter on Systematic Research Synthesis.)

In the computer system example, four design problems have been identified. Because this example is more complex, it is not presented here, but rather in Figure 5. The computer system found to be most

FIGURE 4. Design articulations regarding cognitive procedures.

Since interventions based on cognitive learning principles are considered to be especially relevant for intervention with depression such interventions should be included in the intervention plan. These interventions should be used to modify the effect of maladaptive cognitions on behaviors.

Intervention with depressed clients should include an assessment of maladaptive cognitions; use of techniques to dispute or disrupt the maladaptive thought process; development of a means to help the client understand and control maladaptive thoughts and resulting inappropriate behaviors; provision for teaching of appropriate skills and behaviors, as necessary including problem-solving and/or coping skills; and provision for practice and rehearsal of new skills and behaviors, as needed.

Interventions with depressed clients should not be limited to cognitive techniques but rather they should be combined with other elements including the use of accurate empathy as well as psychopharmacological agents.

FIGURE 5. Expert system example–design problems, generalization and guidelines.

Design Problem 1:

What systematic coding system will be used for representing the knowledge to be included in the computer program? (e.g., production rules, predicate logic, or structured objects).

Summary Generalization:

Based on a review of the literature the following generalization was formed.

Knowledge representation is an area of considerable research activity. According to Fischler and Firscheim at least 10 distinct representation systems of broad generality are currently employed at AI research (*AI Expert*, December, 1988, 44). They note that each representation has advantages and disadvantages and that selection should be goal directed taking into account the characteristics of the knowledge domain to be represented and the decision requirements. In expert systems work production systems or rule-based representations have been most common although frame-based representations are increasingly used. Selection of the representation should be influenced by the familiarity of the developer with the representation, the expert-system shells available to the developer, the characteristics of the knowledge domain, as well as other requirements. Citrenbaum, Geissman, and Schultz propose that the development tools used (e.g., expert system shell) should permit the use of several knowledge representations. They suggest that during early stages of modelling of a domain representations should be relatively transparent or intuitive. In knowledge domains where the knowledge is not extensive, rule-based systems may be sufficient.

Practice Guideline:

Based on this summary generalization the following guidelines illustrate the conversion to prescriptive statements.

In the area of expert system development in social work since the knowledge domains will usually not include an extensive amount of knowledge, rule-based representations will generally be adequate.

Since the expertise of social work developers usually will be relatively limited, complex representation systems may not be appropriate.

Since expert system development in social work and social welfare is at a very early stage, the representation should be fairly intuitive and transparent to permit easy access to the knowledge base.

So as to permit selective use of other representations, expert system shells should be used which permit use of other representation schemes as desired, especially frames.

FIGURE 5 (continued)

Moving from conversion to design specification guidelines would be developed applicable to the particular application.

Since the domain of assessing risk-of-harm for abuse and neglect is a new area of expert system development and since the knowledge in the domain is probably not extensive, a rule-based representation is adequate for purposes of the initial prototype.

Should the initial work on the prototype indicate that rule-based representation is inadequate then experimentation with other representations should be considered.

An expert system shell should be used that permits use of several representation systems such as rules and frames.

Design Problem 2:

What method of knowledge acquisition should be used—should the program learn by being fed new knowledge propositions (e.g., new rules) or should the program be capable of generating and modifying knowledge propositions (e.g., rules) in interaction with an expert or should the program be capable of discovering new concepts and relationships?

Practice Guidelines:

In situations where experts are readily available yet their knowledge is not explicit, the use of knowledge engineers to interview the experts and formulate the knowledge of the experts in the required form should be considered. The knowledge engineers should formulate the new rules to be included in the expert system. This applies to the risk-of-harm situation and therefore the expert system should be designed to learn by being told new rules.

Design Problem 3:

Should the system be capable of reasoning from antecedents to consequences as well as reasoning from a goal or conclusion to determine whether or not the facts exist to support the conclusion (e.g., both forward and backward chaining)?

Practice Guideline:

When the knowledge base contains a small number of rules, forward chaining methods are adequate for most expert system applications. Backward chaining methods are useful when there is a large number of rules. Since the risk-of-harm system is anticipated to require a small number of rules, forward chaining methods are sufficient.

appropriate is an expert system, and the example uses expert system technical terms which may be unfamiliar to the average reader.

FROM DESIGN TO PRODUCT

Guidelines like those illustrated are assembled to form a complete and cohesive intervention design. In Mullen's work with personal intervention modeling, the assemblage is called a personal model. The complete model is expected to include guidelines that are inclusive and compatible. The guidelines developed through the personal modeling process are inherently user ready since they have been developed by the practitioner who will be using the intervention. At the core of the model design are guidelines which specify a range of procedures which can guide intervention in a variety of practice situations.

In the case of designs for general use such as in the example of the computer program, the final design concept should include clearly specified procedures of relevance to multiple potential users. The design stage ends with such guidelines. These guidelines or prescriptive statements set the agenda for development activity. Rossi and Freeman (1985) have stated that design and development work should produce an intervention model which specifies the relationship between a program and the program's goal as well as the strategy for attaining the goal (72).

In the case of the computer program example, the design specifications are that a computer program should be developed for assessing risk of harm and that the system should use a rule-based knowledge representation system, capable of reasoning from antecedents to consequences (i.e., forward chaining), and learning by being told new rules. These were the design problems. In addition, the system would need to have the characteristics specified in the design requirements including capability of explaining conclusions reached and capability of providing information about the certainty of conclusions reached. The requirements also specify that the system should include information typically used by protective service investigators and that the system should be usable by child welfare investigators. Similarly, for the clinical intervention, the design specifications would include the initial requirements and the practice guidelines. Developmental work follows. In development, the design concept is turned into bricks and mortar. Pilot testing, formative evaluation, simulation analysis, and other developmental activities are carried out such that initial design concepts are used, modified as needed, and reused. In this sense design not only permeates the prior stages of intervention research, but it continues into the subsequent work of development. As characterized by Rothman (1980), design is tentative and exploratory, requiring further application, testing, and validation.

DISCUSSION OF DESIGN ISSUES

A number of design issues have been mentioned which merit further attention. Reference has been made to two different types of technology on a dimension of abstractness. Both Egea (1975) and Haeffner (1973) suggest that technologies include both tangible as well as abstract products. How design methods might differ with these types of applications merits consideration.

Munson and Pelz's (1980) ideas regarding levels of innovation also deserve further analysis in terms of implications for design methods. Clearly, design methods will be quite different depending on whether the innovation involves origination, adaptation, or borrowing.

This chapter has only touched on the important design work of generating and selecting among alternative design concepts. The literature makes reference to such techniques as brainstorming and so forth. It is clear that the generation and comparison of alternative concepts is central to creative and productive design. This area also requires further work.

An additional issue in design has to do with how the designer can confidently move from broad generalizations of the type that emerge from the retrieval stage to specific design guidelines. The conceptual processes have been referred to as involving creativity and artistic skills. A better understanding of this process is required.

Two additional issues merit further review. Both address the origins of the design process. The first issue has to do with the centrality of problem-solving in social intervention research and design work. That is, does design work begin with identification of a social problem? Or, can interventions be designed prior to identification of a social problem application? Weiss (1977) has distinguished knowledge-driven (information in search of a user), problem-driven (a need in search of a solution), and reciprocal process (interaction between the user and the information source) approaches to knowledge use. Similarly, Thomas (1984) refers to domain-driven and problem-driven approaches. It seems that the centrality of a focal social problem within the cycle of intervention research design may vary depending on the particular framework used to guide the work as well as where the designer enters into the intervention research process. For example, experience with personal intervention modeling suggests that one might begin with a problem of concern and seek to develop an appropriate intervention–or, one could reverse the order and begin with a particular intervention technology of interest and look for appropriate applications. It is not unusual to find that social intervention research is technology focused rather than social problem focused. For example, Reid's (1987) work in the area of task-centered practice often begins with task-centered technologies and pursues their development with particular problems. In one report, Reid writes that the purpose of the developmental research project was " to test and develop a task-centered family treatment model" (20). (See chapter 11 for an illustration of the approach.) Similarly, in Mullen and Schuerman's (1990) work with expert systems there is an assumption that expert systems technology can be used to address several problems in social welfare. Mullen's interest originates with the technology, and he has subsequently looked for relevant problem areas.

An additional issue requiring work is the extent to which design should begin with identification of intended users of the innovation. That is, is the design to satisfy a consumer need? It is often said that applied research should begin with the user in mind. Is this the origin of design work? An instructive illustration of this issue is presented in the work of Tanenbaum (1987), who describes the development of the Boston Elbow, an arm prosthesis designed to minimize the disability associated with loss of an arm. Tanenbaum demonstrates how the design of the Boston Elbow was influenced by a particular understanding of disability as experienced by disabled people. In this instance the innovator "does something new to sustain an old identity . . . (allowing) users to confirm their identities by restoring a part of them that has been lost" (3). Tanenbaum asks why prosthesis designers do not simply set out to replicate the human arm since this is what might on first glance be expected of medical technology. She poignantly observes that "replacing the natural limb necessarily alters the body system radically and precludes, by definition, real replication of the natural arm" (3). She notes that a device will "embody only a subset of functions and meanings of what was lost"(3). Choices must be made in design and these choices are normative since design reflects a series of human choices. Values enter into this decision process and, because functional loss is contextual and idiosyncratic, Tanenbaum argues that consumers should be involved in these choices and consumer requirements should be central in design choices. In the case of the Boston Elbow, Tanenbaum believes that lack of consumer involvement would have lessened diffusion, increasing the probability that the technology would not have been responsive to consumer need.

In contrast to the idea that design should begin with consumer requirements, an alternate notion is that design begins with the seed of an idea. From this perspective, design is seen as dependent on a creative seed or idea which grows and is formed by design methods. The seed or idea grows and is subsequently adapted to the needs of a variety of possible users. An interesting example of this latter approach is the formulation presented by Long in his description of how the laser was developed in the Western Electric Company (1976). As described by Glaser, Abelson, and Garrison (1983), the stages evolved over more than a dozen years from curiosity (unfolding of the discovery in the laboratory), seed (questioning utility for allocation of developmental resources), fundamental (building knowledge for industrial application), and, maturity (updating) (159). This example of laser development indicates that the origin is basic curiosity leading to the seed of an idea which subsequently is connected to possible applications.

An issue which remains to be clarified is the extent to which the design of intervention can be separated from the needs of the potential user. How do design methods differ across the "knowledge-driven" and the "problem-driven" approaches (Glaser, Abelson, and Garrison 1983:166)? It is probable that both have a place and may describe differing situations. A new idea or product will more than likely be picked up by designers and developers, and applications will be found. Alternatively, a need or pressure for change will often instigate a process of clarification of the nature of the need, which in turn will stimulate creative thinking, leading to the design of alternative solutions or interventions.

Cutting across these various formulations, there would probably be agreement that design is most fundamentally a process of reasoning intended to produce a well-conceptualized intervention plan. Developmental work transforms this conceptual plan into action. The issues of design are the issues of how to think clearly about how to intervene. How can problems be understood sufficiently so that appropriate objectives can be specified? How can feasible interventions be determined? How can intervention requirements be formulated such that the intervention will fit the situation? What are the intervention alternatives from which a choice needs to be made? What criteria can be used to select among these alternatives? In the domain of social intervention, these questions do not have easy answers. But the questions help to focus toward issues needing attention.

REFERENCES

Anderson-Ray, S. 1980. *Personal Practice Model: Technologies and Techniques for Microsystem and Mezzosystem Interventions*. Unpublished manuscript, University of Chicago, School of Social Service Administration.

Costello, T. W. 1968. *Change in Municipal Government: A View from Inside*. Paper presented to 76th Annual Meeting of American Psychological Association, San Francisco, CA.

Edwards, W., M. Guttentag, and K. Snapper. 1975. A decision-theoretic approach to evaluation research. In *Handbook of Evaluation Research*, edited by E. L. Struening and M. Guttentag. Beverly Hills: Sage Publications, 1, 139-182.

Egea, A. N. 1975. Multinational corporations in the operation and ideology of international transfer of technology. *Studies in Comparative International Development, 10*:1,11-29.

Fischler, M. A. and O. Firschein. 1986. Intelligence and the computer. *AI Expert*, December: 43-49.

Glaser, E. M., H. H. Abelson, and K. N. Garrison. 1983. *Putting Knowledge to Use*. San Francisco: Jossey-Bass.

Haeffner, E. A. 1973. The innovation process. *Technology Review, 75*:5, 18-25.

Hargreaves, W. A. and M. Shumway. 1989. Effectiveness of services for severely mentally ill. National Institute of Mental Health. *The Future of Mental Health Services Research*, edited by C. A. Taube, D. Mechanic, and A. Hohnmann. (DHHS Publication No. ADM 89-1600). Washington, DC: U.S. Government Printing Office, 253-284.

Havelock, R. G. 1969. *Planning for Innovation through Dissemination and Utilization of Knowledge*. Ann Arbor: University of Michigan, Institute for Social Research, Center for Research on Utilization of Scientific Knowledge.

Long, T. P. 1976. A case study: Laser processing–from development to application. *Research Management, 19*:1, 15-17.

Mahoney, M. J. and D. Arknoff. 1978. Cognitive and self-control therapies. In *Handbook of Psychotherapy and Behavior Change*, edited by S. L. Garfield and A. E. Bergin. New York: Wiley & Sons, 689-722.

Mullen, E. J. 1978. The construction of personal models for effective practice: A method for utilizing research findings to guide social interventions. *Journal of Social Service Research*, 2:1, 45-63.

Mullen, E. J. 1981. Development of personal intervention models. In *Applied Social Work Research/Evaluation*, edited by Richard M. Grinnell, Itasca, IL.: F. E. Peacock Publishers.

Mullen, E. J. 1983. Personal practice models in clinical social work. In *Handbook of Clinical Social Work*, edited by Aaron Rosenblatt and Diana Waldfogel. San Francisco: Jossey-Bass.

Mullen, E. J. 1988. Using research and theory in social work practice. In *Social Work Research and Evaluation*, edited by Richard M. Grinnell, Jr. Itasca, IL: F. E. Peacock Publishers.

Mullen, E. J. and J. R. Schuerman. 1990. Expert systems and the development of knowledge in social welfare. In *Advances in Clinical Social Research*, edited by L. Videka-Sherman and W. J. Reid. Silver Spring, MD: National Association of Social Workers.

Munson, F. C. and D. C. Pelz. 1980. *Innovating in Organizations: A Conceptual Framework*. Ann Arbor: University of Michigan, School of Public Health and Institute for Social Research.

Patti, R. J. 1981. The prospects for social R&D: An essay review. *Social Work Research and Abstracts, 17*:2, 38-44.

Reid, W. J. 1987. Evaluating an intersection in developmental research. *Journal of Social Service Research, 11*:1, 17-37.

Rossi, P. H. and H. E. Freeman. 1985. *Evaluation: A Systematic Approach*. Beverly Hills: Sage Publications.

Rothman, J. 1974. *Planning and Organizing for Social Change: Action Principles for Social Research*. New York: Columbia University Press.

Rothman, J. 1980. *Social R&D: Research and Development in the Human Services*. Englewood Cliffs, NJ: Prentice-Hall, Inc.

Rothman, J. 1989. Intervention research: Application to runaway and homeless youths. *Social Work Research and Abstracts, 25*:1, 13-18.

Shelton, R. C., S. D. Hollow, S. E. Purdon, and P. T. Loosen. 1991. Biological and psychological aspects of depression. *Behavior Therapy, 22,* 201-228.

Tanenbaum, S. 1987. *Engineering Disability: Public Policy and Compensatory Technology.* Philadelphia: Temple University Press.

Thomas, E. J. 1978. Generating innovation in social work: The paradigm of developmental research. *Journal of Social Service Research, 2*:1, 95-115.

Thomas, E. J. 1984. *Designing Interventions for the Helping Professions.* Beverly Hills: Sage Publications.

Thomas, E. J. 1985. The validity of design and development and related concepts in developmental research. *Social Work Research and Abstracts. 21*:2, 50-55.

Weiss, C. H. 1977. *Using Social Research in Public Policy Making.* Lexington, MA: Lexington Books.

Wolman, B. B. (ed.) 1990. *Depressive disorders: Facts, Theories, and Treatment Methods.* New York: Wiley & Sons.

Zaltman, G. 1979. Knowledge utilization as planned social change. *Knowledge, 1*:1, 82-105.

Chapter 9

Intervention Design for Practice–
Enhancing Social Supports
for High Risk Youth and Families

James K. Whittaker
Elizabeth M. Tracy
Edward Overstreet
John Mooradian
Steven Kapp

INTRODUCTION

This chapter describes the application of an intervention design project in a large, midwestern agency serving troubled youth and their families. The goal of the project was to design and test the clinical utility of social network interventions as a means of aiding clinical supervisors and program staff in addressing the social support needs of this group. We were interested, as well, in the compatibility of our tool, the Social Network Map (Tracy and Whittaker 1990), with the agency's well-developed practitioner-oriented information system (Grasso and Epstein 1987 and 1989). Throughout this present effort and a predecessor project (Whittaker, Tracy, and Marckworth 1988), we were guided by the vision of research-in-service of practice so ably articulated by Rothman (1980) and Thomas (1984). Their pioneering conceptions of "social R&D" and "intervention design and development" (D&D) provided both a catalyst and a framework for organizing our research and development activities.

Our intervention design effort was stimulated by the recognition that the resources of neighborhood and extended family networks are frequently associated with successful service outcomes in youth care. Treatment efforts can apparently be made more enduring through the supportive assistance of kin, friends, neighbors, and other informal helpers who assist youths and families in consolidating the gains made in professional services. While techniques for assessing and strengthening these network resources are not numerous, some pilot efforts have shown promising results (Gaudin et al. 1990/91; Tracy and Whittaker 1987). We were clear at the outset that network interventions offered no panacea. They were seen as a necessary, but not sufficient component of a comprehensive service plan which likely included family treatment, parent education, case management, and related services. Nor did we assume that network members were always supportive. Kin and friends can be the source of excessive demands and expectations as well as support, and they sometimes reinforce such self-injurious behavior as drug use. Indeed, we believed the potential negative effects of network members on client treatment goals was itself a powerful reason for better understanding the strengths and liabilities for the families and youth with whom the agency routinely worked.

We believed that the network mapping instrument developed in our earlier intervention research with Homebuilders (Whittaker, Tracy, and Marckworth 1988) offered a clinically useful and practical tool for assisting therapists in obtaining network information and putting it to good clinical use in a case plan. We were interested in refining our proficiency in training staff in basic skills in social network and social support assessment and in identifying a range of interventions designed to augment and reinforce supportive resources within clients' personal networks. Finally, we were interested in obtaining a clearer picture of network resources and challenges among client families served. The efficacy of these interventions, indeed the usefulness of the basic network assessment itself, awaits future empirical validation.

The project was designed to address a number of obstacles common to conducting research in agency settings. These include:

• Distance often perceived between the academic world and the world of clinical practice

- Researcher's focus on the "average" client versus the practitioner's concern for the needs of individual clients
- Lack of consensus on the objectives of research that often exists between academics and practitioners (Wells and Whittaker 1989)

These obstacles were overcome through the use of D&D methodology, in which the emphasis is on the design, development, field testing, and diffusion of new practice technology (Thomas 1978, 1984; Rothman 1989). This methodology offers a number of advantages as a research tool for intervention development (Whittaker and Pecora 1981).

First, it is oriented toward creating a specific solution, strategy, or answer to a specific problem. The primary research question is "how to" rather than "why." One worker aptly expressed this point: "We could find new ways to do things rather than being evaluated on what we've already done." Second, this methodology actively and meaningfully involves practitioners in all phases of the project. Clinical judgment, practice wisdom, and subjective evaluations of practitioners are viewed as valid and important pieces of information, informing research questions and design. Finally, D&D efforts can lead to a better conceptualized and more testable body of technology for rigorous field experiments.

The following sections describe the tasks and activities undertaken at Boysville in designing procedures for social network interventions in the context of intensive family preservation services. A brief synopsis of a predecessor project conducted with Homebuilders is presented first, since this project was instrumental in completing early phases of the D&D model, such as identification of critical practice issues and retrieval and synthesis of relevant information. The present intervention design project conducted at Boysville of Michigan is presented next in order to illustrate the major phases and steps common to the design phase (Thomas 1984; Mullen, Chapter 8). The final product which emerged from our efforts to date is a set of practice guidelines suitable for more rigorous field testing.

PRELIMINARY WORK
WITH THE HOMEBUILDERS PROJECT

The present Boysville project builds on an earlier effort–the Family Support Project (Whittaker, Tracy, and Marckworth 1988) which sought to identify practical strategies for assessing and enhancing social support resources for families at risk of disruption through out-of-home placement. This project was implemented from April 1987 through September 1988 in conjunction with Homebuilders, an intensive family preservation program located in the State of Washington. The project was funded through a grant from the Edna McConnell Clark Foundation.

The time period just prior to the initiation of the Homebuilders project was devoted primarily to the identification and analysis of critical practice issues related to social support. This phase is generally referred to as an analysis phase; it is a necessary prerequisite to the design phase, and will be briefly discussed here as it related to the Boysville project.

During the analysis phase of an D&D effort, the main tasks are to (a) identify and analyze the social problem and (b) select information sources from which to generate innovations. The product generated during this phase typically includes a state of the art review of existing information. Among information sources which we consulted during this phase were:

- Basic research on the mediating effects of social support
- Applications of social support interventions with specific client populations
- Descriptive and correlational studies of the social network characteristics of various client groups
- Social policy as in "reasonable efforts" to support and maintain children in their own homes mandated by PL 96-272
- Practice examples via case record review of existing practice and a staff survey

A review of the evidence base from existing social science literature suggested that much of the current state of knowledge regarding social support did not easily convert to concrete practice principles (Tracy and Whittaker 1987). Few guidelines existed to aid practitioners in planning and implementing social support interventions. While the research evidence on social support was compelling, much was correlational in nature. It was not clear, for example, whether practitioners should seek to create support systems for clients, improve existing supports, or enable clients to generate their own support. Guidelines to aid practitioners in making these decisions as well as clinically relevant social support assessment tools had been lacking.

Another information source was a staff survey with Homebuilders which yielded additional important information on practitioners' knowledge of social support, how useful they perceived social support to be in helping families, and how frequently they utilized social support in their work with families. The majority of staff surveyed viewed family social support as often influential in overall clinical work.

A number of activities led to the design and adaptation of instruments for assessing a client's informal helping resources. These activities included review of existing tools and procedures, brainstorm sessions with staff about ways in which they currently gathered information on social networks and the types of information they would find useful, and consultation with a research team, which consisted of representatives from each of the Homebuilder programs in Washington State. A variety of training sessions and clinical seminars were conducted during this phase for the dual purposes of sharing information and contributing to the formulation of new social support assessment techniques. Ultimately, two measures were selected: one, the Social Network Map, developed specifically for this project, patterned after several earlier network mapping techniques (Fraser and Hawkins 1984; Biegel, Shore, and Gordon 1984); and one adapted from an existing instrument, the Community Interaction Checklist, developed by Wahler (1980).

While findings from the use of these social support assessment tools have been fully reported elsewhere (Tracy 1990), several findings were critical to our initiation of the Boysville project. Network data generated were analyzed in terms of social network characteristics (network size and composition, frequency of contact, and length of relationships) and perceived availability of social support (type and source of support, reciprocity, and criticalness). In addition, relationships between social network characteristics and perceived support were examined. Some important practice implications emerged from these analyses.

1. Both structural and functional aspects of social networks were important to assess.
2. Network composition was an important factor to consider.
3. It is important to consider the negative as well as positive aspects of social networks. Not all social ties were found to be supportive.
4. Finally, our findings show that *reciprocity* was positively related to some types of support. Teaching reciprocal social skills might be an effective means to increase social support within a network.

As a result of the analysis of these information sources–literature, staff surveys, and data collection with families–a number of critical practice challenges were identified. These constituted our primary objectives in initiating the Boysville project:

• To develop intervention techniques to build, mobilize, and sustain social support resources in order to assist families in their parenting efforts
• To identify practice approaches to bridge the gap between formal and informal helping resources
• To develop and pilot test a training module on social support and social network intervention for family preservation workers

BOYSVILLE INTERVENTION DESIGN PROJECT

Agency Context

The Social Networks Project was begun in June 1989 and completed in November 1990. Boysville of Michigan, that state's largest youth-serving agency, served as host site for the project and, in conjunction with the Skillman Foundation, funded the applied research effort.[1]

Long a pioneer in residential services for troubled and delinquent youth, Boysville has developed an impressive spectrum of services including therapeutic foster care, intensive family preservation services, reunification services, and other community-based programs from inner city Detroit to more rural counties in Michigan and Ohio. An innovative family work program initiated in the early 1980s for youth in residence exemplifies a trend in the agency toward more community-based, family-centered services. In addition, Boysville has made a sizable investment in implementing a computerized information system designed to serve data-based decision making at all levels of management and practice (Grasso and Epstein 1987, 1989). Information about children and families and about the services they receive is collected at regular intervals during intervention and follow-up. The system is capable of providing individual and aggregate data across a wide range of variables and has been the source of considerable research within the agency.[2] In the context of our Social Networks Project, we were keenly interested in the integration of social network and social support assessment within the overall information system. Boysville, in addition to providing a stimulating environment for family practice and research, offered a special opportunity to learn about culturally specific patterns of social support given the rich racial and ethnic mix represented in the client population.

Design Objective

During this phase, relevant information from the analysis phase is applied to the generation and design of an intervention innovation or product. The design is articulated in sufficient detail so as to be usable in the real world; this may involve the formulation of a set of procedural guidelines as an aspect of the design.

---

1. A limited number of staff from a sister agency in Detroit, The Ennis Center for Children, participated as part of the research team.

2. For an up-to-date bibliography of Boysville research projects, contact: Edward Overstreet, Associate Executive Director, Boysville of Michigan, 17117 W. 9 Mile Road, Suite #445, Southfield, MI 48075.

Our design objective was to develop a set of practice guidelines for social network interventions with high risk families. These practice guidelines would help workers more effectively assess and intervene with social networks by providing a conceptual framework and a decision-making guide. The guidelines would provide options for intervention. As such, they would help translate research findings into practice principles.

Design Criteria

During this phase, it is also helpful to identify preliminary design specifications to guide the scope and boundaries of the developmental effort (Thomas 1984).

While the social network data provided an empirical base for our thinking about the design that social network interventions would ultimately take, we were also influenced by the very nature of the intensive family preservation service model. The practitioners and supervisors with whom we worked were clear that social network interventions should enhance the already existing goals of family preservation services. Social network interventions must be congruent with the following goals:

- to help maintain the child safely within the home;
- to defuse the precipitating crisis;
- to prevent future crises from occurring; and
- to foster maintenance of change over time.

Since intensive family preservation programs provide services for a brief, limited period of time, their program goals and objectives are necessarily limited in scope. The same was true for social network interventions. Practitioners felt that unless a clear relationship could be demonstrated between the social network intervention and the existing agency goals of family preservation, they would have neither the time nor the inclination to engage in implementing additional interventions.

Some other important design criteria imposed on the shaping of interventions included the staff's beliefs that social network interventions:

1. Should be individualized to meet each family's unique social support needs
2. Should be congruent with the theoretical stance of the program
3. Should be able to address concerns and needs of the parents, children, and/or entire family
4. Should build on family strengths
5. Should be sensitive to culturally defined patterns of help seeking and giving

In summary, the design criteria specified that social network interventions must be congruent with explicit agency values, philosophy, practice techniques, and goals of intensive family preservation services. Interventions designed and developed within a different program context may look very different from those described here.

Design Problems

In our initial analysis of existing information, we identified a number of unresolved design issues (Whittaker 1986; Tracy and Whittaker 1987; Maluccio 1989). Some design problems stem from social service organizational and administrative concerns, while others are more closely related to the nature of social support, and our limited knowledge of the exact processes through which social supports exert beneficial effects:

- What are the institutional barriers and complexities of introducing nonsalaried informal helpers into formal service plans? Agency liability, accountability for services rendered, and client confidentiality were all expressed concerns of workers and supervisors.
- How will workers respond to the sharing of power and authority with informal helpers implied by social network practice?
- How can workers overcome "person-oriented" training models and adopt an environmental focus to their practice?
- What types of support are most appropriate for a given client group experiencing a given stressor?
- What variables influence a person's perception of and satisfaction with social support?

- What variables influence a person's willingness to use social network resources? For example, what is the relationship between social support and social skills? Is it best to mobilize social support for clients, or to teach them skills to mobilize support on their own? Or is some combination of strategies more appropriate?
- How do well-functioning families use social network resources?
- How can we ensure that social network interventions will be sensitive to diverse cultural groups and culturally defined patterns of help seeking and giving?

In sum, our review of the available evidence on social support, the nature of the dominant practice orientation of the clinicians, and the administrative demands of the agency all posed challenges to the design process.

User Participation and Design Formulation

The Social Network Project employed case consultations to develop and evaluate the impact of various packages of social support intervention strategies. Case consultation sessions were held regularly (generally monthly) with individual teams of practitioners. The goal was to track the development, planning, and implementation of social support interventions with individual youths and families. When a case was discussed at case consultation, the social support assessment information was reviewed to determine what types of goals would most appropriately address the family's needs. A format was developed to guide these discussions. Implementation strategies would then be considered. Over a period of time what worked, as well as what did not work, was noted. In this way, staff became more knowledgeable about interventions. The project's task was to provide workers with a framework for conceptualizing social support interventions. The objective was to help practitioners individualize social support interventions so as to enhance the overall service goals for each family.

This also meant that standardized approaches to social support assessment and intervention were not favored. Staff felt that the timing and introduction of the tools depended greatly on the crisis facing the family. In some cases, staff did not feel that social support assessment was indicated. Time limitations, the presence of severe crisis, and safety issues generally took priority over social support planning. While this is a disadvantage from a strict research perspective, it is an advantage for intervention design, as an understanding of obstacles and barriers is an important factor in planning real world applications.

In addition to the case consultation sessions, a number of other means were utilized for design formulation. Clinical seminars were conducted, in some cases with outside consultants. These sessions provided a means to discuss the use of the assessment tools and the implementation of specific interventions. For example, staff members were asked to brainstorm social and communication skills that they considered key to accessing and maintaining supportive relationships. One session focused specifically on the social support resources of minority families. These discussions yielded rich information for the development of intervention guidelines. Each team member was also responsible for developing training materials. This ensured high levels of involvement and feelings of ownership of the process. Throughout this critical phase of the project, the two principal investigators communicated weekly to keep track of emergent design issues and directions.

Generation of Practice Guidelines

The intervention design proceeded in at least three distinct stages. The first phase involved articulating a rationale for including social network interventions as part of intensive family preservation services. A number of reasons were proposed for looking at social networks and social supports. The most important of these were:

1. To better understand culturally specific patterns of help giving;
2. To identify potential sources of support to aid in the maintenance of treatment gain;
3. To gain an appreciation of the client's perception of support;
4. To pinpoint sources of conflict within the personal social network;
5. To identify patterns of reciprocal helping; and

6. To identify relevant others who may participate in future network interventions (Tracy, Whittaker, and Mooradian 1990).

These rationales were developed with and agreed upon by all participants in the Social Networks Project, and they became part of the training module prepared on social support. They explicitly state the reasons underlying the use of social network interventions.

The second phase involved developing guidelines for use of the assessment tool, the Social Network Map previously described. The assessment tool enabled workers to identify and describe the client's social network, to identify problems in the network as well as favorable features, and to discern ways to strengthen the network. It was our expectation that through the sensitive use of this tool clients as well as workers would be able to:

1. Identify the *structure* of the network;
2. Identify various *types of support* (emotional, informational, concrete) as well as *patterns of support/conflict*;
3. Identify at least one *reciprocal relationship* for each type of support;
4. Identify at least one *multiplex reciprocal* relationship;
5. Pinpoint *sources of conflict* and identify a strategy for dealing with one of them;
6. Assess the *adequacy* of the network for providing support;
7. Identify support for *maladaptive* and life threatening behaviors and identify three ways of replacing them;
8. Track one network structural or functional change from intake to closing;
9. Identify one *positive* agent (e.g., giving or receiving support) daily for five consecutive days; and
10. Visualize an *"ideal"* network, i.e., as the client would like it to be. (Tracy, Whittaker, and Mooradian 1990).

Again, as with the rationales, these guidelines became incorporated in the training manual as practice competency objectives.

With this framework in place–the rationales, clinical goals, and taking into account the design criteria mentioned above–we were able to generate and agree upon a set of strategies for social support interventions. Social support strategies, in our view, might include any one or any combination of the following:

1. *Increase sources of emotional support,* e.g., people who support and reinforce positive change efforts, people who listen to you without making judgment
2. *Increase sources of concrete assistance,* e.g., people who will help you out or give you a break
3. *Increase sources of information and advice,* e.g., people who teach, model, or give constructive advice
4. *Increase skills in dealing with people in the network,* e.g., how to deal with people who do not reinforce change efforts, who do not provide social support, or balancing relationships which are not reciprocal

Implementation of these strategies might mean changing the structure of the network, the skill level of the client–or both. For example, in order to effect structural changes in social networks, the following three strategies were proposed:

1. Increase or decrease size of social network
2. Change composition of social network (e.g., decrease reliance on formal services)
3. Increase or decrease frequency of contact with others

To increase client skill level in dealing with network members, the following were proposed:

1. Develop or increase skills in making friends
2. Decrease negative beliefs about self (if this is a barrier to developing/maintaining supportive relationships); increase positive self-statements and increase ability to identify personal strengths
3. Develop strategies for handling criticism from others
4. Increase assertive skills (if this is a barrier to developing or maintaining supportive relationships)
5. Increase communication skills (if this is a barrier to developing or maintaining supportive relationships)
6. Teach reciprocity skills (if this is a barrier to developing or maintaining supportive relationships)
7. Develop a plan to reach out to others during a crisis period

(Tracy, Whittaker, and Mooradian 1990; Whittaker, Tracy, and Marckworth 1988)

These strategies were generated from focused staff discussion of the existing research base on social support and social skills and the data on agency clients generated by the pilot use of the network map (Tracy and Whittaker 1987, 1990). The principal investigators organized the information and circulated it through the staff team for clarification and consensus.

In general, two types of social support strategies were most common. One type of strategy was structural in nature, to create or supplement the social network. For example, the social support strategy for an isolated mother who exhibited poor social skills was to increase the size of her social network and the frequency of social contacts. A single parent father was provided a copy of his social network map, so that he would be reminded of who might be available to help. The second type of strategy was to improve or enhance the functioning of relationships within the network. For example, the parents of a ten-year-old boy with a developmental disability were taught ways of establishing more productive relationships with the child's special education personnel. The potential usefulness of social network resources in working with substance abusing families was also considered. Social network assessment was a key factor in arranging for child care and safety. Workers actively sought the assistance of previously unused network members who could help provide structure and supervision for the child during the intervention period.

CONCLUSION

On the basis of the Social Networks Project and earlier efforts, we remain convinced of the value of an intervention design and development approach to improving practice technology in the agency context. This is notwithstanding the fact that D&D is a time-consuming and labor-intensive research process. If one truly elevates what Thomas and Rothman have called "practice wisdom" to a major knowledge source, then adequate time must be allotted to "hearing the story." For us, this meant innumerable case conferences, conference calls, supervisory sessions, and staff focus groups to explore the workings of our technology as we were creating it.

There were many times when we experienced conflicts between our desire as researchers to be rigorous and our commitment as colleagues to be responsive. For example, in both the Boysville and Homebuilders' projects the implementation of the assessment tool was extremely varied according to specific preferences of practitioners and needs of families. While this limited us somewhat–for example, in compiling pre- and post-network data–we believe we learned a tremendous amount about the *meaning* of our tool in the practice situation: the various ways it could be used, its clinical importance, and its diagnostic significance.

As a consequence, we believe staff developed a sense of ownership of the project that was ultimately reflected in the use of the products. We took as significant, for example, that in both agency settings, our network mapping tool and intervention guidelines continued to be used long after the "official" project had ended. Our major lesson in all of this is the need for the researcher to be crystal clear about the particular purpose of each phase of the process and to effectively communicate this to the staff team. For example, at a certain point it was essential that all workers implemented the tool in the same manner so that we could obtain baseline network data on families. This need momentarily superseded our general stance about flexible application. In making these shifts, we benefited greatly from strong administrative support from Boysville department heads. We view such support as a critical intervening variable in the implementation of D&D.

Finally, we think it is important to be constantly on the lookout for ways in which the D&D process can create new opportunities for reinforcing existing agency goals and objectives–and to capitalize on these. In our recently completed project, for example, social network interventions turned out to provide a conceptual bridge between family preservation programs operating from very different theoretical orientations: structural and cognitive-behavioral. This fact served to increase the interest of the director of clinical staff training who placed high value on staff learning from each other's differing theoretical orientations and often used project team meetings to discuss differing interpretations of family network data. From a slightly different perspective, the director of research seized on favorable reaction to the use of the assessment tool to illustrate the potential of the data system for informing practice and, more generally, to underscore the importance of systematic data collection and analysis as a basic support to the practice task.

From an educational point of view, D&D methodology is extremely useful for practitioner training. The process of conceptualizing and designing the assessment and intervention protocols yields a significant amount of training material. This makes it easier to implement follow-up training programs and increases the likelihood of consistent application and adoption. We also believe the Boysville Social Networks project illustrates the utility of D&D methodology as an organizing framework for applied intervention research in agency settings. The model was highly appropriate for our projects goals and objectives and consistent with the agency philosophy of staff participation and involvement. Much work remains to be done.

We also learned that implementation of D&D methodology is an ever-changing process. The phases do not always follow a lockstep fashion, and "regressions" to earlier stages are a distinct possibility. Each stage informs the others, and therefore each stage is capable of changing those remaining, as well as those already completed. For example, in our project, we only became aware of one design problem–the theoretical stance of the program–when we were well into the design phase. This issue had not been identified or uncovered during what we felt was an exhaustive analysis phase. We also cannot stress enough the "art" inherent in this process. Such factors as group dynamics, agency culture, supervision styles, and worker personalities and energies are very real issues in intervention design research. These factors are less tangible but, based on our experience in two different agency settings, they appear to be very influential to the resultant design.

The nature of our effort precluded experimental testing of interventions. Thus, while the final empirical test of the effects of network interventions remains to be done, clinical supervisors did gain a valuable understanding of the introduction and timing of network assessments and interventions. Our future research agenda includes further work on the nature, intensity, and treatment integrity of network interventions; the requisite knowledge and skill base for line workers; and the organizational and service delivery requirements of the network interventions that were designed.

REFERENCES

Biegel, D. E., B. K. Shore, and E. Gordon. 1984. *Building Support Networks for the Elderly: Theory and Application*. Beverly Hills, CA: Sage.

Fraser, M. W. and J. D. Hawkins. 1984. The social networks of opioid abusers. *The International Journal of Addiction*, 19(8): 903-917.

Gaudin, J. M., J. S. Wodarski, M. K. Arkinson, and L. S. Avery. 1990/91. Remedying child neglect: Effectiveness of social network intervention. *Journal of Applied Social Sciences*, 15(1), 97-123.

Grasso, A. and I. Epstein. 1987. Management by measurement: Organizational dilemmas and opportunities. *Administration in Social Work*, 2, 89-100.

Grasso, A. and I. Epstein. 1989. The Boysville experience: Integrating practice decision making, program evaluation and management information. *Computers in Human Services*, 4, 85-95.

Maluccio, A. N. 1989. Research perspectives on social support systems for families and children. *Journal of Applied Social Sciences*, 13(2), 269-292.

Rothman, J. 1980. *Social R&D: Research and Development in the Human Services*. Englewood Cliffs, NJ: Prentice-Hall.

Rothman, J. 1989. *Creating Tools for Intervention: The Convergence of Research Methodologies*. Unpublished manuscript, UCLA School of Social Welfare, Center for Child and Family Policy Studies.

Thomas, E. J. 1978. Generating innovation in social work: The paradigm of developmental research. *Journal of Social Service Research*, 2(1), 95-116.

Thomas, E. J. 1984. *Designing Interventions for the Helping Professions*. Beverly Hills, CA: Sage.

Tracy, E. M. 1990. Identifying social support resources of at-risk families. *Social Work*, 252-259.

Tracy, E. M. and J. K. Whittaker. 1987. The evidence base for social support interventions in child and family practice: Emerging issues for research and practice. *Children and Youth Services Review*, 9, 249-270.

Tracy, E. M. and J. K. Whittaker. 1990. The social network map: Assessing social support in clinical social work practice. *Families in Society* (formerly *Social Casework*).

Tracy, E. M., J. K. Whittaker, and J. Mooradian. 1990. *Training Resources on Social Networks and Social Support*. Available from authors.

Wahler, R. (1980). *The Community Interaction Checklist*. Unpublished paper.

Wells, K. W. and J. K. Whittaker. 1989. Integrating research and agency based practice: Approaches, problems and possibilities. In *Group Care of Children: Transition Toward the Year 2000*, edited by E. Balcerzak. Washington, DC: Child Welfare League of America, 351-367.

Whittaker, J. K. 1986. Formal and informal helping in child welfare services: Implications for management and practice. *Child Welfare*, 65, 17-25.

Whittaker, J. K. and P. Pecora. 1981. The social "R&D" paradigm in child and youth services. *Children and Youth Services Review, 3,* 305-317.

Whittaker, J. K., E. M. Tracy, and M. Marckworth. 1988. *The Family Support Project: Identifying Informal Support Resources for High Risk Families.* Seattle, WA: University of Washington, School of Social Work.

EARLY DEVELOPMENT
AND PILOT TESTING

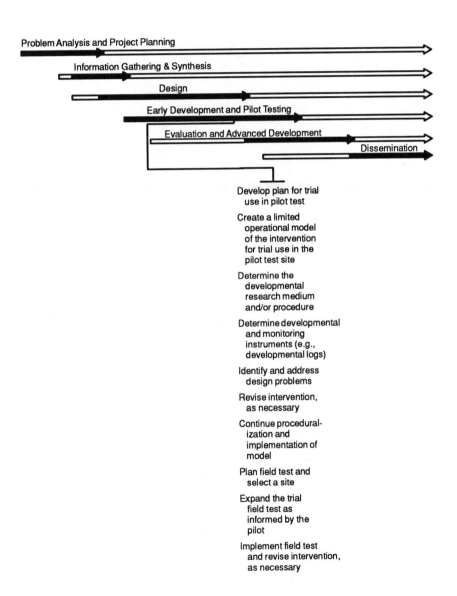

Problem Analysis and Project Planning

Information Gathering & Synthesis

Design

Early Development and Pilot Testing

Evaluation and Advanced Development

Dissemination

Develop plan for trial
  use in pilot test

Create a limited
  operational model
  of the intervention
  for trial use in the
  pilot test site

Determine the
  developmental
  research medium
  and/or procedure

Determine developmental
  and monitoring
  instruments (e.g.,
  developmental logs)

Identify and address
  design problems

Revise intervention,
  as necessary

Continue procedural-
  ization and
  implementation of
  model

Plan field test and
  select a site

Expand the trial
  field test as
  informed by the
  pilot

Implement field test
  and revise intervention,
  as necessary

Chapter 10

Pilot Testing and Early Development of a Model of Case Management Intervention

Jack Rothman
Anita Tumblin

This discussion is concerned with early development of an intervention to aid long-term, severely impaired clients. The study was conducted through the Center for Child and Family Policy Studies at UCLA, in collaboration with the Los Angeles County Department of Mental Health. Because of the varied definitions of case management and the multiple extant forms of practice, the Department requested the Center to aid in constructing a clear-cut, coherent model of case management functions. An early step involved establishing an information base to guide the work. Initial information gathering included comprehensive retrieval and synthesis of existing research on case management (Chapter 7 and Rothman 1992). Concurrently, 48 case managers were interviewed intensively in a field survey concerning the functions they performed, the sequencing of these functions, and interrelationships among the functions (Rothman 1987). Based on these findings, the research staff, working with agency representatives, designed an initial model of case management functions (Rothman 1991). See Figure 1 for the working formulation of the original model.

The task then was to pilot-test the model as an intervention design to determine whether it could be implemented by case managers in natural agency settings, and to otherwise examine its viability and utility as a practice tool. It was intended that this would

FIGURE 1. Schematic model of case management intervention.

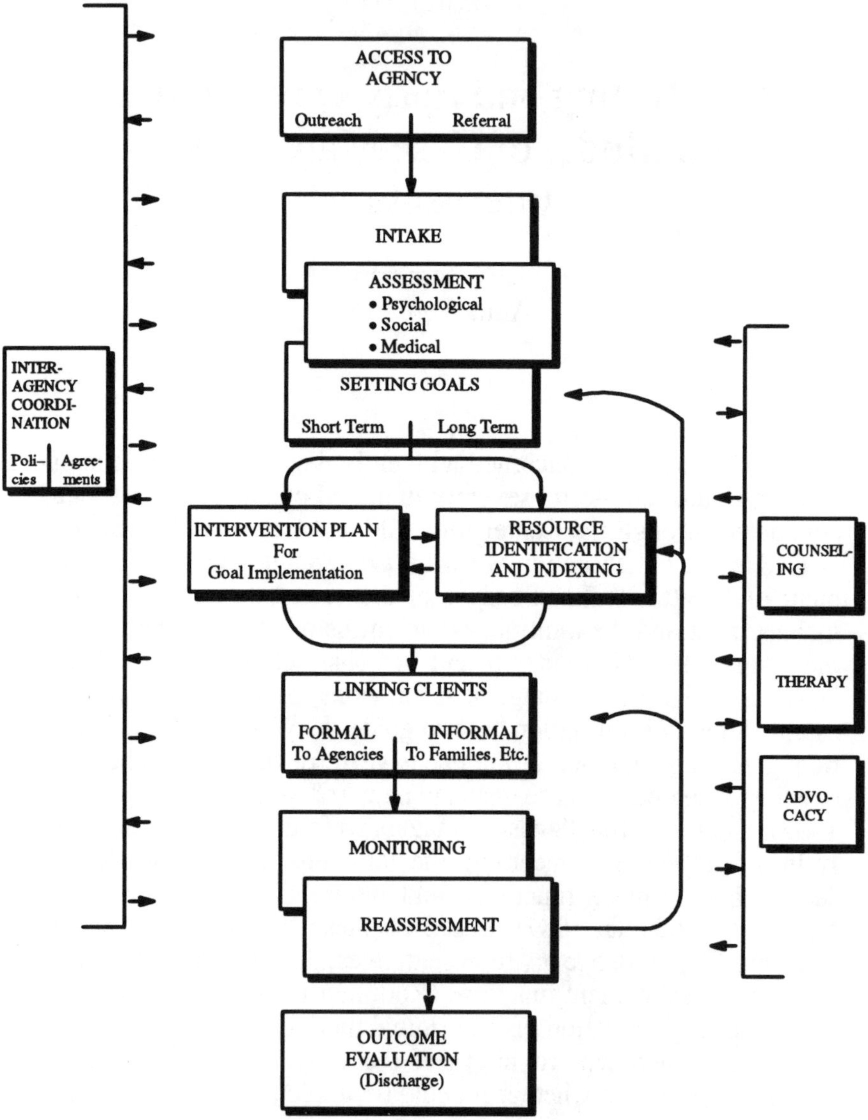

THE FUNCTIONS OF CASE MANAGEMENT

All functions are central to intervention. The middle set are somewhat sequential, though cyclical. The functions depicted on the sides enter intermittently at various times and at different points in the sequence.

result in the refining and detailing of the intervention, leading to subsequent outcome evaluation of a more crystallized practice vehicle. The discussion here will set forth and analyze the early development process.

Considerable effort had gone into the design of the model. In describing the model development approach, Paine et al. (1984) state: "Precise description of the components of a model and details of their use is a logical prerequisite for establishing either effectiveness or comparative utility" (23). Riecken and Boruch (1974) indicate that social experimentation is untenable if "the program is characterized by ill-defined or very heterogenous activities which are difficult to document or measure" (138).

Specifying the program or treatment is critical in design and development research because the intervention comprises the independent variable in the evaluation of effects, and is the focal point of attention. If the independent variable is amorphous or indeterminate, there is no way to know if the designated independent variable (or intervention) was causal in the outcome implicated in the dependent variable.

These factors initially enter in the design phase. Once the design is adequately constructed it must be piloted in a real world context under close surveillance. Questions to be examined are these: Can the intervention design be brought into being or actualized under conditions approximating the ultimate application setting (in functioning agencies with typical participants)? How does it work in action? What are the procedures and conditions of implementation? Does it bring about the results expected of it? Are clients or policies changed as intended? Can the means of operationalization be set down or codified in a form that is conducive to their dissemination with reasonable ease to other practitioners?

These concerns are typically addressed through process evaluation and monitoring. Honnard and Wolkon (1985) articulated the task as follows: "Process evaluations examine what happens during treatment. . . to determine if 'good case management' is being applied. . . [and] the extent to which accepted [prescribed] case management practices are used" (105). Rossi and Freeman (1989) refer more generally to "measuring the degree of congruence between a plan for providing services and treatments (program elements) and the ways they are actually provided" (170). They also observe that close attention to implementation is important because the design is frequently carried out in a way that is faulty, incomplete, or muddled; i.e., the intervention/independent variable either cannot be or has not been made operative.

There were two aspects to pilot work in the case management project. One was normal operational testing in a trial implementation. A small number of case managers in a regional facility of the Mental Health Department were trained to use the model and employed it experimentally with a portion of their normal caseload. Their intervention behavior was closely monitored.

The other aspect of model testing was supplemental and might be termed *cognitive testing*. Field interviews were conducted with a sample of the case managers who originally participated in the survey upon which the model was based. The model that had been constructed was presented to them, and they were asked to indicate whether it represented practice as reflected in their own experience and as they had tried to convey in the original survey. This was meant to constitute a conceptual reality check by practitioners on the accuracy of the model. The particulars of the overall methodology will be elaborated in the sections that follow.

TRIAL IMPLEMENTATION

The basic purpose of the pilot trial was to test the implementation of the model of case management functions that was constructed from the earlier study findings, consistent with intervention research methodology. Although the model had been constructed on a retrospective basis through case managers recalling how they had conducted their practice (together with evidence from previous research), this aspect of the study was concerned with how it might be implemented on a prospective basis by selected practitioners who use it to guide their evolving practice with clients. The emphasis was on examining proceduralization, which delineates the sequential steps involved in an intervention design (Thomas 1985).

Through consultation with relevant agency supervisors, a site was selected for this pilot work. It was a district mental health center engaged in typical case management tasks with a particularly diverse cross-section of clients, and where the director was open to innovation in service delivery. Within the setting, three case managers were willing to voluntarily participate and were considered by supervisors to be appropriately competent in their practice behavior and capable of recording for research purposes. A second site was selected; however, the staff was highly reluctant to participate, leading to an alternate mode of piloting the intervention design, the cognitive testing field survey previously mentioned.

The Study Plan

Rossi and Freeman (1989) suggest four basic sources of data for process evaluation studies: information from service providers, participant observation, use of agency service records, and responses from targets of intervention. The first three of these were employed, particularly information from case managers implementing the model. This involved what Reicken and Boruch (1974) refer to as retrospective reporting. These authors indicate that this form of monitoring is particularly useful when the intention is to understand the process and dynamics of a program, including the reasons for its success or failure. They indicate that the data gathered is subject to distortion due to memory loss. However, these deficiencies are mitigated when a multimethod format is employed, as in the present case. The use of a variety of methods in process evaluation studies generally is advocated among researchers who study program implementation (Sonnichsen 1989).

Each case manager in the study selected a set of three "project cases" for implementation of the model. The practitioners already had heavy case loads, and this was the maximum extra recording and close tracking that could be expected of them. This highly focused approach is consistent with other exploratory practice research of this nature. For example, Rosen and Mutschler (1982) tracked six practitioners who each served four study clients.

Selection criteria for project clients were established in advance, such that about half of the project cases would be new clients (and therefore able to provide information in detail about the model's "early" functions such as access, intake, assessment, and so forth), and the other half would be clients who had some previous history with the case manager and were engaged in later functions. By splitting the client pool in half, opportunity to examine all functions in the sequence of the model was assured. Those selected were to represent the broad middle-range client grouping and excluded extremes of age or severity of illness. The trial was conducted for a 16-week period, and, with client turnover in caseloads, 16 clients were included in the study.

Following client selection, data collection proceeded; case managers submitted forms on a weekly basis for each of their project clients, and they participated as well in regular interviews concerning each clients' progress–including how the model reflected it. These interviews, conducted every week, monitored each project client individually, and resulted in both practitioner and researcher-generated recordings on the intervention process. The four basic forms used in the pilot study (Appendix A) are described below.

Forms Completed by the Case Manager

1. A chronological log of every personal contact with each project client and of all other related contacts and activities with others performed on behalf of the client.

These are very brief notes giving a running account of case management activities. The log also indicates the particular function associated with the contact or activity and whether the activity in that context is consistent with the case management model. This log was also supplemented by service notes ordinarily kept by the practitioner using standard agency procedures.

2. A weekly review and analysis of case management activities performed for each client, according to the model functions.

This begins with a brief, narrative, open-ended overview of case managers' activities related to each project client. It is followed by a summary of actions according to functions performed. Since functions were already coded on the log form, it is relatively easy to aggregate them for the week. The practitioner also checks again whether the actions were consistent with the model.

Forms Completed by the Researcher

1. The Researcher Weekly Reporting Form is based on an interactive interview and discussion between the researcher and case manager.

This is partially descriptive, giving greater detail and dimension to activities carried out according to function. It is also highly analytical in terms of providing the rationale for a given action, facilitating and hindering factors in the practice environment, and any other contextual variables related to the practitioner, the client, the client's family, the organization, or the community. This interview also notes whether the activities conformed to the model and, if not, why a variation occurred.

2. The weekly Critical Incident Reporting Form was completed by the researcher, following a review of all actions carried out on behalf of a client during the previous seven-day period.

A critical incident is defined as any action or event that is a departure from the process delineated by the intervention design (Thomas et al. 1987). The researcher indicates the nature of the alteration (skipping ahead, reverting back, combining functions, simultaneous execution, etc.). There is also an indication of whether the variation seems appropriate or inappropriate and why. Specific implications are stated regarding revision of the model, its implementation, training of case managers, etc. The critical incident form is an important check on the fidelity of model implementation. It also suggests points at which it is not feasible to implement or not effective to do so. There are positive aspects to divergence from a model. In their study, Rosen and Mutschler (1982) found that practitioners did not perform half of the strategies that they had designated in their pre-treatment plans. Better judgment may have emerged in the doing. Rossi and Freeman (1989) state that discrepancies "may lead to efforts to move project implementation closer to design or to a respecification of the design itself" (220).

These forms were supplemented in several ways. At the conclusion of pilot work, a retrospective semi-structured interview was conducted with each of the case managers, in which they were asked to reflect generally on the implementation experience: how well the model worked in action, what its defects were, and what changes are suggested.

The researcher developed a close relationship within the facility and engaged in participant-observer functions. These informal observations supplemented the formal procedures and were an *in vivo* check on practitioner performance. In addition, the normal on-the-job recording and service reporting forms that the case managers filled out were used to augment pilot project reporting. The use of both quantitative and qualitative approaches for process evaluation is strongly supported by the literature (Mocniak and Hegarty 1989; Reid 1987).

The recording and data collection instruments that were developed seem to have appropriately matched the research objectives. In interviews, the pilot practitioners concurred with this observation. The procedures, however, required intensive, focused attention and commitment, and, thus, may not be applicable in every situation. Staff need to be especially cooperative and motivated; researchers need to be especially sensitive and collegial; and the entire process is extremely time consuming and labor intensive.

Initiating Trial Implementation

Start-up activities were important for a proper trial. An early meeting was called to bring together members of the research project team and the case managers at the pilot site who had elected to participate in the study. Purposes were severalfold. The practice group needed a chance to meet and become acquainted with both research project personnel and the time and task requirements of the research protocol. It was essential to acquaint case managers with the practice model to be employed, and to give at least a partial overview or history of the previous project phases and results obtained to date. Aims were to create a climate of collaboration and, by respecting the need of practitioners for information and involvement, to give them a stake in the undertaking. In addition, this meeting was the first opportunity to distribute and review the case management handbook that had been composed to present, and aid in implementing, the model.

The meetings with the entire group offered opportunities to unobtrusively monitor early data collection activities, and to discuss any problems about how to categorize client activities correctly within the model, or to resolve other recording issues that might have been encountered. Role-playing was employed to demonstrate procedures. The handbook was used as a reference resource throughout the pilot, and training was ongoing through the field researcher's close contacts with the practitioners.

Results of the Pilot Implementation

The practitioners in the pilot trial stated in their concluding open-ended interviews that the model was useful and relevant. Their comments indicated overall positive support for its veracity as a case management tool.

One case manager felt that "it covers all of the bases" and that "the picture here manages to express things very well." The others concurred, commenting that "yes, it is an accurate way of showing case management," and "the depiction of the whole process has been done accurately here, I feel."

A common view was that fluidity built into the model (through feedback loops and overlapping functions) aided in providing a true representation. One respondent stated this as follows:

> The flexibility incorporated in the diagram is important too: different sorts of clients and different sorts of problems require case management 'handling' to be individualized to an important extent, and yet though we do individualize our actual service provision case-by-case, the depiction of the whole process has still been done accurately here I feel.

When asked if they had to depart from the model in practice, all three responded in the negative. This was conveyed as follows:

> I can't think of anything about my job of case management or the way I do it that wasn't on here; there's nothing really missing in or wrong about the drawing of it here.

All three respondents further cited as important the fact that the model diagram could be conveyed succinctly yet still maintain both accuracy and flexibility. As stated by one, it is "a special plus that it fits on a single page." (Other open-ended comments of the respondents will be discussed shortly.)

The same conclusion about the utility of the model in guiding and reflecting practice was demonstrated in the weekly reporting forms completed by the practitioners and the field researcher. There were only two variations from this in the recordings. The first six functions seemed more concentrated and overlapping than they appeared in the model. This is because in the pilot facility that phase is conducted in an accelerated way, referred to as "orientation." Staff join together to move clients rapidly through the process. This procedure appears to be peculiar to this facility rather than common in the Department or the field generally. It was identified by the researchers as a matter to receive continued investigation in further and broader field-testing and development. In any additional work in this agency, these early functions will be bracketed in the diagram to indicate their possible compression.

The other apparent variation that appeared in the weekly reports was sequential linking. Linking a client to an agency is not a single event, as several linkages to different agencies often take place following intervention planning and any one linkage may involve a number of sequential activities. Upon analysis, this was not seen as a variation from the model as much as an explication of its mode of implementation.

Also, in field observations it appeared that the therapy and counseling functions overlapped a great deal or were not clearly distinguishable. Therapy when so designated was often focused on concrete problem solving and here-and-now emotional support. For this reason, the diagrammed model will be redrawn so that these two functions are overlayed, similar to the way some others had been portrayed.

The research staff was surprised by the degree of fidelity to the model reflected in the trial. This may be accounted for by the intensive initial and ongoing training that was provided. Also, in the training sessions, the pilot group had been told that the most valuable thing they could do for the study is report accurately. It is possible they did not heed that injunction. The pilot practitioners may have wished to accommodate the researchers and thus reported in comformity with what they thought would be favorably received. Parenthetically, this would be in contrast to a common pattern in agency-based field research, where practitioners often contest researchers rather than try to please them.

In the concluding open-ended interviews, some additional reflections on the model were expressed that were not evident in the weekly reports. For example, one respondent indicated that practice is more dynamic and disorderly than the "lifeless" representation in the model.

> I would say that all-in-all the whole thing doesn't really seem alive somehow; although I do see and agree that the picture does describe case management rather accurately and I can use it to guide my work as we have done in this project along the past weeks, I still can't get all the way past feeling that it misses some quality of life somehow, or maybe energy. It leaves a rather more sterile picture than I think is what it really seems like to do the job.

Having voiced this concern, however, she stated that this may be a characteristic of models generally, which reflect dynamic processes without duplicating them in all their nuances:

> Since I don't know of any way to really change it and make it reflect that 'quality.' There's really nothing to do about this, it's accurate about the basic technical aspects of the case manager's responsibilities.

This comment suggested the idea of explanatory notes appended to the model diagram, which elaborate or clarify aspects which could not be depicted directly. This included the notion that the functions often overlap and blend into each other, and that the process of case management is highly time consuming. The concurrent field interview survey had essentially similar results and led to an expanded set of such explanatory notes.

SURVEY OF THE ORIGINAL CASE MANAGER INFORMANTS

In this survey we selected for intensive interviewing approximately one-third of the case managers (15 of the 48 who originally participated in the earlier field study, and whose responses provided the basis for formulating the working case management model).

Jain (1989) found it highly useful in studying intervention to ask for "feedback from and assessment of the target group [practitioners]" (171). The second round of respondents were situated in nine different department facilities. We returned to this sample, presented them with the model, and asked whether it represented what they collectively told us. As with the trial implementation group, we inquired about whether the model as constituted accurately reflected case management practice as they experienced it (the specific functions, their sequence, and whether any should be added or deleted). If the model was not accurate, we asked them to indicate changes in the functions and sequential process.

Research staff began each field interview with the following preliminary comments:

> You will remember that one of our research team came out last spring and interviewed you and other staff members about the functions of case management. Based on what you and about fifty of your colleagues told us, we have constructed a diagrammed model of case management functions. Now we are coming back to ask you whether we have accurately captured and put down on paper what was told to us. We want to know whether the diagram gives a true reflection of the flow of activity in the practice of case management.
>
> To start, please think about the functions of case management you ordinarily carry out in working with clients. Think about the sequence of steps you usually go through from when you first learn of a case to when you close the case.
>
> I know there is a lot of variation in detail from case to case, but try to picture the broad pattern. Maybe bringing to mind a typical case or two would help.
>
> O.K., now I'd like you to look at this case management diagram (offer brief explanation and invite questions). Can you tell me whether it depicts your own experiences with case management?

The questionnaire contained a combination of closed and open-ended items, and generally took just under an hour to complete.

Analysis Methods

Analysis of the open-ended questions was time consuming, requiring researchers to responses and construct sets of categories on an inductive basis from raw responses, and to arrive at a consensus on these through joint analysis by a team of research assistants. The project director then conducted further independent analysis. Discrepancies were resolved through joint decision making.

Findings

A substantial majority of the respondents reported that the model faithfully reflected case management practice. In the responses 11 of the 15 felt this was "an accurate way" to depict case management, 12 indicated that they would eliminate none of the functions, and 13 stated that they would add no functions to the diagram. Among the few who varied from this view, there were no consistent or common trends, i.e., particular difficulties or suggestions mentioned predominantly reflected only one individual, and were thus highly idiosyncratic. Some reflected conceptual difficulty in comprehending the model. Those variations that were indicated, upon analysis, embodied elaborations or needed clarifications of the model, rather than a basic change in its structure. Again, this suggested the need for a set of explanatory notes to accompany the diagram–for example, that in a large service agency linkage can be internal to the organizational system as well as external. The findings of the two sub-studies are presented in the set of notes that were developed to incorporate the results.

Explanatory Notes on the Case Management Schema

Flexibility. The diagram is meant to be flexible rather than rigid, allowing for individualized use of the feedback loops and the overlapping functions. By having the arrows loop back into the process, service provisions can be tailored to the varying needs and goals of particular clients. Also, functions often overlap in various ways. Thus the sequence is approximate and suggestive rather than a precise progression.

Time. There is an explicit time element involved in the case management process. First, the entire process with any client can be highly time consuming, sometimes measured in years. Second, when caseloads are high, there exist time pressures and priority decisions in providing care across a caseworker's full client group. Third, each individual function may vary in its time demands. Thus, differing periods may be needed in moving from one function to another. Finally, the administrative tasks related to carrying out these functions, including the filling out of forms and attending meetings, require a heavy time allotment.

Non-Clinical or Administrative Discharge. The diagram, in normative fashion, indicates the possibility of an occasional therapeutic discharge as a case management function, based on a positive evaluation by the practitioners. However, nonclinical administrative discharges can take place at any time. These are client-initiated acts rather than case manager-initiated acts. The client may voluntarily withdraw from service, move out of town, become deceased, change to another agency, etc. The case manager reacts to these rather than carrying out a purposive function.

Cyclical Process. Case management is a cyclical process. The diagram represents one sequential experience with a client. However, in those relatively few instances when a chronic patient is evaluated as well enough to receive a therapeutic discharge, the commitment to continuing care does not terminate. New circumstances may require reestablishment of services, with a looping back to the Access or Intake functions.

Dynamic Character of Case Management. Case management is a process with much vitality. It is alive with human and organizational relationships, pressures, successes, and disappointments. The diagram does not explicitly depict this quality, but recognizes and acknowledges it. The diagram provides the structure, not the drama, of case management. It is like a road map that gives you a route to your destination, but cannot convey your experience of enjoyment, frustration, or boredom along the way. While the diagram may seem stiff or routine on its surface, this is an artifact of conceptual models. It is assumed that robust human factors animate all functions.

Some Functions not Implemented. The diagram shows a range of functions that are carried out by the preponderance of case managers. However, in certain situations a case manager may not, nor be expected to, include a particular function, such as outreach, inter-organizational relations, therapy, or advocacy.

Internal Linkage. Linkage in the diagram ordinarily refers to connecting clients with external services and supports. However, in some large mental health service systems in metropolitan areas, internal linkage (to other units or regions in the county department) may involve complex, informal processes equivalent in character to linking with external agencies. Within a particular service unit, linkage (or referral) may be quite informal. Internal linkage is carried out at any point in the case management sequence, including referral for intake, collateral diagnosis, service planning, etc. A very common form of internal linking involves making arrangements with another unit of the organization for medical dispensing.

DISCUSSION AND CONCLUSIONS

The logic of this study involved designing a case management model from: (a) field interviews by case managers about their work; and (b) existing empirical research knowledge about case management. This design concept was then tested in the field by having case managers use it in their practice and by obtaining reactions to it by experienced case managers, who originally contributed to its conception. The model was evaluated in terms of whether, as constructed, it: was useful, as is, as a practice tool; was useful, but needed to be refined or reformulated; or was not useful and should be discarded.

It is clear that an empirically-based model can be designed by synthesizing information given by practitioners about their functions, together with a synthesis of existing research findings. It is also clear that case managers found such a model to be reasonably coherent and reflective of the essentials of their practice. The field studies suggested qualifications and refinements which were incorporated into explanatory notes. This aspect of development is portrayed by Reid (1987): "The purpose is not merely to make a statement about the characteristics of the intervention-in-use, as might be the goal in conventional process research but rather, to apply the data to developmental purposes . . . the design may need to be modified" (22). In this instance, the modifications were re-finements rather than fundamental changes.

This study has set forth one means of conducting pilot-testing and early development. It is not the only method available for this, or necessarily the most effective. In this early stage in the emergence of intervention research, varied means need to be experimented with and assessed for design and development.

The use of dual piloting procedures in triangulation fashion is a promising concept to be considered by others. The findings in the pilot implementation and interviews usefully overlapped and reinforced each other.

The methods used in the pilot implementation were demanding of time and energy. They provided a rich and voluminous source of information about the case managers' facility in using the model, and problems or confusions in the model itself. A great deal of sensitivity was involved in the weekly research interviews. In particular, it is important that the interviewer not put words into the mouths of these case managers during follow-up probes. Questions eliciting additional information or factual details regarding the week's events are necessary, but questions leading to doubt or untruthful responses by case managers must be avoided. This work demands a subtle touch; as much information as possible is desired, however, overzealous, intrusive questioning or brusque follow-up probes can create serious problems with some practitioners who may interpret information-seeking as criticism, and respond defensively or compliantly thereafter. It is extremely important, therefore, that interviewers use tact and be alert to unspoken clues from case managers that need to be pursued.

A disciplined approach is a route for walking this fine line. For example, there was initially a tendency for the researcher to engage immediately in a discussion of the week's data just received; it was useful, however, to allow a week's lag between receipt of material and interview follow-up, thus permitting the interviewer an opportunity to organize queries and for things to "sink in" for the case manager.

In the pilot trial we discovered that practitioners found it difficult to follow a formal conceptual model in shaping their work. They had a tendency to use the model to analyze activities they had already performed, rather than as a guide for forward planning. Also, they sometimes had difficulty in conceptualizing their activities in terms of the functional categories of the model. For this reason, it is necessary to conceive of training for implementation as an active process over time, rather than a discrete initial occurrence.

Implementation of a conceptual model is not easy and requires continuing reinforcement and training. Also, recurring encouragement and guidance is needed to use the model systematically as a forward planning tool. Absorption of a new model may be easier to accomplish with new workers coming into the field rather than with experienced workers, whose modes of performance are firmly established. Thus, tentatively, one of its strongest assets may be in providing a training framework for orienting employees who are new to the agency, or in serving as an educational medium in professional schools in the human services.

There have been certain positive side effects of model implementation. Staff have become more reflective of their practice. Some have expressed a sense of increased professionalism in their work. By taking time to describe and analyze more precisely what they do, they have come to realize how complex their job actually is, and to place greater value on their performance and contribution.

Certain organizational preparation issues are worth recounting. The agency was in the midst of important structural changes, and under these circumstances, research-related activities are less salient and can become postponed or disrupted. The agency had to be given time to resolve its organizational and programmatic concerns before research could proceed with some ease. There were issues about who would be the appropriate agency liaison and contact person for the project, how the previous year's report should be disseminated and discussed in the agency, what kind of facility would be suitable and accessible for a pilot project, and how to gain participation in the pilot sites.

In addition, a new special pilot approach to case management was concurrently and unexpectedly initiated in the department. In some ways this diverted a measure of attention and energy away from the ongoing pilot. Overlapping relationships and distinct features of each of the pilots had to be investigated, and an understanding reached about the best way to proceed. It was decided that the projects should be separate and parallel, with communication between the two. The director of the other project sat as a member of the steering committee of our project as a way of maintaining some degree of interrelationship.

We found it important for there to be top-level support and advocacy for the research project to gain proper grounding in the agency. The problems, pressures, and expectations faced by agency staff are multiple and intense. Staff need to clear cognitive and emotional space to deal with a research project, which typically has less immediacy and urgency than front-line client and organizational issues. We had to call on the offices of the executive director on various occasions to gain the authorization and attention necessary to proceed. These kinds of organizational factors will likely effect any pilot study having an action or research focus with an evaluation component.

In brief, the pilot work gave support to the formulation of the case management intervention model that had been designed. Certain points of confusion or incompleteness were identified, which suggested refinements. These have been codified into a set of explanatory notes to be appended to the diagram of the model. Rossi and Freeman (1989) point out that there is no basis for moving between pilot testing and wider implementation "without reasonable evidence the appropriate treatments [can] be delivered to the intended targets" (171). The modified model formulation was appraised to be ready to continue into expanded field-testing for purposes of rigorous outcome evaluation and advanced development.

REFERENCES

Jain, P.S. 1989. Monitoring of rural development programmes. *Evaluation and Program Planning, 12*, 171-177.

Honnard, R. and G. H. Wolkon. 1985. Evaluation for decision making and program accountability. In *Case Management in Human Service Practice,* edited by M. Weil, J. M. Karis and Associates. San Francisco: Jossey-Bass, 94-118.

Mocniak, N. L. and T. W. Hegarty. 1989. Evaluating a pilot program and designing it, too. *Evaluation and Program Planning, 12*, 291-293.

Paine, S. L., G. T. Bellamy, and B. L. Wilcox. 1984. *Human Services that Work.* Baltimore: Paul H. Brookes.

Riecken, H. W. and R. F. Boruch. 1974. *Social Experimentation: A Method for Planning and Evaluating Social Intervention.* New York: Academic Press.

Reid, W. J. 1987. Evaluating an intervention in development research. *Journal of Social Service Research, 11*(1), 17-36.

Rosen, A. and E. Mutschler. 1982. Correspondence between the planned and subsequent use of interventions in treatment. *Social Work Research and Abstracts, 18*(2), 28-34.

Rossi, P. H. and H. E. Freeman. 1989. *Evaluation: A Systematic Approach.* Newbury Park, CA: Sage.

Rothman, J. 1987. The practice of case management: A study of case managers' experiences and views. Los Angeles: Center for Child and Family Policy Studies, School of Social Welfare, University of California, Los Angeles.

Rothman, J. 1991. A model of case management: Toward empirically based practice. *Social Work,* 36:4.

Rothman, J. 1992. *Guidelines For Case Management: Putting Research to Professional Use.* Itasca, IL: F. E. Peacock Publishers, forthcoming.

Sonnichsen, R. C. 1989. Methodology: A bridge or barrier between evaluators and managers? *Evaluation and Program Planning, 12,* 287-290.

Thomas, E. J. 1985. The validity of design and development and related concepts in developmental research. *Social Work Research and Abstracts, 21*(2), 50-55.

Thomas, E. J., J. Bastien, D. R. Stuebe, D. E. Bronson, and J. Yaffe. 1987. Assessing procedural descriptiveness: Rationale and illustrative study. *Behavioral Assessment, 9,* 43-56.

APPENDIX A

Forms for Pilot Trial of Case Management Model

IMPLEMENTATION FIELD TEST SUB-STUDY

FORMS COMPLETED BY PILOT PRACTITIONERS

Chronological Log

All Client Contacts and Client-Related Activities

Week of _____   Case Manager # _____

Client # _____

Date	Brief Description of Contact or Activity	C.M. Function Code (1-15)	Activity Consistent With C.M. Model — Yes	Activity Consistent With C.M. Model — No

Weekly Review and Analysis
Self-Reporting Form of Case Management Activities and Functions

Week of _____   Case Manager # _____

Client # _____

General overview of the case during the past week–Open-ended comments. Any changes in client's situation or psychological state. What was the general direction of your efforts? Any changes in your assessment or intervention approach, etc., etc.

In the next section note your activities this week according to the different categories of case management functions.

Client # _____

Week of _____

C.M. Function	Activities (Time-ordered within function)	Activity Consistent with C.M. Model Yes	No
1 Access Activities			
2 Intake Activities			
3 Assessment Activities			
4 Setting Goals			
5 Intervention Planning			
6 Resource Identification and Indexing			
7 Linking Clients to Agencies			
8 Linking Clients to Families			

C.M. Function	Activities (Time-ordered within function)	Activity Consistent with C.M. Model Yes	No
9 Monitoring			
10 Reassessment			
11 Outcome Evaluation			

(Intermittent Functions)

12 Counseling			
13 Therapy			
14 Advocacy			
15 Interorg. Coordination			

A. Other functions:

B. Key client outcomes or problems this week:

C. No contact this week _____ Reason for no contact:

FORMS COMPLETED BY RESEARCHER

Researcher Weekly Reporting Form

Function: _____   [A Separate Sheet for Each Function Applied During the Previous Week]

1. Describe your main _____ activities for this client this week in some detail.

2. Why did you engage in these activities at this time?

3. Did the activities follow the format of the model?
   Yes _____   No _____

4. Was it a natural flow or forced?   6. Variation _____
   Natural _____   7. Why did it go that way?
5. Explain: _____   _____
   _____   _____
   _____   _____
   _____   _____

Facilitating and hindering factors in use of the model:

	8. Facilitating Factors	9. Hindering Factors
Yourself		
Client		
Family		
Organization		
Community		
Other		

10. Total time doing Access function with the client this week:
    hours _____   minutes _____

11. Remarks and reflections: Problems, insights, external influences, pressures, resource issues, etc.

    Yourself
    Client
    Organization
    Community

Critical Incident Reporting Form

Weekly Changes in Implementing Model Functions

Week of _____   Case Manager # _____

Client # _____   Researcher _____

1. Describe change

    Skipped ahead _____   from _____   to _____

    Reverted back _____   from _____   to _____

    Combining   _____   _____

    Simultaneous
    Impl.   _____   _____

    Other   _____   _____

2.. The variation seems *appropriate* _____

    2a. Reason   _____

                   _____

                   _____

3.. The variation seems *inappropriate* _____

    3a. Reason   _____

                   _____

                   _____

    3b. Practitioner aspects _____

                   _____

                   _____

4. Implications for Model–Revision, implementation, training, etc.

                   _____

                   _____

                   _____

                   _____

COGNITIVE FIELD TESTING SUB-STUDY
UCLA/DMH Case Management Study

Date of Interview: _____   Interviewer: _____

Facility: _____   CM: _____

1. Is this an accurate way of showing your own experience with the case management process?

    _____ YES

    1:1 Are there any variations at all from the diagrammed pattern? _____ yes _____ no

    1:2 If yes, what are they? _____

    _____

    _____

    1:3 How often, and under what circumstances do variations occur? _____

    _____

    _____

    1:4 Are there any ways to improve on the diagram in depicting case management? _____ yes _____ no

    1:5 If yes, how? _____

    _____

    _____

    [Go on to Question 5]

_____ NO

1:6 What specific changes would you make to give a more accurate picture of the process? _____

_____

_____

1:7 Is this an occasional variation on the diagram or a different general pattern? _____

_____

_____

_____ VARIATION

1:8 How often does the variation occur? _____

_____

_____

1:9 Under what circumstances does it occur? _____

_____

_____

_____ DIFFERENT GENERAL PATTERN

1:10 Let us try to change the diagram to reflect the different pattern.

(Modify Diagram)

Notes _____

_____

_____

2. Would you eliminate any of the functions?

    _____ YES

    2:1 Which ones? _____

    _____

    _____ NO

3. Would you add any functions?

    _____ YES

    3:1 Which ones? _____

    _____

    _____ NO

4. Would you change the sequence?

    _____ YES

    4:1 Describe this: _____

    _____

    _____

    _____

    _____ NO

5. Which three functions do you spend the most time at, in order of time involvement?

    Most _____

    Next _____

    Least _____

6. Which three functions do you spend the least time at, in order of:

     Very Least Time _____

     Next Least Time _____

     Next Least Time _____

7. In addition to assisting individual clients, what other case management activites or roles do you engage in? _____

_____

_____

_____

_____

_____

Chapter 11

Field Testing and Data Gathering on Innovative Practice Interventions in Early Development

William J. Reid

In this chapter I present and illustrate a strategy for field testing in early development. The strategy is concerned with the development of a single intervention (as opposed to the development of an intervention model or service program).

In brief, an intervention is first piloted and shaped through single case studies. When a sufficient number of these studies has been accumulated, their data are aggregated and further analyzed. The aggregated analysis will hopefully yield additional results that will inform the development of the intervention. The case study/aggregation cycle can then be repeated or more rigorous designs–e.g., controlled single case or group experiments–can be conducted to provide more definitive results on the effectiveness of the intervention. Because my interest is in early development, I shall consider only a first round of case studies and aggregation.

Combining separate and aggregate analyses of case studies has shown promise in practice research (Benbenishty 1988, 1989). In the present strategy, this approach is focused on a single intervention and is applied within a developmental research framework.

The strategy I have outlined is well suited to development that is a part of ongoing agency programs in which service goals have priority and in which controlled experimental research may be diffi-cult to implement. The case study methods, which provide a basis for direct modification of the intervention as well as for the aggre-gate analyses, are unobtrusive and practioner friendly. The benefit from using the strategy is not only to ready the experiment for more stringent testing but to produce an intervention that has been improved through a systematic process of trial and modification–what Thomas (1990) has called "developmental practice." Pending a more rigorous evaluation, the improved intervention can serve as a useful addition to the practitioner's repertory.

This strategy will be illustrated by the development of a particular intervention: the Family Problem-Solving Sequence (FPSS). This work was conducted as a part of a larger effort–the Task-Centered Family Treatment Project (Reid 1985; Reid and Hanrahan 1988). A more detailed report of the FPSS and its development can be found in Reid 1987a, 1987b.

THE FAMILY PROBLEM-SOLVING SEQUENCE

In its simplest form, the FPSS consists of two tasks. The first task (session task) involves two or more clients in face-to-face efforts in the treatment session, working toward the resolution of a family problem. These efforts culminate in the second task (home task), which consists of an action plan to be implemented at home during the week between sessions.

The practitioner serves not only as a facilitator and coach but also assumes a collaborative role in the development of the action plan. For example, in one case a major problem was the wife's smoking, which the husband opposed. In a session task the wife agreed to limit her smoking to certain rooms and her husband agreed, in response to the practitioner's suggestion, to become involved in social activities which his wife desired. The plan was thus accomplished through tasks at home. In another case, a teenage daughter and her parents, with the practitioner's help, negotiated a conflict concerning sleep-in visits by the daughter's boyfriend. The agreement, which restricted his visiting to one night, was implemented the following week. This intervention was part of a broader task-centered approach that made use of other methods, including "free standing" session and home tasks that were not combined into sequences (Reid 1985).

The FPSS draws from problem-solving, communications, and decision-making models to help family members resolve real-life issues during treatment sessions (Thomas 1977; Jacobson 1981; Jacobson and Margolin 1979; Robin 1981; Stuart 1980). Work on the FPSS has added to these previous endeavors with close attention to specific aspects of intervention process and outcome within an intervention research context.

THE CASE STUDY

Developmental work begins with trials of the intervention in a series of case studies. The idea for the intervention may be derived from theory, earlier work, or may have occurred serendipitously in a previous case. A set of procedures for practitioners to use in applying the intervention is developed as well as instruments for them to record its use. A more objective though less accessible record is provided by tape recordings of the case. Retrospective baselines are obtained on the problems to which the intervention will be applied. Practitioners supply assessments of weekly problem change, which are checked against judgments made from the audio tapes. Data on various dimensions of client functioning and change are gathered through pre- and post-administrations of standardized instruments. Client assessments of change are obtained in a structured terminal or follow-up interview conducted by the practitioner and through questionnaires independently completed by the clients. These case study procedures were followed in developmental work on the FPSS.

The case study can provide preliminary data about the intervention under study: how it is actually carried out, what problems practitioners are having in applying it, how well it appears to achieve its immediate goals, what are its apparent longer range effects. Answers to such questions help identify areas requiring improvement. The kinds of tools and structures that facilitate pursuit of these questions in early developmental work will now be considered.

INFORMATIVE EVENTS

A systematic method of obtaining data from cases is a form of critical incident, referred to as an "informative event" (Reid 1985; Reid and Davis 1987; Davis and Reid 1988). Informative events are incidents or episodes that have both factual and generative aspects. They provide specific facts which by themselves are of interest. For example, a particular method fails to work in a particular situation. The generative value is in what they suggest. An instance of failure may raise questions about the method being used or the assumptions on which it is based. The use of an innovative variation may suggest ways in which the innovation may be varied or may suggest other applications of it. The generative aspect is an essential ingredient. It is what makes an event informative. Thus failures or successes must in some way be instructive. That is, they must offer ideas for improvement to whatever method or model is being tested.

Informative events may be obtained from a review of records and tapes or case presentations by project practitioners. Practitioners themselves may supply them through special recording forms.

To take an illustration from the development of the FPSS, an informative event occurred when a practitioner took a creative tack in working with a family in which a child was having difficulty with a classmate. Instead of having the parents and child discuss the problem following our usual format, the practitioner used a role play in which the father, taking the role of the child, modeled how the son might handle his antagonist. The outcome was quite successful. The incident suggested a range of possibilities for using parents to model behavior for their children.

Some informative events, such as the one just illustrated, have value as single occurrences. An innovation that produces results deserves to be tried again. Events that reveal a failure in a treatment component may point to immediate corrective action while with other informative events, a pattern of occurrence over a number of cases may be needed to provide an adequate base for action. After the initial event has been analyzed, the developer can look for similar occurrences or specify that practitioners record them.

For example, a common problem in early stages of development is what McMahon (1987) has referred to as "shifts in intervention," that is, "any consistent deviation from a written, explicit procedure or a plan recognized implicitly for treating the presenting problem" (13). A single occurrence of a deviation may be of little consequence, but repeated occurrences would be a source of concern. To illustrate, session tasks in the FPSS were to consist primarily of structured communication among family members with the practitioner serving as coach, facilitator, etc. A pattern of informative events revealed that a particular intervention shift was occurring: practitioners frequently moved in too quickly and too intrusively, either on their own initiative or in response to a question or comment from a client. This pattern of events, together with information as to why it occurred (to be discussed subsequently), led to revisions in the intervention protocol and training procedures.

SIGNED CAUSE ANALYSIS

More systematic analysis of intervention outcomes can also be employed in the single case phase through what we call, following Cook and Campbell (1979), "signed cause analysis." According to Cook and Campbell (1979), a cause may operate with such specificity that it leaves a unique "signature" in its effects. Or as Gilbert, Light, and Mosteller (1975) argue, certain effects of intervention are sufficiently large and immediate to be readily apparent. The notions of "signed causes" (Cook and Campbell 1979) and "slam bang" effects (Gilbert, Light, and Mosteller 1975) enable the researcher, as these writers suggest, to make assessments of treatment effectiveness under certain circumstances even in the absence of controlled designs. Because the effects are either so obvious or strong (or both), alternative explanations are not likely to arise: hence, control devices are not needed to rule them out.

In applying a signed cause analysis to the FPSS, the following criteria were developed: (1) the intervention had to yield a home task designed to make a specific, immediate, and significant impact on a durable problem; (2) the home task had to be successfully implemented; (3) there had to be immediate, positive problem change following predictably from the task (the signed cause); (4) the change had to persist and be a clear contribution to positive change in final outcome measurement (based on practitioner and client ratings of problem change). For example, in one case a session task involved three siblings whose fighting was part of a target problem. At the end of this task one of the siblings, a twelve-year-old boy, agreed (as the oldest) to take responsibility for keeping peace by not hitting his siblings. He carried out this task assiduously. The fighting which had occurred on an almost daily basis ceased abruptly during the week following and did not recur during the treatment period.

A coding scheme incorporating these criteria was developed and applied by two independent judges to all FPSSs in project cases. Judges were instructed to identify those FPSSs that, in their opinion, substantially met all four criteria for the presence of a signed cause. Interjudge agreement for occurrence (that is, disregarding agreement on nonoccurrence) averaged 67 percent, a less than satisfactory but still encouraging figure for preliminary trials of a complex scale. Considering only the FPSSs in which both judges agreed that a signed cause was present, it was found that approximately 10 percent of the FPSSs examined revealed this effect.

The analysis provided a way of systematizing judgments about effectiveness that a model developer makes in evaluating the use of an intervention in single case studies. With respect to the FPSS, evidence resulting from signed cause analysis appeared positive enough to warrant continued development. Moreover, it pointed to specific uses that seemed especially promising, such as its use with sibling conflict in the example given.

This kind of analysis does not, however, yield conclusive evidence about the effectiveness of an intervention. It cannot completely rule out such factors as maturation and contemporaneous events that might also be operative. In addition, if the proportion of signed cause occurrences is low, as in the present case and as it might be generally, interpretation of the extent of effectiveness becomes quite dubious. For example, does the 10 percent we found represent well-documented "pure strains" of effectiveness of a potent technique or just the isolated results of a technique of inconsistent or questionable efficacy? Unfortunately, there is no way to answer these questions. Given these limitations, signed cause analysis is best seen as a preliminary guide to what appears to be working or as a part of a larger base of evidence bearing on the effectiveness of an intervention.

STRUCTURAL CONSIDERATIONS

Early developmental work requires more than tools for data collection and analysis. It must also be conducted in the kind of project structure that facilitates both implementation and modification of the intervention. The practitioners need to be comfortable with the intervention and sufficiently skilled to carry it out. Sufficient training must be given so that initial trials show enough conformity to the intervention design to permit use for developmental purposes. Once case applications begin, the flow of cases should ideally be slow enough to allow the developer to apply to later cases what has been learned from earlier ones. There needs to be a structure for monitoring the practitioners' efforts, as well, to enable sharing of information among practitioners and researchers. Weekly seminars or meetings, in which cases are discussed and presented, can serve this purpose.

Developmental work on the FPSS was conducted largely as part of an advanced practice seminar at the School of Social Welfare, the State University of New York at Albany. Students, who were at both the master's and doctoral levels, served as project practitioners. Cases were drawn from cooperating agencies, usually those in which the student received field training or was employed. The seminar, which met weekly, provided a vehicle for case presentation and discussion as well as for considering and implementing modifications of the intervention. For example, the seminar was used to explore reasons why practitioners found it difficult to adhere to the session task procedures (in the illustration given earlier). The reasons, including lack of confidence in the family's ability to do its own problem solving and reluctance to appear unresponsive to family members who wanted to involve the practitioner, emerged in the group discussion, and corrective steps were determined.

Although the project was university-based, it was conducted as part of ongoing agency service programs. The same structure can be adapted to agency-based projects. A seminar consisting of agency practitioners becomes the means of organizing developmental work.

AGGREGATE ANALYSIS

When a sufficient number of single case studies has been accumulated, an aggregate analysis can be performed. A study of aggregated data can reveal statistical characteristics and associations that cannot be discerned from a case-by-case approach. The decision about when to aggregate involves a trade-off: the more cases you have the more you are likely to learn; however, the longer you wait to accumulate cases, the longer you delay the research-based feedback that can improve the intervention. As a rule, aggregation begins to make sense when the pool of cases studied is in the 25 to 60 range. Obviously, the rate at which cases are accumulated is an important factor in this kind of decision. Another issue has to do with case comparability. The single case studies have resulted in changes, hopefully improvements, in the intervention. If significant, systematic changes have been implemented, then one may need to wait until the intervention stabilizes before single cases are aggregated.

The aggregation provides basic data on characteristics of the intervention (e.g., how often used, with what variations and outcomes, including immediate and longer-term effects). It is useful to do a comparative analysis in which application of the innovative intervention is contrasted with a baseline condition, the application of some alternative intervention, or of the intervention package without the innovation. Comparative cases can be drawn from a period prior to the introduction of the innovation, or one can make use of practitioner variation in use of the innovation in current cases.

In the present program the initial aggregation consisted of single case studies. A critical feature of this aggregation was an ex post facto comparison of the FPSS, with a close alternative, called "home tasks only." These are tasks that were planned in the session but are not the outgrowth of face-to-face problem solving by family members. Although practitioners were strongly encouraged to use the FPSS, it was not set forth as the only method of intervention. Consequently, there was a good deal of use of home tasks only. Table 1 presents illustrative findings resulting from the initial aggregation of case studies.

CHARACTERISTICS OF USE
AND DESIGN SPECIFICATIONS

A basic set of questions in evaluating an intervention concerns how the intervention is actually used and the relationship of its use

TABLE 1. Findings on performance of FPSS based on an aggregation of 47 case studies.

Variable	Findings	
1. Characteristics of Use		
Frequency of use of FPSS	Overall n=94; Mean per case, 2.0	
Types of home tasks in FPSS*	Shared–34%	
	Reciprocal–25%	
	Individual–40%	
2. Immediate Outcomes		
Successful Completion of		
Home Task		
Overall	FPSS	68%
	Home Tasks Only	58%
Reciprocal	FPSS	68%
	Home Tasks Only	31%
Families with Adolescents	FPSS	40%
in Trouble	Home Tasks Only	37%
Postive Problem Change	FPSS	51%
Week Following	Home Tasks Only	33%
	Baseline Session	39%

* = 111

to whatever is specified by the intervention design. Included here are questions relating to frequency and characteristics of use, variations between what was done and what the design called for (intervention shifts or fidelity in application), obstacles to implementation, and aspects of the intervention not anticipated by the design. The purpose is not merely to make a statement about the characteristics of the intervention in use, as might be the goal in conventional process research, but rather to apply the data to developmental purposes. One may find that the practitioners do not follow the intervention design because guidelines may lack sufficient completeness, specificity, and so on (Thomas et al. 1987). In other instances the guidelines may be clear but may not take certain practice realities into account.

In this evaluation, quantitative methods can be used to provide counts of usages, and other descriptive data. However, at an early stage of a developmental effort, obtaining extensive quantitative data derived from fine-grained content analyses of records or tapes may not be feasible. Even if such data are available, a close qualitative analysis of the complex details of actual application provides perhaps the most efficient means of fashioning the host of specific modifications needed to improve the intervention.

Frequency

How frequently an intervention is used must be established in order to put subsequent evaluations in proper perspective. Does the intervention occur only now and then in a series of cases, or is it a central feature of most cases? How does actual frequency compare with what is called for by the treatment design? Thus, if an intervention is supposed to be used in every case but occurs only in some, consideration of "why here, but not there?" becomes a logical next step.

In the present model, it was expected that the FPSS would be used in most middle phase sessions (roughly from the second to the seventh) in a typical eight-session course of treatment. The FPSS was used a total of 94 times–at least once in all but three of the 47 cases. The mean use per case was two, with a maximum of eight uses in one case. Since the median number of sessions in the cases was eight and active interventions tended to be concentrated in the middle phase, the intervention was a more dominant feature of most cases than it first might appear. On the whole, frequency of use was judged to be adequate though somewhat less than expected.

Type of Use

Another simple and informative technique is to classify the intervention according to one or more categories and determine the frequency of the use of these types. The FPSS was classified into three types depending on the form of the home task: shared (two or more family members doing one task, such as spending time together); reciprocal (a quid pro quo exchange); or individual (family members performing separate tasks).

The distribution in Table 1 revealed a higher proportion of individual tasks than expected given the emphasis on shared and reciprocal tasks in written guidelines and training. A qualitative examination of individual tasks suggested that most made sense in the framework of this form of family treatment–for example, doing chores, ignoring rather than punishing a particular behavior of a young child, making requests of family members not involved in treatment, and so forth. This analysis suggested that individual tasks provide a valid means for family members to take independent actions within a family context or with external systems. It was apparent that their function was generally more family-oriented than the term "individual" suggests.

Effectiveness

In a design and developmental research context, preliminary assessments of the effectiveness of an intervention serve at least two purposes. First, there is interest in learning if the intervention shows sufficient potential to warrant further developmental effort. If it does, then one wishes to learn under what conditions it may or may not be effective and to identify obstacles to effectiveness. In this analysis it is helpful to view the effectiveness of an intervention in relation to both intermediate and final goals.

Intermediate Outcomes

Two kinds of intermediate outcomes of an intervention can be distinguished. The first measures whether or not an intervention achieved whatever "process" goal it is specifically designed to attain. The second measures immediate change in a target symptom or problem that should result if the process goal is achieved. Thus if a cognitive procedure works as intended with a depressed client, the intervention should change the client's cognitions–the process goal. These changes in turn should have at least a short-term effect on the client's depressed mood. Assessing intermediate outcomes not only provides preliminary evidence on effectiveness, but it also serves to trace the process by which an intervention produces change (Barlow, Hayes, and Nelson 1983).

The major process goal for the FPSS is accomplishment of the home task determined in the session. Although the successful completion of the task should have a positive effect on the problem, this effect may be indirect or represent too small a step to be detected on a session-to-session measure of problem change. Home task attainment was measured on a four-point scale: completely (4) substantially (3) partly (2) or not accomplished (1) (Reid and Epstein 1977).

Although the data reported are taken from the practitioners' records, the practitioner ratings of task achievement agreed quite well (r = .76) with the ratings of independent judges who reviewed audio-taped samples of the interviews. The judges were ignorant of whether the home task was part of a FPSS.

The great majority of the home tasks (68 percent) in the FPSS were either completely or substantially achieved. This figure suggests that the intervention achieved immediate goals in most cases, an encouraging sign. However, one is interested in learning how this rate of achievement (ratings of 4 and 3) would compare with some alternative means of attaining the same objectives. For example, a goal of having a father spend time with his son could be attained by a simple directive. In this study, as discussed earlier, the FPSS was compared against "home tasks only," which may be planned in the session but are not the outgrowth of session tasks involving face-to-face interaction among family members. The comparable attainment rate for home tasks only in the present project was 57 percent. Moreover, the FPSS seemed to be particularly advantageous with reciprocal tasks, or quid pro quo exchanges, perhaps because the session task provided a medium for family members to work out and agree to terms of the exchange.

As has been noted, the FPSS varied in respect to proximate goal achievement. What factors might account for this variation? With initial home task ratings again as the criterion, successful and unsuccessful FPSSs were compared on a number of client and service dimensions.

Various measures of client and service characteristics were employed in these analyses, including initial scores on the Family Assessment Device (FAD), a standardized instrument to measure family functioning (Epstein, Baldwin, and Bishop 1983); ratings of client motivation; various classifications of problems, families, and identified clients; and the timing of the FPSS. The only analysis that proved discriminating involved the isolation of a particular type of referral problem, in which the identified client was an adolescent (13-19) in serious trouble in the community or at home (often both places) for some form of antisocial or unmanageable behavior. Adolescents in trouble (n=15) constituted the single largest type of referral problem. Remaining types of included behavior difficulties of younger children and less serious problems concerning youth (n=11), marital conflict (n=12), and other family problems, such as child protective cases and nonmarital relationship issues involving adults (n=19).

The rate of achievement of the FPSS was only 40 percent for adolescents in trouble, about the same as the rate for home tasks only (37 percent). By contrast, the rate across remaining categories for the FPSS was 84 percent.

Qualitative analysis of cases involving adolescents in trouble suggested that the most frequent reason for difficulties in clients' accomplishing tasks either in the session or at home was overt conflict among task participants. In some instances, session tasks erupted in arguments; in others, conflict at home either between the adolescent and parent or between the parents themselves vitiated attempts to implement the plans worked out in the session.

Effective use of the FPSS should lead to immediate improvement in the target problem. While not all home tasks are designed to effect such short-run changes, most are intended to have such effects, which are expected to accumulate into attainment of the final goal of substantial problem alleviation.

In the present study, evidence on this point was obtained from the practitioners' reviews of changes in specific target problems made in each weekly session. Again there was good reliability (78% agreement) between the practitioner's ratings and those independent judges who reviewed samples of audio tapes.

Uses of the FPSS designed for a given problem were marked. Change in the problem during the week following the use of the FPSS was recorded. A similar procedure was followed for home tasks only. (Excluded were the few sessions in which both types of intervention were used for the same problem.) Another comparison was added: change following sessions prior to the first use of either of these interventions for a given problem. This latter comparison provided an approximation of a baseline condition.

The measure then was an attempt to capture short-run changes that might result from the FPSS. Even though the changes might be transient, they could indicate that the FPSS was able to make inroads in the target problem.

Of uses of the FPSS (n=87), slightly over half (51 percent) were followed by positive change in the relevant problem during the next week. For home tasks only (n=102), the comparable figure was 33 percent; for baseline sessions, 39 percent. Thus, on the whole, the analysis provided evidence consistent with the explanation that the FPSS was a contributing factor in incremental problem change. However, alternative explanations cannot be ruled out, as shall be discussed subsequently.

Contribution to Final Outcome

A larger question concerns the contribution of the innovation to a final measure of outcome, such as improvement in client functioning or positive change in target problems.

On the whole, these measures were uniformly positive. According to practitioner ratings, 81 percent of the cases showed substantial improvements for the overall problem. On independent client questionnaires, 91 percent of the clients reported the main problem had shown some improvement; 67 percent said they were getting along "much better" than when treatment began, and 76 percent said that they were "considerably benefited" by service; 80 percent showed pre-to-post gains on the Family Assessment Device. The client self-report data are more positive than those obtained for similar items on a large scale national survey of family agency cases (Beck and Jones 1973).

As might be expected from earlier findings, the subgroup of cases that did most poorly were those involving adolescents in trouble. Of the 15 cases in this subgroup only six (40 percent) were found to have outcomes at a moderate-or-better level of improvement (on a composite measure of outcome) as opposed to 77 percent in remaining categories. Clearly, adolescents in trouble proved the most difficult not only for the FPSS but for the model as a whole.

However, these findings did not answer questions concerning the contribution of the FPSS to final outcome. Since the intervention was used in almost all cases this determination cannot be made satisfactorily. Only an indirect and inferential assessment is possible. First, the intervention was a central part of an intervention package of which the outcomes were largely positive, as noted. Second, there was evidence that use of the FPSS was associated with immediate change in the target problem. It is not unreasonable to assume that these weekly positive changes were cumulative and made a difference in final outcome measures. Some data support this point: the extent of immediate problem change proved to be correlated (with rs in the .48 to .63 range) with principal measures of final outcome, including practitioner and client assessments of problem change and gain scores in the Family Assessment Device. Finally, the signed-cause analysis, presented earlier, produced instances in which the FPSS appeared to have contributed to the final outcome. Such evidence, while encouraging, falls far short of demonstrating the effects of FPSS on outcome at termination.

Clients' and Practitioners' Perspectives

The perspectives of clients and practitioners may provide valuable input in the evaluation of an intervention. The client's point of view may be elicited through questionnaires or interviews during or at the end of service. In the present study, clients were asked to give their opinions about "negotiating or conferencing" with other family members in the session and "working on assignments or tasks at home." All but a few clients thought that both were at least "of some help." Slightly over half in both instances thought the techniques were "particularly helpful," the highest rating.

Practitioner evaluations were obtained from seminars, individual consultations, and from written critiques of the model. Practitioner evaluations were also positive on the whole. Some expressed difficulties in setting up and sustaining session tasks, as previously discussed. Others noted problems, also mentioned previously, in use of the intervention in cases involving adolescents in trouble.

Utilization Criteria

As can be seen, Table 1 contains no "p" values. In this research strategy tests of significance are not used for two reasons: first, the units of attention, interventions, lack independence which complicates use of tests of significance. Second, and more important, our interest is not in contributing to scientific knowledge but rather to make practical decisions about interventions in a particular practice context. Judgments about apparent magnitude of effects provide a more realistic standard. If type I errors of judgment (taking chance differences seriously) occur, they can presumably be caught in further evaluations of effectiveness of the intervention. Tests of significance were developed as a substitute for replication. In this research mode replication is an essential component.

We concluded that the findings gave a genuine "go" signal for the FPSS. Given the lack of a controlled study, it is possible that the signal was misleading. Using statistical controls, we were able to rule out certain alternative explanations. For example, the home tasks in the "home task only" condition did not differ in type from the home tasks in the FPSS. Also, there was no tendency for the FPSS to be used more with better functioning families as measured by initial scores on the Family Assessment Device. However, random allocation was not used to assign practitioners or families to FPSS or "home tasks only." Nor was there any delineation of the conditions under which these alternative interventions were to be employed. As a result, the use of one or the other of the interventions was a matter of practitioner judgment. Given lack of random assignment, it is quite possible that the FPSS was used to a greater extent by more skilled practitioners or by families more adept at problem solving. Or, practitioners may have been more likely to use the intervention at points when families were showing readiness for change. To the extent that credence can be given to any of these possibilities (and others could be added), then the greater immediate problem change that followed the use of the FPSS might have been explained by other factors—e.g., practitioner skill, family problem-solving adeptness, family readiness for change, etc. Nevertheless, as model developers utilizing our own findings, and with the opportunity for replication, our truth test was perhaps not as strict as it might be in conventional interpretation and reporting of treatment effects. Our question was: Is there enough evidence to suggest that the intervention will contribute to the efficacy of the model? Our answer in this case was "probably," and thus we decided to push on with the FPSS. However, in presenting the model itself for wider consumption, we would want to make clear the evidence used in its development so that potential consumers could come to their own conclusions about its empirical basis.

DIRECTIONS FOR DEVELOPMENT

In conventional research on practice, one usually concludes a study with implications of the findings for practice. The researcher hopes that these suggestions will somehow and someday influence future practice. In contrast, modifications suggested by developmental research are incorporated directly into the intervention under development. For illustrative purposes, I shall summarize some of the modifications in the FPSS that resulted from the case studies and the aggregate analysis. I shall also indicate how these investigations might inform the next phase in the developmental process.

Intervention Shifts

To correct the tendency for practitioners to become prematurely or inappropriately involved in session tasks, we made changes in both treatment protocols and training procedures. For example, we constructed new guidelines to help practitioners handle situations in which clients would address *them* rather than other family members. In training, we placed more emphasis on session tasks generally with greater use of tapes of successful tasks. We also utilized role plays illustrating ways that practitioners could bring session tasks to successful conclusions without premature or inappropriate involvement.

Home Tasks in FPSS

We also made revisions in treatment protocols and in training in respect to the home task part of the FPSS. Individual tasks were given a more important role since they seemed to be used frequently and to good advantage in implementing agreements among family members worked out in session tasks. It was also emphasized that reciprocal tasks at home (quid pro quos) should be part of the FPSS whenever possible.

Adolescents in Trouble

Cases involving adolescents in trouble presented difficulty for the model as a whole, whether or not the FPSS was used. Although the extent of this shortfall was made clear in the aggregate analysis, evidence of it had appeared earlier during the case study phase. Failures in individual cases had caused us to begin to rethink our approach to this kind of family. We concluded that structural changes in the family may be needed before a problem-solving approach could be effective. For example, the parental alliance may need to be strengthened before the parents could cooperate in performing tasks that might reduce the teen's troublesome behavior. Accordingly, we began, in the case study phase, to incorporate elements of structural family therapy into the model (Minuchin 1974; Aponte and Van Deusen 1981). We noted that creators of similar approaches had also moved in a similar direction (Robin and Foster 1989). The aggregate analysis occurred before we had made much progress toward implementing those changes and, of course, served to reinforce our belief that they were in order. Consequently, new guidelines were developed which identified obstacles in family structure that might need to be addressed when applying the FPSS to families with adolescents in trouble (as well as to certain other types of families that seemed to present some of the same issues). The kinds of task strategies that could be used to achieve structural change were also explicated. These strategies were subsequently used in a successful application of the FPSS in a case involving adolescents in trouble (Reid and Donovan 1990).

The next phase in development would call for a more systematic evaluation of the FPSS, ideally one that would take the form of a controlled experiment. The work reviewed here provided some qualified evidence that the FPSS was able to achieve the short-term goal of immediate change in a target problem but could not satisfactorily determine its contribution to final outcome.

A next step might be a controlled experiment that could provide better evidence on the short-term effects of the FPSS as well as some evidence on its longer-term effects. reasonable design might be the kind of "micro experiment" used in developmental research on task-centered treatment of children, (Reid 1975) in which the operation of the experimental variable (the FPSS in the present case) is limited to one or two sessions while controls receive an alternative form of intervention. Should the experiment achieve positive results the use of the FPSS could be extended in a replication. Such an approach would fit with the notion of the FPSS as one of a number of interventions to be used over the course of a case rather than as a self-sufficient method.

The case studies and aggregate analysis have laid the groundwork for whatever experimental design might be used by providing data on what the intervention looks like in practice, the obstacles and contingencies that arise in its use, and its possible short-term effects. These data in turn have resulted in substantial modifications of the intervention itself. As a result the intervention has moved closer toward readiness for an experimental test and should be better able to demonstrate its efficacy when such a test occurs.

REFERENCES

Aponte, H. and John M. Van Deusen. 1981. Structural family therapy. In *Handbook of Family Therapy*, edited by A. S. Gurman and D. P. Kniskern. New York: Brunner/Mazel.

Barlow, D. H., S. C. Hayes, and R. O. Nelson. 1983. *The Scientist Practitioner: Research and Accountability in Clinical and Educational Settings*. New York: Pergamon Press.

Beck, D. F. and M. A. Jones. 1973. *Progress on Family Problems: A Nationwide Study of Clients' and Counselors' Views on Family Agency Services*. New York: Family Service Agency of America.

Benbenishty, R. 1988. Assessment of task-centered interventions with families in Israel. *Journal of Social Service Research*, 11, 19-43.

Benbenishty, R. 1989. Combining the single-system and group approaches to evaluate treatment effectiveness on the agency level. *Journal of Social Service Research*, 12: 31-48.

Cook, T. D. and D. T. Campbell. 1979. *Quasi-Experimentation: Design and Analysis Issues for Field Settings*. Chicago: Rand McNally.

Davis, I. P. and W. J. Reid. 1988. Event analysis in clinical practice and process research. *Social Casework*, 69 298-306.

Epstein, N. B., L. M. Baldwin, and P. S. Bishop. 1983. The McMaster family assessment device. *Journal of Marital and Family Therapy*, 9, 171-180.

Gilbert, J. P, R. J. Light, and F. Mosteller. 1975. Assessing social innovations: An empirical base for policy. In *Evaluation and Experiment*, edited by C. A. Bennett and A. A. Lumsdaine. New York: Academic Press.

Jacobson, N. S. 1981. Behavioral marital therapy. In *Handbook of Family Therapy*, edited by A. S. Gurman and D. P. Kniskern. New York: Brunner/Mazel.

Jacobson, N. S. and G. Margolin. 1979. *Marital Therapy: Strategies Based on Social Learning and Behavior Exchange Principles*. New York: Brunner/ Mazel.

McMahon, P. 1987. Shifts in intervention procedures: A problem in evaluating human service interventions. *Social Work Research and Abstracts*, 23:(4):13-17.

Minuchin S. 1974. *Families and Family Therapy*. Cambridge: Harvard University Press.

Reid, W. J. 1975. An experimental test of a task-centered approach. *Social Work*, 20, 3-9.

Reid, W. J. 1985. *Family Problem Solving*. New York: Columbia University Press.

Reid, W. J. 1987a. Developing an intervention in developmental research. *Journal of Social Service Research*, *11*, 17-39.

Reid, W. J. 1987b. The family problem-solving sequence. *Family Therapy*, 14:135-146.

Reid, W. J. and P. Hanrahan. 1988. Measuring implementation of social treatment. In *Evaluating Program Environments*, edited by K. J. Conrad and C. Roberts-Gray. San Francisco: Jossey-Bass.

Reid, William J. and I. P. Davis. 1987. Qualitative methods in single case research. In *Perspectives on Practitioners as Evaluators of Direct Practice*, edited by Naomi Gottlieb. School of Social Work, University of Washington, Seattle, June 16-18, 1987.

Reid, W. J. and T. Donovan. 1990. Treating sibling violence. *Family Therapy*, 71:49-59.

Reid, W. J. and L. Epstein. (eds.) 1977. *Task-Centered Practice*. New York: Columbia University Press.

Robin, A. L. 1981. A controlled evaluation of problem solving communication training with parent-adolescent conflict. *Behavior Therapy*, 12:593-609.

Robin, A. L. and S. L. Foster. 1989. *Negotiating adolescence: A behavioral family systems approach to parent-adolescent conflict*. New York: The Guilford Press.

Stuart, R. B. 1980. *Helping Couples Change: A Social Learning Approach to Marital Therapy*. New York: The Guilford Press.

Thomas, E. J. 1977. *Marital Communication and Decision Making: Analysis Assessment and Change*. New York: Free Press, 59, 182, 185, 186, 194.

Thomas, E. J. 1990. Modes of practice in developmental research. In *Advances in Clinical Social Work Research*, edited by L. Videka-Sherman and W. J. Reid. Silver Spring, MD: NASW Press.

Thomas, E. J., J. Bastien, D. R. Stuebe, D. E. Bronson, and J. Yaffe. 1987. Assessing procedural descriptions: Rationale and illustrative study. *Behavioral Assessment*, *9*, 43-56.

EVALUATION
AND ADVANCED DEVELOPMENT

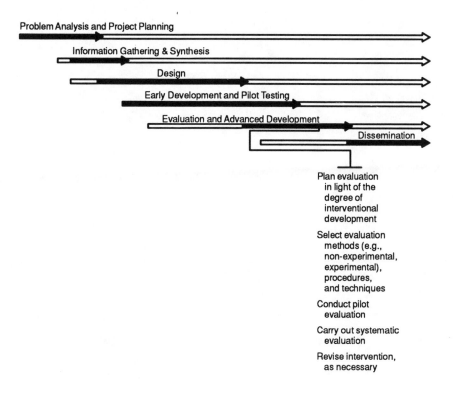

Problem Analysis and Project Planning

Information Gathering & Synthesis

Design

Early Development and Pilot Testing

Evaluation and Advanced Development

Dissemination

Plan evaluation
in light of the
degree of
interventional
development

Select evaluation
methods (e.g.,
non-experimental,
experimental),
procedures,
and techniques

Conduct pilot
evaluation

Carry out systematic
evaluation

Revise intervention,
as necessary

Chapter 12

Evaluation, Advanced Development, and the Unilateral Family Therapy Experiment

Edwin J. Thomas

Evaluation in intervention research is empirical inquiry directed toward determining the effects of the intervention, including its effectiveness. Although there is typically some evaluation of aspects of the intervention at most points of the D&D process, major emphasis is placed on systematic outcome evaluation in the phase of evaluation and advanced development. As an integral part of the innovation process, evaluation should provide the necessary results to determine whether the innovation should be retained and utilized more or less as it was designed or should be redesigned and developed further. Satisfactory results in evaluation generally provide a basis for moving ahead into the subsequent phase of dissemination.

This chapter presents some of the main steps involved in evaluation and advanced development, using the research of the author and his associates on unilateral family therapy (UFT) for alcohol abuse to illustrate various points. Rigorous and systematic evaluation would generally be premature in early development, but becomes critical in later stages when the intervention is sufficiently well formed to justify the time and expense required to conduct an appropriate evaluation. Although evaluation can be carried out with a developed intervention without also undertaking additional development, it is rarely the case in human service that interventions are sufficiently well developed so that additional improvements cannot be made. Repeated application of an already developed intervention generally provides many occasions to detect limitations that were or could not be addressed earlier, and to achieve more skillful and refined application. While it is possible at any point to prohibit further development and focus exclusively on evaluation, the gains of allowing selective development to occur concurrently with evaluation generally outweigh possible limitations.

Advanced development presupposes that initial design and pilot testing have been carried out with the intervention and that what has been learned in the earlier trial use is sufficiently positive to justify more systematic appraisal of intervention outcomes. Trial use provides occasions for developmental testing in which an innovation is systematically tested, revised, or redesigned (Thomas 1984). Advanced development thus involves further developmental testing of the intervention. Such testing provides for the replicated use of interventions that do not need to be revised when they are utilized in essentially the same way as they were designed to be used. As the process of development progresses, the practitioner-researcher moves from innovation to innovation and from case to case until most or all interventions in the domain of design and development have been implemented successfully without needing major alterations or redesign. If performed appropriately, the additional developmental testing of the intervention should extend the depth of development and thus enhance its developmental validity (Thomas 1985).

OVERVIEW OF THE UNILATERAL FAMILY THERAPY EXPERIMENT

The purpose of the research summarized here was to develop and evaluate a treatment program whereby spouses of alcohol abusers unmotivated for treatment could be assisted to influence the drinker to enter treatment, reduce drinking, or both. There has been increasing use by alcohol counselors and therapists of confrontive interventions that are carried out by the alcohol abuser's family or significant others (e.g., see Johnson 1986). Case reports and some nonexperimental studies have shown that such confrontive interventions may help induce the abuser to enter treatment (e.g., Liepman, Nirenberg, and Begin 1989; Logan 1983) and that family members can promote treatment of problem drinkers (e.g., see Sisson and Azrin 1986). However, there have been few experimental studies of this type of intervention, and no prior experimental evaluations of the more general unilateral approach to alcohol abuse.

In the unilateral approach, a spouse or other cooperative family member is assisted to mediate change in an uncooperative family member (Thomas and Santa 1982). Although the therapist intervenes with the participating person alone, the objective is to change the behavior of an uncooperative person or other aspects of the marital or family system through changes mediated by the influence of the participating person or persons. The assumption that inducing change in an individual can lead to change in the system of which that person is a part has precedence in clinical outcome research (e.g., Szapocznik et al. 1983; Szapocznik et al. 1988), systems theory (e.g., Bowen 1974; Carter and Orfanidis 1976), and other conceptions of addressing marital problems through one spouse (e.g., Bennun 1984). The assumption underlying this experimental approach to treatment was that although spouses cannot be viewed as responsible for their partner's drinking they can often be engaged to function as a critical point of leverage to reach and help change the previously inaccessible alcohol abuser.

The main emphases of the treatment were designed and developed in an earlier, three-and-a-half year pilot project in which 26 spouses of uncooperative drinkers received a unilateral spouse treatment program lasting 4 to 6 months. Some two-thirds of the abusers of these spouses who received full spouse treatment entered treatment for their alcohol abuse, stopped drinking, or reduced their drinking appreciably; and the treatment was significantly associated with positive gains in affection and sexual satisfaction and reduced life distress for the spouses (Thomas, Santa, Bronson, and Oyserman 1987). The positive results in this development phase led to further funding for the four-year experimental evaluation described below.[1]

1. The research reported in this chapter was supported in part by grants 1 R01 AA04163-03 and 5 R01 AA04163-07 of the National Institute on Alcohol Abuse and Alcoholism, Edwin J. Thomas, Principal Investigator. I wish to acknowledge the contributions of Denise Bronson, Cathleen Santa, Joanne Yaffe, and Daphna Oyserman in the pilot phase of the research and Richard D. Ager, Marianne Yoshioka, Kathryn Betts Adams, and David Moxley in the evaluation phase.

Based on methods developed in the pilot project, spouses of alcohol abusers unmotivated for treatment were recruited by newspaper advertisements to participate in an experimental treatment program to help them do something about their partner's drinking. All spouses were screened by telephone for eligibility with approximately 1 in 5 meeting all criteria (e.g., no alcohol abuse on the part of the cooperative spouse, and the absence of serious domestic violence and other drug abuse for both partners). One in each successive pair of eligible spouses was randomly assigned to either the Immediate ($n=27$) or Delayed ($n=28$) Treatment Condition in which spouses received 6 months of unilateral treatment. A No-Treatment Condition consisted of 14 otherwise eligible spouses whose alcohol abusing partners were unwilling to give consent for their spouses to receive this type of treatment. Research assessments were given to all spouses before treatment and subsequently at 6-, 12-, and 18-month intervals (see Table 1 for the research design). The research assessment battery consisted of some 20 instruments, including new spouse assessment inventories developed on this project (e.g., the Spouse Enabling Inventory).

TABLE 1. Design of the evaluation of unilateral family therapy for alcohol abuse, by experimental condition and times of research assessment.*

Experimental Conditions	Assessments			
	Time 1 (Project Entry)	Time 2 (6 months)	Time 3 (12 months)	Time 4 (18 months)
Immediate Treatment ($n=27$)	(1) Pre 1	(2) Post 1	(3) Post 2	(4) Post 3
Delayed Treatment ($n=28$)	(5) Pre 1	(6) Pre 2	(7) Post 1	(8) Post 2
No Treatment ($n=14$)	(9) Pre 1	(10) Pre 2	(11) Pre 3	(12) Pre 4

*Assessments were completed by all spouses and those abusers who gave their consent to participate in assessments.

As indicated, the focus of the treatment program was on preparing the spouse to function as a mediator of change with the uncooperative alcohol abuser. Among the main areas of the program were treatment orientation for the spouse, clinical assessment using the spouse as a sole informant, and spouse role induction to assist the spouse to become a positive rehabilitative influence. The treatment components of the spouse role induction included unilateral relationship enhancement (Thomas et al. 1990), reduction of the spouse's customary drink control behavior (Yoshioka, Thomas, and Ager 1992), and spouse disenabling (Thomas, Yoshioka, and Ager 1993). The treatment program also contained abuser-directed interventions as central features (e.g., a programmed confrontation or request by the spouse [Thomas and Yoshioka 1989]), and maintenance (e.g., spouse sobriety support). Further details are also given elsewhere (Thomas, Santa, Bronson, and Oyserman 1987; Thomas 1989b; Thomas in press; Thomas and Ager in press).

By way of a brief overview of the results, it was found that there were positive changes relating to the spouse role induction that were directly associated with spouse participation in the treatment program. Among these changes for spouses were reductions in nagging and other dysfunctional drink-related spouse influence behaviors, in enabling, psychopathology, and life distress, and improvements in marital adjustment and satisfaction.

There were also significant changes in drink-related outcomes for the abusers associated with the spouse treatment program. For example, treatment entry of abusers was significantly higher following spouse treatment, and abusers reduced their drinking from Time 1 to 4 by 68 percent in the treatment conditions, versus 20 percent in the No-Treatment Condition. Although there were some improvements through time in drink-related outcomes for all abusers, the improvements associated with spouse treatment were notably greater (Thomas et al. 1993).

In addition to the experimental findings as briefly noted above, the outcomes included further developments of the UFT approach. Among these advances were several new inventories intended for research as well as clinical purposes. These instruments were the Life Distress Inventory, the Spouse Treatment Mediation Inventory, the Spouse Enabling Inventory, and the Spouse Sobriety Influence

Inventory. Practice procedures for the use of the inventories in assessment and change were evolved for such areas as spouse enabling (Thomas, Yoshioka, and Ager 1992) and customary spouse drink control (Yoshioka, Thomas, and Ager 1992). Among the principal advances, however, were those relating to each of the main treatment components of the UFT program identified earlier. In addition to developments in the UFT program cited earlier, other developments are currently being prepared for publication.

An important conclusion of the research was that spouses can be assisted to become a positive rehabilitative influence with an uncooperative drinker. The spouse treatment program served to enhance the skills of the spouse to cope with an alcohol abusing marital partner and to assist the spouse in inducing the abuser to enter treatment and/or to achieve moderated drinking or abstinence. Success in such spouse treatment also depends, of course, upon how amenable the uncooperative alcohol abuser is to change in response to inductions mediated by the cooperative spouses. The findings of this study are necessarily restricted to the present sample as selected by the eligibility criteria.

Requirements of Evaluation and Advanced D&D

Considered more generally, evaluation and advanced D&D in intervention research have three related requirements. The first is that the evaluation should constitute a fair test of the outcomes of the intervention. As indicated, the evaluation requirement was met by conducting an outcome experiment of the UFT approach consisting of three experimental conditions and four time periods of research assessment (see Table 1). In this experiment, experimental control for the treatment conditions was achieved in two ways. First, the spouses assigned to the Delayed Treatment Condition did not receive treatment for six months during which time their spouse counterparts assigned to the Immediate Treatment Condition received treatment. The cells of the research design in the Delayed Treatment Condition between treatment entry (cell 5) and the six-month assessment at Time 2 (cell 6) provide a before and after contrast without treatment. When the results for these cells are compared with the results obtained by comparing cells 1 and 2 for the Immediate Treatment Condition, a basis is provided for determining the initial effectiveness of treatment.

The second type of control was made possible by having the No-Treatment Condition. Assessments were also given to these spouses at time points comparable to those at which assessments were given for the spouses in the treatment conditions. For reasons having to do with the right to treatment of subjects participating in treatment research, human subjects regulations did not allow for a pure spouse No-Treatment Condition in which fully eligible spouses could be randomly assigned to this condition or to one of the treatment conditions. Even so, the spouses in the No-Treatment Condition had met all the eligibility requirements the other spouses met except the one mentioned, and they did not receive treatment. When compared with the spouses in the treatment conditions on demographic and other characteristics measured at Time 1, the spouses in the No-treatment Condition were not found to be significantly different.

The availability of a No-treatment Condition provided for making important additional comparisons which strengthened the design. Thus, contrasts across various assessment times made possible additional comparisons to examine the initial and follow-up effects of treatment, the effects of being placed on a waiting list in the Delayed Treatment Condition (cells 5 and 6 vs. 9 and 10), and of not being involved in any treatment (cells 9-12 vs. 1-4 and 5-8). Simplifying the design would have greatly reduced its rigor whereas increasing the power of the design to rule out other possible threats to internal and external validity would have exceeded the resources and time available to conduct the study.

The second is a service requirement in which the intervention being evaluated should provide the human service for which objectives of the intervention were intended. The service for the spouses in the UFT study was to assist them with coping with the effects of living with an uncooperative alcohol abuser and with helping them to induce the abuser to enter treatment for alcohol abuse and/or to reduce the drinking, including achievement of abstinence. Service for other personal, marital, or family problems of the spouses was not included because it would have gone beyond the scope of the treatment program evolved in the pilot phase and would have taken the service in directions inconsistent with those of the evaluation and of the D&D. This is one of several important ways in which the service in D&D can be different from that ordinarily provided in an on-going agency.

The third requirement is that advancement of the intervention calls for implementing the intervention in the evaluation so that development of the intervention is furthered beyond that which was accomplished in the earlier pilot testing. Based as it is on repeated applications of the intervention with additional cases, advanced development should provide additional opportunities for trial use and additional depth of development along the lines set down in the pilot phase. Advanced development can also enhance the breadth of D&D, but the scope of development should generally not be extended beyond that which was established in the pilot phase, if that extension involves breaking ground in entirely new areas.

In the case of the UFT project, further depth of development was anticipated and fostered for all of the main treatment areas established in the pilot phase (e.g., the several components, such as disenabling, of the spouse role induction and the diverse abuser-directed interventions, such as programmed confrontation), and was expanded to include additional emphasis on maintenance in the form of providing sobriety support for the spouse and alcohol abuser. The program refinements and extensions were directly related to the purpose and focus of the intervention program as evolved in the pilot phase. In addition, the means of client selection, types of therapists, assessment criteria, and methods used in the evaluation were based on and kept very similar to those of the pilot phase.

The service, evaluation, and advanced development requirements noted above are to some extent different such that pursuit of one without reference to the others can cause difficulties. For example, the service requirements, if different from those of the intervention being evaluated or of the domain of advanced development, can interfere with the validity of the evaluation and adequacy of further development. The areas of advanced development need to be coordinated with those of initial development and with the requirements of the evaluation. The challenge is to meet the requirements of service, evaluation, and advanced development while also bringing the three together in a complementary relationship.

THE TASKS OF EVALUATION

The activities of evaluation consist largely of applying established methods and techniques of research to the objectives of the intervention evaluation. Although the research methodology undergirding evaluation is becoming increasingly more sophisticated, its main outlines and methods have been in place now for many years. It is beyond the scope of this chapter to review this large methodology. Rather, attention will be given to some of the main steps that need to be carried out in evaluation and some of the principal issues the researcher is likely to face.

Steps in D&D Evaluation

To meet the requirements of evaluation, a number of tasks need to be completed in more or less stepwise order. These range from formulating the objective of the evaluation on through to refining and redesigning the intervention, as necessary (see Table 2). Although the tasks associated with these steps have their counterparts in other types of research, they are generally implemented somewhat differently in intervention research. For example, human subject procedures in work with patients, clients, and other participants in human service intervention can be more restrictive than their counterparts in other types of research (e.g., see *Federal Register,* 1974, May 30). Intervening with clients and others with human service problems can place special restrictions on what research designs are feasible and appropriate. Therapists and assessors need to be trained and the intervention should be carefully defined and organized. Some of these differences were illustrated in the above description of the UFT evaluation, and other aspects will be highlighted below in connection with discussing some of the evaluation issues.

Some Special Issues in D&D Evaluation

Some of the special issues in D&D evaluation are highlighted below along with some alternatives for resolution and how the issue was addressed in the UFT experiment.

TABLE 2. Steps in D&D Evaluation

---

1. Statement of evaluation objective
2. Determining what is to be evaluated
3. Establishing project organization
4. Selecting an evaluation site
5. Selecting the sample
6. Selecting the research design
7. Selecting measurement and assessment instruments
8. Establishing human subjects procedures
9. Defining and organizing the intervention
10. Selecting and training practitioners/or therapists
11. Selecting and training assessors
12. Assessment of the clients or other subject participants
13. Implementing the intervention
14. Determining intervention integrity
15. Monitoring outcomes
16. Analyzing the results
17. Interpreting the results
18. Drawing conclusions
19. Refining and redesigning the intervention, as appropriate

---

What Is To Be Evaluated

In deciding what is to be evaluated, researchers can focus on such outcomes as effectiveness, efficiency, cost, or quality assurance. Of these, evaluation of intervention effectiveness is fundamental and is generally a major focus of evaluation with other matters such as efficiency, cost, and quality assurance being addressed at later points, providing that the intervention is sufficiently effective. In the case of the UFT evaluation, systematic evaluation of the effectiveness of the treatment approach was clearly the first order of business since the main focus of the pilot phase was on initial development and less so on evaluation. There had been no prior systematic evaluation of the UFT approach. Criteria involving abuser changes, as indicated, involved their entry into treatment or reduced drinking, including abstinence, whereas spouse outcomes included those relating to enabling, life distress, psychopathology, and marital adjustment.

The Degree of Evaluation Rigor

In general, the research design for an evaluation should be as rigorous as possible in the light of available resources, time, and the requirements of the service and D&D associated with the intervention. To this end, experimental designs with appropriate experimental and control conditions are to be preferred in general over non-experimental designs, and periodic follow-up assessments should be provided to examine the effects over time of the intervention.

Because the design of the UFT experiment was relatively rigorous, as described earlier, it made it possible to discern some effects that otherwise would not be observed. For example, despite reductions in abuser drinking associated directly with spouse treatment, there were in addition gradual reductions in drinking through time for all abusers. Also, while spouse treatment was reliably associated with treatment entry of the alcohol abuser, there was a tendency for a few abusers in the No-Treatment Condition to enter treatment as time went by. Further, while most of the positive changes associated with spouse treatment did not revert at follow-up to pretreatment levels, there were small rebound effects from the 6- to 12-month follow-up for a few outcomes (e.g., spouse psychopathology).

The Amount of Advanced Development

As indicated earlier, advanced development should generally be directed toward effort within the initial domain of D&D, with emphasis largely on extending the depth of the earlier development. However, even when appropriately focused, there is the question of how much time and effort should be invested in further development, given the ever-present constraints of time and resources. How much advanced development can be achieved while also carrying out an on-going evaluation?

We found in the UFT project that the day-to-day requirements of the evaluation (e.g., providing the intervention, research assessments, and processing and, later, analyzing the evaluation data) placed a firm limit on the amount of time available for some aspects of development. While refinements of the treatment program were readily discussed, implemented, and documented, there was generally a lag in detailed proceduralization and the preparation of reports and papers on the treatment methods. Had proceduralization been elevated in priority, it would inevitably have displaced some of the on-line requirements of the evaluation. As it was, an important portion of the UFT project effort was set aside for further development which, despite the limits set by the evaluation, was ample enough to refine the treatment program.

Single Case versus Group Experimental Designs

There has been increasing recognition that single-system evaluation is an important class of experimental designs that have widespread application in human service (e.g., see Barlow and Hersen 1984; Berlin 1983; Bloom and Fischer 1982; Blythe and Tripodi 1989; Dean and Reinherz 1987; Gingerich 1979, 1990; Hayes 1981; Jayaratne and Levy 1979; Kazdin 1982; Kratochwill 1978; Kratochwill, Mott, and Dobson 1984; Mutschler 1979; Nelsen 1981; Polster and Lynch 1985; Reid 1983; Richey et al. 1987; Schinke 1983; Thomas 1975, 1978c, 1983; Thyer 1986; Thyer and Curtis 1983; Tripodi 1983; Tripodi and Epstein 1980; Wodarski 1981). Such experimentation has been found to be highly flexible and applicable in clinical and other interventive situations while, at the same time, it is capable of providing a high degree of experimental rigor, depending upon the single-system experimental design chosen. While researchers often differ in their views about whether single-system or group experimentation is to be preferred, the perspective here is that each type, in general, has its own strengths and limitations and that both types have an important place in evaluation (also see Jayaratne 1977). In the present perspective, single-system designs lend themselves particularly well to examination of effectiveness with small samples of individuals or other systems in the earlier stages of D&D. In contrast, group experimental designs (e.g., see Beck, Andrasik, and Arena 1984; Kendall and Norton-Ford 1982; Tripodi 1983) are particularly appropriate for systematic evaluation of interventions that have been shown earlier to be effective in single-system experiments and/or in pilot testing.

It is sometimes possible to evolve an experimental plan that combines single-system and group experimental features, thus capitalizing on some of the advantages of both. In the UFT experiment, the single-system components consisted, first, of before, after, and follow-up evaluations for every case. Second, each successive pair of cases constituted a cross-over experimental dyad in which, as indicated, one spouse was assigned at random to an Immediate Treatment Condition and the other to the Delayed Treatment Condition. When aggregated, the immediate and delayed treatment spouses represent the subjects for the conditions of a group experimental design, as indicated earlier and as shown in Table 1. The main outcomes of the UFT experiment were evaluated using the outcomes of the group design because it afforded contrasts that allowed for drawing the strongest inferences. Even so, however, each constituent cross-over experimental dyad nested in the aggregate design was a legitimate single-system experiment on a smaller scale. When the results were consistent with the aggregate outcomes, selected cross-over dyads were chosen to document quantitative clinical results in reports on particular intervention procedures, such as disenabling (Thomas, Yoshioka, and Ager 1993) and reduction of customary drink control (Yoshioka, Thomas, and Ager 1992).

Outcome versus Field Testing

Field testing involves examining whether the intervention can be implemented appropriately under normal operating conditions. In contrast, outcome testing, as viewed here, is addressed to evaluating the interventional outcomes in settings selected to obtain the best test of the intervention that is not confounded with the operation of extraneous factors. Outcome testing may be conducted in an agency or a special setting, whereas field testing is generally carried out in the appropriate agency in the field with the typical clientele, practitioners, and work and administrative arrangements. While there can be exceptions, field testing is generally most appropriate to conduct after outcome testing has demonstrated that the intervention yields the intended benefits.

Special settings, like the experimental analog, may provide a purer test of outcome but may do so under atypical service conditions (e.g., see Kazdin 1978). In contrast, while evaluating the intervention in the indigenous agency may be a suitable field context, it may provide distorted results because of extraneous or confounding factors that exist in that setting that could be designed out, if found to interfere with the intervention. More generally, if outcome and field testing are combined, unsuccessful results could be due to the confounding of effects of the particular field conditions, inherent ineffectiveness of the intervention, failure to implement the intervention appropriately in the field, or all three. Thus, the separation of outcome testing from field testing can provide for more accurate and interpretable results (for more details, see Thomas 1984). Even so, however, in either case there may be important limitations on the generalizability of the results.

The outcome evaluation of UFT was conducted in a special site of the research project (The Marital Treatment Project) by project practitioner-researchers with the spouse participants obtained through newspaper advertisements and subsequently screened by telephone for eligibility. Eligibility criteria were employed to ensure the relevance of cases to the focus and scope of the treatment program. Whether or not the evaluation had been conducted in an agency setting, criteria such as these would have had to have been employed in order to select clientele appropriate for the intervention.

However, solicitation by newspaper advertisement may have drawn spouses who differ from those to be found in a client population of spouses of uncooperative drinkers. Some studies have shown that there are few differences between treatment outcomes for solicited versus nonsolicited patients (e.g., see Last et al. 1984). More generally, it was concluded from a review of 14 studies that compared solicited and nonsolicited patient groups treated or studied in clinical settings that the data were too limited to permit conclusions regarding generalizability of findings on treatment efficacy based on solicited patient samples (Krupnick, Shea, and Elkin 1986). The issue is made particularly complex in the UFT study because the treatment program was essentially a prototype and the spouses and their uncooperative alcohol abusing marital partners were hard-to-reach clientele about which very little at present is known.

Standardized versus Non-Standardized Intervention

In general, standardized intervention is to be preferred over the nonstandardized inasmuch as standardization provides for uniform treatment of clients using the same intervention procedures. Without sufficient uniformity, an intervention can confound an evaluation and produce uninterpretable results. Standardized interventions make reliable replication possible, are necessary to achieve quality control (Ramp 1984), and are an essential feature of an appropriately designed model of intervention (Paine 1984).

A standardized program may or may not involve individualized application. In the UFT treatment program, all the treatment components contained steps and procedures that were to be uniformly applied, but, in so doing, they were made individually relevant, depending upon the clinical conditions for the spouse and abuser. For example, uniform assessment and intervention planning methods were employed to prepare a plan to reduce spouse enabling, but the plan was applied to the specific enabling behaviors and interventional opportunities for that spouse. Scripting and rehearsal of a programmed confrontation likewise made use of standard procedures, but they were individually implemented in every instance. An important aspect of advanced development on the UFT project was determining, codifying, and retrieving relevant case data concerning the conditions under which particular, individualized applications were or were not feasible.

Assessing Treatment Integrity

Treatment integrity has been defined as a degree to which a treatment is delivered as intended (Salend 1984; Yeaton and Sechrest 1981). Lack of reliability in the delivery of the intervention can represent a serious threat to the internal and external validity of the intervention. The use of treatment manuals can facilitate reliability in interventional delivery (e.g., see Dobson and Shaw 1988), as can the use of videotaped recording of intervention sessions.

A variety of means were used in the UFT project to endeavor to ensure the integrity of the treatment program. The treatment methods were written, described, or illustrated on audiotape, clinical records of each treatment session were promptly prepared after the contact, these records and audiotapes of the treatment sessions were regularly reviewed by the author (as the project director), and regular staff meetings were held to review, analyze, and refine treatment procedures.

Addressing Potential Confounds

Because intervention research is typically conducted with clientele having real difficulties by practitioners or others who deliver an intervention applicable in life situations, more than the usual number of potentially confounding variables may bias the results. Some of the potential sources of bias in a D&D evaluation are given in Table 3. Consider, for example, a shift in intervention which McMahon has defined as "any consistent deviation from a written, explicit procedure or plan recognized implicitly for treating the presenting problem" (1987:13). McMahon has indicated that lack of treatment integrity may be due to a shift in intervention in which the procedure takes on a new, consistent form. One version of intervention shift is intervention maturation in which the intervention is modified and improved through time. Clearly, intervention maturation could be a likely result of successful advanced development. However, such maturation could represent an important confound in the evaluation that needs to be considered in the analysis of results.

Comparisons in the UFT experiment of the Delayed with the Immediate Treatment Conditions over time and of other time-related contrasts did not disclose any treatment maturation effect in

TABLE 3. Some potential sources of bias in evaluation research.

Differences in therapist proficiency

Differences in measurement (e.g., measurement procedures, instruments, and/or assessors)

Noncomparability of experimental conditions

Subject attrition

Variations in intervention dosage (e.g., number of treatment sessions)

Treatment shift and/or maturation

Lack of treatment integrity

---

the outcomes. Even so, special analyses were conducted to examine the possible effects of treatment maturation. In one, the date of treatment for the spouse was used as an indicator of treatment maturation, with later cases presumably receiving more refined treatment methods than earlier cases. The date of treatment was employed as a covariate in an analysis of covariance of quantitative measures of abuser drinking, with the results indicating no relationship between the date of treatment and the drinking variable. In another analysis, a measure of therapist experience on the project was examined on the assumption that therapists more experienced on the project could have used more mature treatment methods. The indicator of therapist experience consisted of rankings of the dates of treatment entry of each of the spouses in treatment with them, with the higher rank indicating greater therapist experience. These rankings, in turn, were then correlated with selected treatment outcomes for these spouses, with the results again indicating no relationship. The other potential confounds listed in Table 3 were also examined and not found to be sources of bias that had to be taken into consideration in the final analysis of the outcomes.

Clinical versus Statistical Significance

The outcome results of an evaluation typically and appropriately involve findings expressed statistically. Such findings are of course critical to appraising the effectiveness and other outcomes of the intervention. However, the rendering of the outcomes of an evaluation in terms of statistical averages which provide no information on the effects of the intervention for the individuals involved and which are based upon tests of statistical significance may have little direct clinical relevance (e.g., see Jacobson 1988; Jacobson, Follette, and Revenstorf 1984). For example, one indicator of clinical significance is the proportion of clients who benefit from the treatment by some clinical standard. In the UFT study, this was illustrated by the proportion of abusers in the various experimental conditions who entered treatment for alcohol abuse. As indicated earlier, there was a clear positive effect of the treatment using this criterion.

There was also a 68 percent reduction in drinking from Time 1 to

Time 4 for abusers in the treatment conditions, as mentioned before. While this was statistically significant, this result would not be sufficiently clinically relevant for many practitioners. It is possible for a heavy drinker to reduce his or her drinking by a given percentage and still be heavily addicted to alcohol, whereas some reductions in drinking short of abstinence can be clinically meaningful. To make the drinking reductions more relevant clinically, the amount by which each abuser reduced his or her alcohol consumption was converted into four categories of levels of ounces of 86-proof equivalent alcohol consumed per week. These categories were heavy drinking (more than 42 ounces), controlled drinking (21 to 42 ounces), moderate drinking (more than 0 to 21 ounces), and abstinence (0 ounces). Percentages of abusers who reduced their drinking levels using these categories were then calculated with the result that 73 percent of the abusers of spouses who received the UFT treatment achieved and maintained clinically meaningful reductions in their drinking levels by the last follow-up at Time 4, with many becoming abstinent. Considering both the change criteria of entry into treatment and a reduction in drinking levels, it was found that 79 percent of the abusers had achieved one or the other criterion by the final follow-up assessment at Time 4.

THE TASKS OF D&D

Some of the tasks of D&D to be performed concurrently with those of evaluation are reviewed below along with some of the major issues. The methodology of D&D also goes well beyond that which can be touched on here. For more details, the reader is referred to other chapters of this volume and to other sources (e.g., Azrin 1977; Fairweather 1967; Fawcett in press; Fawcett, Mathews, and Fletcher 1980; Mullen 1978, 1983; Paine, Bellamy, and Wilcox 1984; Reid 1979; Rothman 1980, 1989; Thomas 1978a, 1978b, 1984, 1985, 1989a, 1990).

The Steps of D&D

Many of the tasks of D&D, like those of evaluation, lend themselves best to being carried out in a certain order. Some of the major steps in advanced D&D are given in Table 4. The reader will note that some of these are also aspects of the steps of evaluation (e.g., selecting the intervention site, selecting clients or other participants). For these overlapping activities, questions of D&D need to be considered along with those of evaluation. More generally, the steps of D&D must be coordinated and closely linked with those of evaluation so that meeting the requirements of one does not interfere significantly with meeting those of the other. Once the intervention is implemented and data concerning the success in implementing the intervention are coming in, these and other data relating to the D&D aspects of the intervention are analyzed, the intervention is refined and redesigned, as necessary, proceduralization is undertaken, and there is further D&D, as appropriate (as indicated in steps 8-11 of the table). These later steps of data analysis, redesign, proceduralization, and further D&D are generally not carried out just once, but rather are repeated with each aspect of the intervention being developed, often at different points in time. Proceduralization, for instance, may be performed at many different points to capture progress with the different interventional components and with each resulting version of the procedure then being employed as a tool in conducting subsequent D&D.

TABLE 4. Some major steps in advanced D&D.

---

1. Selecting the intervention site[a]
2. Selecting clients or other participants[a]
3. Determining the scope of advanced D&D
4. Determining the mode of practice or intervention
5. Selecting interventionists[a]
6. Selecting the method of developmental testing
7. Establishing procedures to retrieve innovation data
8. Analyzing the data
9. Refining and redesigning the intervention, as necessary[a]
10. Proceduralization
11. Engaging in further D&D, as appropriate

---

[a]These are also steps in evaluation, as indicated in Table 1.

Some Special Issues

Some of the tasks of D&D that involve special issues are discussed below along with some alternatives for resolution and illustrations of how the issue was handled in the UFT evaluation.

Concurrent versus Delayed D&D

In the foregoing discussion of advanced D&D, it was assumed that, at least to some extent, developmental testing and other aspects of D&D would be carried out concurrently with implementing the intervention in the evaluation. As has been indicated, there are many benefits to taking advantage of the opportunity to extend development when implementing the intervention. However, there are also possible disadvantages, particularly for maintaining strict uniformity in implementing an intervention. If a completely standardized intervention is required and variations due to intervention refinements cannot be tracked and addressed in the research design or through post-evaluation data analysis, then further D&D, if needed, should not be made until after the evaluation. In this alternative, possible changes could be noted and logged during the evaluation, and processed afterward when final procedures and treatment manuals are prepared. Delaying refinements in this way loses the gains of ongoing developmental testing but, in some cases, its benefits for the evaluation could make it the best alternative. As indicated, the emphasis here is on D&D concurrent with evaluation, assuming the advantages of the D&D outweigh the limitations.

Establishing the Area of Service

As was noted earlier, the area of human service addressed in the evaluation should ideally be closely related to, or be the same as that of, the domain of D&D. This was achieved in large measure in the UFT project by restricting the domain of service to essentially that which involved the treatment program and its objectives. The participating spouses understood this from the outset, which meant that other problems than those relating to the drinking (e.g., child management, sexual difficulties in the marriage) were not addressed, and the spouses were steered elsewhere for service if the matters seemed to be particularly pressing. While many of the spouses did indeed have other personal or marital and family concerns, in virtually all cases the problem of the abuser's drinking was paramount and the spouses were able to put aside the other concerns during their treatment on the project or to seek help for the concerns elsewhere.

Establishing the Domain of D&D

The domain of design is a function of the number of design problems and the number of components of the intervention strategy open for design (Thomas 1984). As noted earlier, the domain of development in advanced D&D should generally not exceed the domain of design of the earlier pilot work. However, as indicated, advanced development usually involves extending the depth of development along the lines of development initially established. If the breadth of development is also extended, it should be restricted to that which pertains directly to the principal objectives of the intervention.

In the UFT project, the domain of D&D was limited, first, by selecting spouses who met specific eligibility criteria (e.g., absence of domestic violence and other drug use, history of severe mental disorder). Relaxation of any of these criteria in the evaluation would have expanded the domain of D&D inappropriately. Thus, if abusers had been included who were also mentally ill, the requirements of also addressing the mental illness would have taken the project into treatment programs for dual diagnoses which would have gone beyond the capability of the treatment program as initially developed. The second method of restricting the domain of further development was by applying the components of the treatment program in the evaluation that were pilot tested earlier and by not introducing new developments that went beyond the initial objectives of the program. While restricting the domain in these ways necessarily limits the generalizability of the findings from the evaluation, it is essential in keeping the domain of D&D appropriate and manageable.

Determining the Mode of Practice

In D&D involving human service, the medium by which the intervention is implemented is generally practice or some other aspect of service. The intervention may be implemented by means of conventional practice of one type or another, following the requirements of the particular practice approach in question. Opportunities for ongoing advanced development in carrying out the practice would generally be foregone in this instance, leaving possible refinements and redesign, if undertaken at all, to some later point following the completion of the evaluation.

In contrast, developmental practice would allow for addressing appropriate opportunities for advanced D&D as they occur (or shortly thereafter) in the process of implementing the interventional innovation. Developmental practice is a mode of practice in which the practitioner is also a developer of interventions.

> *Developmental practice* differs from conventional practice in that, in addition to the use of relevant practice methods, methods of design and development are followed, cases are selected according to the criterion of developmental relevance, innovations are introduced and developmentally tested in practice, the outcomes of the testing are monitored in the context of a larger design and development process of which the particular practice endeavor is a part, and the outcomes of such practice include innovative interventions, as well as possible gains in service. (Thomas 1985:54)

As has been discussed in more detail elsewhere (Thomas 1989a; Thomas 1990), developmental practice is the mode that would appear to be most appropriate for implementing interventions in D&D.

In following this mode of practice in the UFT project, every important clinical event was treated as a D&D opportunity in one of three different but related ways: replicating the particular procedure being developed, providing it was appropriate; redesigning an aspect of the procedure, if necessary; or, designing new methods and procedures when they were needed and were directly on the mainline of development. By this means, most all aspects of the UFT treatment program were subjected to repeated and trial replication many times, particularly those in the role induction segment (e.g., unilateral relationship enhancement and disenabling were essentially replicated with every spouse). At the same time, most procedures were refined at least to some degree and, throughout, conditions under which the procedures were judged to be applicable or inapplicable were logged, described, and explicated. Among the additional areas designed and developed, as indicated, were sobriety support and maintenance procedures.

Establishing Methods of Developmental Testing

Many of the relevant methods of developmental testing in D&D were noted and illustrated earlier. Some of these are summarized below along with some others: (a) selection of relevant spouses and abusers accomplished by eligibility screening at the outset, as mentioned; (b) systematic implementation of the intervention components, thus making possible the repeated application of the assessment and the intervention methods being developed; (c) systematic gathering of data on D&D processes and outcomes through such means as developmental logs (Rothman 1974; Thomas 1984; Yaffe 1987), critical incidents (e.g., Reid and Davis 1987; Thomas, Bastien, Stuebe, Bronson, and Yaffe 1987), examination of failures of implementation or outcome (e.g., see Barlow, Hayes, and Nelson 1984; Foa and Emmelkamp 1983), and the use of systematic methods of retrieval (e.g., clinical and developmental recording and description of procedural innovations); (d) solving problems using D&D methods (e.g., with a D&D team); (e) testing the innovations through repeated trial use, as described before; and (f) proceduralization of the interventions, making it possible to have successive refinement of the procedures when repeated.

When and How Much to Proceduralize

The documentation and explanation required to describe a new intervention procedure in writing so that an appropriately trained individual can understand it and carry it out can be challenging and very time consuming. In the face of many intervention components simultaneously being developed, an important issue is when and how much to proceduralize. The cost in time and effort to proceduralize ongoing interventions must be weighed against the advantages of noting important new developments and having them clearly described and made explicit for purposes of refinement and guiding further implementation. In any case, it is not always feasible or possible to prepare intervention procedures in final form until late in the D&D process, often only after trial use has been completed. Even so, there needs to be some means by which advances in intervention procedures are systematically recognized, captured, and recorded as D&D progresses.

Other issues such as what innovation retrieval procedures to use and how to enhance the generalization of the results are also relevant, but go beyond the scope of the present discussion.

EPILOG

A single evaluation, especially an appropriately conducted experiment, can be very important in determining the fate of an innovation. However, a single evaluation, whether or not it involves concurrent development, is best viewed as part of a larger process of ongoing D&D rather than as an end in itself. In the larger process, many investigators, generally from several fields, are involved over time in different aspects of the D&D activities of a given intervention area. And, as has been indicated, an intervention found to be effective should be evaluated in terms of other outcome criteria, such as efficiency and cost, and outcome evaluations should be followed by field tests. To enhance the generality of the findings, the intervention should be conducted with different client populations and under different conditions to determine the limits of its applicability.

Such is the case with unilateral family therapy for alcohol abuse. While the results to date have been very promising, further research is needed. Thus, this approach must be evaluated in field tests, to be examined with different populations of alcohol abusers than those selected for the UFT experiment, and, more generally, to be applied with different populations of uncooperative substance abusers and other types of hard-to-reach clientele.

REFERENCES

Azrin, N. H. 1977. A strategy for applied research: Learning based but outcome oriented. *American Psychologist, 32,* 140-149.

Barlow, D. H. and M. Hersen. 1984. *Single-Case Experimental Designs: Strategies for Studying Behavior Change,* 2d ed. New York: Pergamon

Barlow, D. H., S. C. Hayes, and R. O. Nelson. 1984. *The Scientist Practitioner: Research and Accountability in Clinical and Educational Settings.* New York: Pergamon.

Beck, J. G., F. Andrasik, and J. G. Arena. 1984. Group comparison designs. In *Research Methods in Clinical Psychology,* edited by A. S. Bellack and M. Hersen. New York: Pergamon.

Bennun, I. 1984. Marital therapy with one spouse. In *Marital Interaction: Analysis and Modification,* edited by K. Hahlweg and N. S. Jacobson. New York: Guilford, 356-374.

Berlin, S. 1983. Single-case evaluation: Another version. *Social Work Research and Abstracts, 19,* 3-11.

Bloom, M. and J. Fischer. 1982. *Evaluating Practice: A Guide for Helping Professionals.* Englewood Cliffs, NJ: Prentice-Hall.

Blythe, B. J. and T. Tripodi. 1989. *Measurement in Direct Social Work Practice.* Newbury Park, CA: Sage Publications.

Bowen, M. 1974. Alcoholism as viewed through family systems theory and family psychotherapy. *Annals of the New York Academy of Science, 223,* 115-122.

Carter, A. E. and M. M. Orfanidis. 1976. Family therapy with one person and the family therapist's own family. In *Family Therapy: Theory and Practice,* edited by P. J. Guerin. New York: Halsted Press.

Dean, K. and H. Reinherz. 1987. Psychodynamic practice and single-system design: The odd couple. In *Perspectives on Direct Practice Evaluation,* edited by N. Gottlieb, H. A. Ishisaka, C. A. Richey, and E. R. Tolson. Seattle, WA: Center for Social Welfare Research, School of Social Work, University of Washington.

Dobson, K. S. and B. F. Shaw. 1988. The use of treatment manuals in cognitive therapy: Experience and issues. *Journal of Consulting and Clinical Psychology, 56,* 673-680.

Fairweather, G. 1967. *Methods for Experimental Social Innovation.* New York: John Wiley & Sons.

Fawcett, S. B. In press. Some emerging standards for community research and action. In *Researching Community Psychology: Integrating Theories and Methodologies,* edited by P. Tolan, C. Keys, F. Chertok, and L. E. Jason. Washington, DC: American Psychological Association.

Fawcett, S. B., R. M. Mathews, and R. K. Fletcher. 1980. Some promising dimensions for behavioral community technology. *Journal of Applied Behavior Analysis, 13,* 508-518.

Federal Register. May 30, 1974. Protection of human subjects: Policies and procedures. Washington, DC: Department of Health, Education, and Welfare, 39(105), 2.

Foa, E. B. and P. M. Emmelkamp. 1983. *Failures in Behavior Therapy*. New York: Wiley.

Gingerich, W. J. 1979. Procedure for evaluating clinical practice. *Health and Social Work, 4,* 104-130.

Gingerich, W. J. 1990. Rethinking single-case evaluation. In *Advances in Clinical Social Work Research*, edited by L. Videka-Sherman and W. J. Reid. Silver Spring, MD: National Association of Social Workers.

Hayes, S. C. 1981. Single-case experimental design and empirical clinical practice. *Journal of Consulting and Clinical Psychology, 49,* 193-212.

Jacobson, N. S. 1988. Defining clinically significant change: An introduction. *Behavioral Assessment, 10,* 131-133.

Jacobson, N. S., W. C. Follette, and D. Revenstorf. 1984. Psychotherapy outcome research: Methods for reporting variability and evaluating clinical significance. *Behavioral Therapy, 15,* 336-352.

Jayaratne, S. 1977. Single-subject and group designs in treatment evaluation. *Social Work Research and Abstracts, 13,* 35-42.

Jayaratne, S. and R. Levy. 1979. *Empirical Clinical Practice*. New York: Columbia University Press.

Johnson, V. E. 1986. *Intervention: How to Help Someone Who Doesn't Want Help*. Minneapolis, MN: Johnson Institute Books.

Kazdin, A. E. 1978. Evaluating the generality of findings in analogue research. *Journal of Consulting and Clinical Psychology, 46,* 673-686.

Kazdin, A. E. 1982. Single-case experimental designs. In *Handbook of Research Methods in Clinical Psychology*, edited by P. C. Kendall and J. Butcher. New York: John Wiley and Sons.

Kendall, P. C. and J. D. Norton-Ford. 1982. Therapy outcome research methods. In *Handbook of Research Methods in Clinical Psychology*, edited by P. C. Kendall and J. Butcher. New York: John Wiley and Sons.

Kratochwill, J. R. 1978. Foundations of time-series research. In *Single-Subject Research: Strategies for Evaluating Change*, edited by T. R. Kratochwill. New York: Academic Press.

Kratochwill, J. R., E. Mott, and C. L. Dobson. 1984. Case study and single-case research in clinical and applied psychology. In *Research Methods in Clinical Psychology*, edited by A. S. Bellack and M. Hersen. New York: Pergamon Press.

Krupnick, J., P. Shea, and I. Elkin. 1986. Generalizability of treatment studies utilizing solicited patients. *Journal of Consulting and Clinical Psychology, 54,* 68-78.

Last, C. G., M. E. Thase, M. Hersen, A. S. Bellack, and J. M. Himmelhoch. 1984. Treatment outcome for solicited versus non-solicited unipolar depressed female outpatients. *Journal of Consulting and Clinical Psychology, 52,* 134.

Liepman, M. R., T. D. Nirenberg, and A. M. Begin. 1989. Evaluation of a program designed to help family and significant others to motivate resistant alcoholics into recovery. *American Journal of Drug and Alcohol Abuse, 15,* 209-211.

Logan, D. G. 1983. Getting alcoholics to treatment by social network intervention. *Hospital and Community Psychiatric, 34,* 360-361.

McMahon, P. M. 1987. Shifts in intervention procedures: A problem in evaluating human service interventions. *Social Work Research and Abstracts, 23,* 13-18.

Mullen, E. J. 1978. The construction of personal models for effective practice: A method for utilizing research findings to guide social interventions. *Journal of Social Service Research, 2,* 45-65.

Mullen, E. J. 1983. Personal practice methods. In *Handbook of Clinical Social Work,* edited by A. Rosenblatt and D. Waldfogel. San Francisco, CA: Jossey-Bass Publishers.

Mutschler, E. 1979. Using single-case evaluation procedures in a family and children's agency: Integration of practice and research. *Journal of Social Service Research, 3,* 115-134.

Nelsen, J. C. 1981. Issues in single-subject research for non-behaviorists. *Social Work Research & Abstracts, 31,* 31-37.

Paine, S. C. 1984. Models revisited. In *Human Services that Work: From Innovation to Standard Practice,* edited by S. C. Paine, G. T. Bellamy, and B. L. Wilcox. Baltimore, MD: Paul H. Brookes Publishing Co.

Paine, S. C., G. T. Bellamy, and B. Wilcox. 1984. *Human Services That Work: From Innovation to Standard Practice.* Baltimore, MD: Paul H. Brookes Publishing Co.

Polster, R. A. and M. A. Lynch. 1985. Single-subject designs. In *Social Work Research and Evaluation,* edited by R. M. Grinnell. Itasca, IL: F. E. Peacock Publishers.

Ramp, K. K. 1984. Effective quality control for social service programs: One piece of the puzzle: In *Human Services that Work: From Innovation to Standard Practice,* edited by S. C. Paine, G. T. Bellamy, and B. L. Wilcox. Baltimore, MD: Paul H. Brookes Publishing Co.

Reid, W. J. 1979. The model development dissertation. *Journal of Social Service Research, 3,* 215-225.

Reid, W. J. 1983. Developing intervention methods through experimental designs. In *Handbook of Clinical Social Work,* edited by A. Rosenblatt and D. Waldfogel. San Francisco, CA: Jossey-Bass Publishers.

Reid, W. J. and I. P. Davis. 1987. Qualitative methods in single-subject research. In *Perspectives in Direct Practice Research, Monograph 5,* edited by N. Gottlieb, H. A. Ishisaka, J. Kopp, C. A. Richey, and E. R. Tolson. Center for Social Welfare Research, School of Social Work, University of Washington: Seattle, WA.

Richey, C. A., J. Kopp, E. R. Tolson, and H. A. Ishisaka. 1987. Practice evaluation in diverse settings. In *Perspectives on Direct Practice Evaluation,* edited by N. Gottlieb, H. A. Ishisaka, C. A. Richey, and E. R. Tolson. Seattle, WA: Center for Social Welfare Research, School of Social Work, University of Washington.

Rothman, J. 1974. *Planning and Organizing for Social Change: Action Principles for Social Science Research.* New York: Columbia University Press.

Rothman, J. 1980. *Social R&D: Research and Development in the Human Services*. Englewood Cliffs, NJ: Prentice-Hall.

Rothman J. 1989. Intervention research: Application to runaway and homeless youths. *Social Work Research & Abstracts, 25* (1), 13-18.

Salend, S. J. 1984. Therapy outcome research: Threats to treatment integrity. *Behavior Modification, 8*, 211-222.

Schinke, S. P. 1983. Data-based practice. In *Handbook of Clinical Social Work*, edited by A. Rosenblatt and D. Waldfogel. San Francisco, CA: Jossey-Bass Publishers.

Sisson, R. W. and N. H. Azrin. 1986. Family member involvement to initiate and promote treatment of problem drinkers. *Journal of Behavioral Therapy and Experimental Psychiatry, 17*, 15-21.

Szapocznik, J., W. M. Kurtines, F. H. Foote, A. Perez-Vidal, and O. Hervis. 1983. Conjoint versus one-person family therapy; some evidence for the effectiveness of conducting family therapy through one person. *Journal of Consulting and Clinical Psychology, 51*, 889-899.

Szapocznik, J., A. Perez-Vidal, A. L. Brickman, F. H. Foote, D. Santisteban, O. Hervis, and W. M. Kurtines. 1988. Engaging adolescent drug abusers and their families in treatment: A strategic-structural systems approach. *Journal of Consulting and Clinical Psychology, 56*, 552-557.

Thomas, E. J. 1975. Uses of research method in interpersonal practice. In *Social Work Research: Methods for the Helping Professions*, edited by N. A. Polansky. Chicago, IL: University of Chicago Press.

Thomas, E. J. 1978a. Generating innovation in social work: The paradigm of developmental research. *Journal of Social Service Research, 2*, 95-116.

Thomas, E. J. 1978b. Mousetraps, developmental research, and social work education. *Social Service Review, 52*, 468-483.

Thomas, E. J. 1978c. Research and service in single-case experimentation: Conflicts and choices. *Social Work Research and Abstracts, 14*, 20-31.

Thomas, E. J. 1983. Problems and issues in single-case experiments. In *Handbook of Clinical Social Work*, edited by A. Rosenblatt and D. Waldfogel. San Francisco, CA: Jossey-Bass Publishers.

Thomas, E. J. 1984. *Designing Interventions for the Helping Professions*. Beverly Hills, CA: Sage Publications.

Thomas, E. J. 1985. Design and development validity and related concepts in developmental research. *Social Work Research and Abstracts, 21,* 50-58.

Thomas, E. J. 1989a. Advances in developmental research. *Social Service Review, 63*, 578-598.

Thomas, E. J. 1989b. Unilateral family therapy to reach the uncooperative alcohol abuser. In *Behavioral Family Therapy*, edited by B. A. Thyer. Springfield, IL: Charles C Thomas Publishers.

Thomas, E. J. 1990. Modes of practice in developmental research. In *Advances in Clinical Social Work Research*, edited by L. Videka-Sherman and W. J. Reid. Silver Spring, MD: National Association of Social Workers.

Thomas, E. J. In press. The spouse as a positive rehabilitative influence in reaching the uncooperative alcohol abuser. In *Cognitive and Behavioral Social Work Treatment*, edited by D. K. Granvold. Belmont, CA: Wadsworth Publishing Co.

Thomas, E. J. and R. D. Ager. In press. In *Marital and Family Therapy in Alcoholism Treatment*, edited by T. O'Farrell. NY: Guilford Press.

Thomas, E. J., K. B. Adams, M. R. Yoshioka, and R. D. Ager. 1990. Unilateral relationship enhancement in the treatment of spouses of uncooperative alcohol abusers. *American Journal of Family Therapy, 18*, 334-344.

Thomas, E. J., J. Bastien, D. R. Stuebe, D. E. Bronson, and J. Yaffe. 1987. Assessing procedural descriptiveness: Rationale and illustrative study. *Behavioral Assessment, 9*, 43-56.

Thomas, E. J. and C. A. Santa. 1982. Unilateral family therapy for alcohol abuse: A working conception. *The American Journal of Family Therapy, 10*, 49-60.

Thomas, E. J., C. A. Santa, D. Bronson, and D. Oyserman. 1987. Unilateral family therapy with spouses of alcoholics. *Journal of Social Service Research, 10*(3), 149-162.

Thomas, E. J. and M. R. Yoshioka. 1989. Spouse interventive confrontations in unilateral family therapy for alcohol abuse. *Social Casework, 70*, 340-347.

Thomas, E. J., M. R. Yoshioka, and R. D. Ager. 1993. *Drinking Enabling of Spouses of Uncooperative Alcohol Abusers: Assessment and Modification.* Manuscript submitted for publication.

Thomas, E. J., M. Yoshioka, R. D. Ager, and K. B. Adams. 1993. *Experimental Outcomes of Spouse Intervention to Reach the Uncooperative Alcohol Abuser: Preliminary Report.* Manuscript submitted for publication.

Thyer, B. A. 1986. Single-subject designs in clinical social work: A practitioner's perspective. In *Social Work Policy and Practice: A Knowledge Driven Approach*, edited by H. R. Johnson and J. E. Tropman. Ann Arbor: University of Michigan, School of Social Work.

Thyer, B. A. and G. C. Curtis. 1983. The repeated pre- post-test single-subject experiment: A new design for empirical clinical practice. *Journal of Behavioral Therapy and Experimental Psychology, 14*, 311-315.

Tripodi, T. 1983. *Evaluative Research for Social Workers*. Englewood Cliffs, NJ: Prentice-Hall.

Tripodi, T. and I. Epstein. 1980. *Research Techniques for Clinical Social Workers*. New York: Columbia University Press.

Wodarski, J. S. 1981. *The Role of Research in Clinical Practice: A Practical Approach for the Human Services.* Baltimore, MD: University Park Press.

Yaffe, J. 1987. *The Developmental Log: A Method for Assisting in the Development of Innovations*. Unpublished doctoral dissertation, University of Michigan, Ann Arbor, MI.

Yeaton, W. H. and L. Sechrest. 1981. Critical dimensions in the choice and maintenance of successful treatments: Strengths, integrity and effectiveness. *Journal of Consulting and Clinical Psychology, 49*, 156-168.

Yoshioka, M. R., E. J. Thomas, and R. D. Ager. 1992. Nagging and Other Drinking Control Efforts of Spouses of Uncooperative Alcohol Abusers: Assessment and Modification. *Journal of Substance Abuse, 4*, 309-318.

Chapter 13

Intervention Research as an Interorganizational Exchange

Yeheskel Hasenfeld
Walter M. Furman

INTRODUCTION

Intervention research entails a process of innovation (e.g., Thomas 1985; Rothman 1980) which frequently involves the coordinated effort of several participating organizations. Each organization, separately or jointly, is responsible for some key phases of the process; for example, one organization may provide the funding, another may contribute research competency, and still another may offer the experimental site. Most commonly, intervention research, especially in its development phase, involves the collaboration between a university-based researcher or research unit working with a service-based agency on the design and implementation of improved service modalities.[1] (This is illustrated in Chapters 9, 10, and 11.) Consequently, the success of this effort, measured in part by the actual adoption of the innovation, is in no small measure a function of the interorganizational coordination between a university and a social agency. The purpose of this chapter is to present the process and outcomes of this research endeavor, not in terms of the research

---

1. There are obviously other organizational models for intervention research–such as labs or service programs run by a university (as described by Thomas in the previous chapter), or a research and development unit within a social agency–but consideration of the inter-organizational dynamics of those models of R&D is beyond the purview of the present chapter.

or program design methods per se, but rather as an example of an interorganizational exchange. The typical intervention research project entails a sustained relationship between a university and a service agency. We propose that an understanding of that relationship, and attention to the interorganizational issues which arise from the collaboration, are essential for successful intervention research.

The analysis that follows will draw upon three recently concluded research and development projects of the Center for Child and Family Policy Studies of the UCLA School of Social Welfare. The first such project is the Runaway Adolescent Pilot Project (RAPP), a program development initiative of Los Angeles County Department of Children's Services in conjunction with university staff from our Center (Rothman and David 1985; Rothman et al. 1987; Rothman, Furman, and Weber 1988). This program is an attempt by the county child protective services agency to extend assistance to runaway and homeless teenagers, a group clearly identified as a local social problem, but recently largely excluded from services by the mainstream public agencies. The second project to be used as an example involved the GAIN welfare reform program in Los Angeles County (Schneiderman et al. 1987). The core of this work was an in-person survey with a random sample of 1,046 recipients of Aid to Families with Dependent Children (AFDC–often known as "welfare"), in order to develop planning estimates for needed service programs. Third, we will draw from an effort of the Center, in conjunction with the Los Angeles County Department of Mental Health, to define and improve case management services for chronically mentally ill clientele of that unit (Rothman 1987a; Rothman 1987b; Rothman 1988a; Rothman 1988b). That program entailed a series of research steps in order to conceptualize and field test a model of case management that would assist mental health service agencies with their case management functions.

The overarching objective of this analysis is to offer practical guidance, based upon the precepts of interorganizational analysis and our recent experience in such projects, for successful intervention research projects. How can the agency and the university-based researchers work together, and what helps and hinders the collaboration? While the difficulties inherent in the endeavor are marked, applying knowledge gleaned from an interorganizational analysis can allow the diverse participants to openly address thorny issues of how the university and the social service agency can work together cooperatively.

We believe that intervention research (IR) presents some special challenges for interorganizational relations that are generally not presented by other types of academic research in the human services. At the core of the difficulty is the very objective of this research: development of procedures that may restructure the service system of the agency and redefine the job activities of its staff. Clearly, the approach touches on a core issue of autonomy: the university is concerned about preserving its academic autonomy, while the agency is apprehensive about its autonomy in defining its service functions. We argue that for IR to be successful both organizations must forego some of their respective autonomies. To do so requires establishing interorganizational relations that can compensate for the perceived loss.

AN ORGANIZATIONAL DEFINITION OF INTERVENTION RESEARCH

We start with an apparently straightforward issue of definition. What characterizes a good IR project? Does it have to do with how happy the two sides of the relationship are with the project, that is, the university and the agency? Does it matter if the innovation was adopted or diffused, or whether the technological innovation or adaptation when rigorously tested was of use to clients? Should diffusion beyond the context of any single agency or milieu be a criterion of useful IR?

A successful venture should encompass all of the features noted above–satisfaction by participants, adoption of the innovation, effectiveness of the innovation, and eventual diffusion. At its core, the process by definition entails the development of tested intervention procedures and techniques that improve the effectiveness of the service delivery system. This definition has several implications. It implies, first that the design of the intervention was correct (either initially or as modified) so that the procedures or techniques do indeed ameliorate the presenting problem; second, that the innovation has been tested (perhaps refined if necessary) and has been found to work; and, third, that some ongoing agency practices have adopted the innovation, thereby aiding service delivery in some operational sense. Thus, it would seem such a project should ultimately benefit agency clients, and indeed this should be its foremost criterion of success.

Such an outcome is not easily accomplished, and is predicated on two interorganizational conditions: extensive exchange of resources (Cook 1977), and effective patterns of coordination (Rogers et al. 1982). A development project is conceptualized in our framework as an interorganizational exchange because it involves the exchange of valued resources between two organizations–the university and the social service agency. The university controls such resources as knowledge and expertise, while the agency controls such resources as funding, staff, and clients. As in exchange relations, each organization seeks to optimize its interests using the resources it controls, and its ability to do so is a function of the power-dependence relations that develop between them (Pfeffer and Salancik 1978). These relations determine how much influence each organization can exert on the other in order to protect and optimize its interests.

IR presents an inherent incompatibility of interests between the university and the social service agency which is expressed in the potential conflict between research and development components. Development–the perspective of the social service agency–focuses on solving a specific service delivery problem within the unique organizational context. Research–the traditional perspective of university–focuses on knowledge development which can be generalizable, and on a research design which enhances validity and reliability by isolating the research from the organizational context. While IR methodology is geared to lessen the impact of this split at the conceptual level, it cannot erase the tension at the organizational level. Put differently, while IR articulates procedures to foster the integration between knowledge development and service delivery, one cannot assume that these procedures are also applicable to integrating the divergent organizational interests, ideologies, and reward systems of the university and agency.

An example of the tension between the agency's needs to solve a specific service problem and the university's commitment to knowledge development is demonstrated in the evaluation phase of the

RAPP project. The university team, which earlier had participated in intervention design, was engaged in the evaluation of the development phase of the program. The evaluation had undertaken to understand this pilot program for runaways from a community perspective, from an organizational perspective, as well as from a client processing perspective. We presented a comprehensive report with what seemed to us well-grounded criticisms, appreciations, and recommendations for program improvements. In meeting with the new program director to review the initial draft report, she stated that it would be highly useful, but she also said that it amused her because it was "so academic." In retrospect, this service operator's view of the report seems related to our team's disposition to state the findings in accordance with acceptable scientific standards, to use a theoretical base whenever we could, and to try to generalize the lessons emerging from the project. Only by a series of informal discussions between research and program staff were we able to convey precisely what we were suggesting for the program.

A second example of this tension can be drawn from our experience with the County Department of Public Social Services (DPSS) in connection with the County's GAIN—or welfare reform—plan. In the early participant needs assessment phase, DPSS stated that they did not want us to have a racial/ethnic identifier variable included in the study. They believed this material to be highly political, and that these statistics in public reports could potentially embarrass them. They also stated that analysis of the racial/ethnic patterns in the data would only serve "academic interests." We, however, concluded that racial and ethnic characteristics are important for planning these services, and in research on welfare dependence generally. Resolving this conflict required negotiation at the highest level, and eventually we persuaded them that the variable was too important to ignore. Still, within that project, DPSS sought to restrict the analyses we were to perform (let alone those that we could publicize) to only those agreed upon specifically in advance. This is an instance in which the university and the agency employed the power-dependence relations between them to shape the outcome of the exchange.

Interorganizational relations must be developed so that the inherently different interests of the university and the agency can be bridged, and through which a mutually acceptable working relationship can be formed to implement the process. Moreover, as noted earlier, such strategies are burdened by the need of each organization to preserve its autonomy. These interorganizational relations may range from an agency-university contract, to joint ventures, depending on the contingencies that both organizations encounter (Oliver 1990). These contingencies include external pressures (e. g., governmental requirements), degree of reciprocity, perceived efficiency of the relationship, environmental stability, and degree of legitimacy. Hence, a joint venture between the university and the social service agency is more likely to occur when neither party is threatened by competition, both are in a balanced bargaining position, the cost of the interorganizational relationship is low, and there is public support for the venture.

Similarly, the interpretive schemes that each organization uses to understand its environment, especially other organizations, will play a key factor in fostering or inhibiting interorganizational collaboration and coordination (Rogers et al. 1982). By interpretive schemes, we refer to perceived need, perceived rewards and costs, organizational ideologies, agreements of domain, and the like. In general, the greater the compatibility of the interpretive schemes between the university and the agency, the greater the likelihood that a collaborative relationship will emerge.

CONDITIONS FACILITATING INTERORGANIZATIONAL COLLABORATION

What are some of the conditions that support developing a successful intervention research project between the university and a social agency? From the framework of interorganizational analysis, and our working examples, we have generated some action guidelines.

Compatibility of Motivations to Enter the Exchange

One of the most important conditions facilitating an interorganizational collaboration is the compatibility of motivations to enter the exchange. Both social agencies and universities can have varying motives for embarking on this venture. For the agency, the motivations might be:

1. Technical–in which a question of effectiveness or efficiency of service delivery is the matter of interest
2. Political–in which a conflict of values or interests motivates a project. This conflict might be around priorities, population to be served, locale of service, or any other important domain issue
3. Managerial–in which the structure and functioning of the organization itself is an issue
4. Resource related–in which the agency views the project as a means to procure augmented resources

For the university, similar, but not identical, motivations to undertake IR projects may exist. One or more of the basic functions of academia–to train, do community service, generate knowledge, or even to augment its own resources–may be paramount. We believe that certain motives for a project on the part of the university and the agency are likely to lead to positive outcomes, but also that it is the compatibility of the motives that controls the collaboration.

When the agency's motive is primarily political, we suspect that a successful undertaking is unlikely. While the university will attempt to create a relatively value-neutral project to review the core issues, it is unlikely that the essential conflict of interest at the agency is soluble by such means. The project then also will be seen as a part of the political conflict, with its methods and findings themselves subject to controversy.

Agency motivation of a technical nature, we believe, is most likely to lead to successful collaboration. When the agency presents a clear means-ends problem, i.e., when it is asking how best to achieve certain ends within a given context, then the IR collaboration is likely to be successful. Under these conditions, it is best if the university is motivated primarily by knowledge development and secondarily by service, and less so by training or even resource acquisition objectives.

Managerial problems may cause an agency to seek university involvement. To the extent that management sciences can be applied to the organizational issues that are presented, the effort may prove successful. However, such organizational problems are also often tinged with political divisions, and so we suspect that projects directed at managerial problems will, again, be viewed as political.

Not infrequently, the motivation for agency-university collaboration is based on acquisition of resources rather than the production of knowledge or a solution to a technical problem. This, however, need not be a hinderance to a successful collaboration. Indeed, when both organizations are mutually dependent on each other to obtain resources, they are motivated to form a coalition which is a necessary condition for a successful collaboration. However, such motivation must be augmented by mutual understanding as to how these resources will be shared. That is, to be productive, research and development must occur in the context of freely negotiated sharing of extra resources resulting from the collaboration.

The Problem to be Addressed by the R&D Must be Clear

A reasonable level of consensus both within each organization and between organizations on the problem to be addressed is necessary for a successful outcome. The relationship of that problem to the missions of the university and the agency may affect the results of the project. When there are contesting interest groups around the issue, it is less likely that effective collaboration will emerge.

The definition of the problem addressed by the IR influences the magnitude of the tension between the research and development components of a project. When the problem is mostly technical and can be isolated from political and economic issues there is less chance for a conflict. When the problems are ideological, political, and economic, but couched in technical terms, the potential for conflict increases.

An example of how problem definition can influence success is afforded by the Runaway Adolescent Pilot Project conducted jointly by our Center at UCLA and the Los Angeles County Department of Children's Services. That agency, known as DCS, is the child protective services agency in this county. Dealing with the problems of abuse and neglect in Los Angeles county is a huge and perplexing concern, and the agency is repeatedly subject to public scrutiny in soul searching cases.

Soon after DCS became a distinct organization (before, it was part of public social services), the organization undertook a joint project to investigate and recommend an approach to services for status offenders. In IR style, the project staff looked at the problem from both the general and particular positions, and made a set of recommendations to the agency. Some recommendations related to needed resources (for example, needed long-term housing options), some related to elements of program that seemed useful (such as in-depth assessment and the use of volunteers), but first and foremost they recommended an organizational strategy of outreach to the population at risk and to the agencies that dealt with these youths on the front line, with DCS then serving as a central intake and referral source to ensure that no youths then "fell through the cracks." After a series of community meetings to air and discuss this idea, a joint agency-university committee met several times, and then the final program design stage was taken over by DCS, with UCLA entering as the evaluator of development field testing of the approach.

The program as implemented was modified in several respects from that which had originally been recommended. Rather than an intake and referral center for all youths to all programs, RAPP served as a linking or bridging mechanism for a narrower band of youths, mostly from shelters, into the offerings of the child protective services agency (services such as foster care placement of medium length, plus more intensive casework services in this pilot than are normally available in DCS) (Rothman et al. 1987).

This example illustrates some of the points about problem definition and the success of the effort. Because runaways are not the central focus of DCS, this pilot program is what we term "loosely coupled" to the main structures of the service agency. This serves to reduce interorganizational conflict about this project. Further, the problem of how best to organize a service response to a particular client type seems to be primarily a technical problem, although we are aware that there were political and resource components operating as well. Still, improved communication between the university and the agency during the period when the agency particularized the proposal to its structure and environment, and even during the later period of university-based evaluation of the demonstration, would have improved the interorganizational relationship, and in all likelihood would have produced a more successful project.

Power Balance Between the Two Organizations

To the extent that there is a relatively even balance of power, so that both parties have an equal voice in the project, trust will increase. This trust is essential for an effective IR project, in the same way that it is vital to any successful interorganizational relations (Levinthal and Fichman 1988).

Of paramount importance is the agency's trust in the expertise of the researchers. How do researchers gain the trust of the service community? This is not easy, but can be influenced by several factors. The reputation of the researchers seems important. Robert K. Merton (quoted in Rich 1981:8) notes that "not only does utilization affect esteem, but esteem also affects utilization." Important also is the quality of information provided and its relevance to the practical problems faced by the agency. Rich (1981) points out that "the quality, precision and accuracy of information (also) affect utilization." Carol Weiss (1980) also found that quality was relevant in policymaker's decisions whether to use policy-related information. "Her study showed that policymakers are sophisticated consumers; they understand issues of quality control and make judgments concerning them" (Rich 1981:9). Our view of the evidence is that for the academics to gain the trust of the agency three factors are needed: (1) substantive expertise in the subject area to be addressed; (2) expression of understanding by the researcher about the nature of the problem faced by the agency; and (3) a recurring flow of information during the project and at its culmination that meets a high standard of both professional quality and utility to the agency.

Conversely, the researcher must trust the agency's ability to define the nature of the problem, and to evaluate the utility of the end product. This too is not easy to achieve, since academic researchers tend to view the problem with a different lens. Of special importance is the need of the researchers to respect the constraints experienced by the social service agency. In this respect, the researcher's professional experience and expertise is invaluable.

Who pays for a project affects the power-dependence relations between the university and the agency, and influences (negatively or positively) the interorganizational dynamics. When the funding source is the social service agency itself, the university may find itself in a power disadvantage and thus under greater pressure to emphasize development rather than research. Under these conditions, the agency's need for the university's expertise will be a major factor in determining the degree of reciprocity that can be developed between the two. The difficulty that the university may experience with such funding is to convince the agency to commit itself to the full range of intervention design and development.

When the funding is secured by the university independently of the agency, the latter may become a passive and even reluctant collaborator. The agency may agree to participate in the enterprise because of the prestige, legitimacy, and resources it may gain from the university. But unless the agency perceives a significant benefit from the collaboration, it may engage in symbolic rather than substantive collaboration to the detriment of the project. The university too, having control over the funding, is more likely to emphasize the research rather than the development component of the project.

The most effective prerequisite for a successful venture is for both the university and the agency to join together in obtaining funding for such a project from a third party. Such a joint venture ensures a level of power balance and trust that can foster substantive collaboration.

The Linking Mechanisms Established Between the Researchers and the Agency

To the extent that the linkages develop at three levels–institutional, managerial, and operational–the more effective will be the collaboration. Institutional linkage refers to the joint commitment by the executive leadership of the organizations. While this linkage is often symbolic, it is importantly so, and signals other organizational levels about the legitimacy of the interorganizational tie; commits the institutions in a general way to a course of action; and affords an opportunity to make general commitments to a project that are critical to later ironing out of details.

The second level of needed linkage is at the program management level. The researchers need routine and regular communication with the program's management. From time to time, while undertaking a project, we have slipped on this dimension temporarily, and have always paid the price in some way such as lessened enthusiasm for the product, lessened cooperation on data collection, or diminished responsiveness to recommendations about the project. A special feature to note is the need for linkage with any specialized research unit at the agency. Even if the agency's research, planning, management information system, or evaluation unit is not to be involved in the project, they will be interested observers, and capable of influencing the receptivity of the organization to the research methods that were used and to innovations that are developed.

Finally, linkage at even the institutional and managerial level is insufficient for success. It is imperative to develop close working relationships with the line staff because they assume the preponderant responsibility for actual implementation. It is line staff who will be required to undertake new role responsibilities, to alter the service procedures they use, and to maintain careful records of their activities. As front line staff, they also have considerable power to either support or hinder the project, and their level of motivation and commitment to the project will play a significant role in its successful execution. Therefore, an effective implementation of a development project requires provision of sufficient inducements and rewards to the staff to make it worthwhile for them to accept the additional costs, burdens, and uncertainties that implementation entails. Forging close working and trusting ties between the researchers and the line staff is fundamental to the success of the interorganizational exchange.

Compatibility of Cultures

Stable interorganizational relations develop when there is a shared system of symbols and norms (Warren, Rose, and Bergunder 1974; Benson 1975). Hence, "cultural compatibility" promotes the interorganizational collaboration between the university and the social agency. Projects that build on shared symbols and language between the agency and the university are more likely to succeed. That is, social service agencies which regularly use information and research in their decision-making processes and which are open for training and innovations are more likely to understand and accept the academic culture. Conversely, academics who have practice experiences reflecting the realities of agency life; who are committed and experienced in training agency staff; and who feel comfortable with applied research and some of the messiness involved in pilot testing innovations are more likely to develop a common language and a shared frame of reference with the social agency and, thus, reduce interorganizational conflict.

INTRAORGANIZATIONAL VARIABLES THAT INFLUENCE INTERORGANIZATIONAL COLLABORATION

Intraorganizational factors also influence the capabilities of the university and the social agency to develop interorganizational collaboration. Our experience points to three important intraorganizational variables: structural stability; fit of the intervention research methodology with the interorganizational structure; and structural centrality of the project.

First, successful collaboration necessitates that the internal structures having responsibility for the project are relatively stable over time. This is so because when the internal structure of the organization is unstable, reflecting conflicts over power, domain, and resources, the more erratic an interorganizational exchange will be. Put differently, interorganizational relations require a degree of certainty and predictability and these cannot be attained when the internal structure of one or more of the participating organizations is unstable (Pennings 1981).

This generalization pertains to both the university and the social agency. At times of escalating service demands, declining resources, retrenchment, and privatization, the world of social service agencies–and, in particular, public agencies–is in some degree of permanent flux. Universities too are not immune from these trends. Reorganizations occur frequently in large public agencies, and therefore an interorganizational exchange that depends upon a stable structure in the agency is vulnerable to disruption.

The project aimed at developing a case management model suffered numerous yet unavoidable mishaps due to intraorganizational instability in the social service agency. And while there has been relative stability and continuity in our relationship with the Department of Children's Services around the Runaway Adolescent Pilot Project, it is true that in the three years of the project it has been housed within two major bureaus of the parent agency, has had three different project directors, and has had three different staff supervisors, in addition to normal line staff turnover. This, however, is business as usual.

Second, the internal structure of the organization needs to respond to the methodological contingencies of the development activities (Van de Ven and Ferry 1980). For example, a project which requires a team approach in which its members can share multiple sources of information and adjust their procedures in light of the information cannot succeed if the agency's working structure is highly hierarchial with vertical lines of communication. Similarly, a project which requires clear and explicit criteria and lines of accountability cannot succeed if the working structure of the research group is too fluid, with overlapping and ambiguous assignments of responsibilities.

The third generalization pertains to the centrality of the project to the organization, and how management structures are best designed for central and peripheral tasks (Astley and Sachdeva 1984). This, too, applies both to the university and to the social agency. When the project requires extensive organizational involvement or addresses core issues in the social organization, it requires a highly centralized and tightly-coupled structure and a strong commitment by the top administrators to support and implement the work. Too often, projects that can demonstrate effectiveness fail to become institutionalized in the agency or the university because they lack the programmatic centrality they should command. This occurs when the project is relegated to peripheral units or deals with marginal concerns in either the agency or the university.

On the other hand, there are advantages to IR projects that can be insulated from other organizational activities. By being "loosely coupled" to other organizational units, the project is protected from failures in other parts of the organization, it becomes less threatening, and other parts of the organization are protected from problems and potential failures in the project (Weick 1976). Hence, those projects that involve high risk, frequent modifications, and a heuristic decision-making structure are more likely to be tolerated when they are more or less insulated from other organizational activities.

A comparison of two of our recent projects may exemplify this generalization. Case management is quite an important function in public mental health, and so the project required substantial support from that department's central level in order to allow the development and field testing of the model which emerged. On the contrary, service to adolescent runaways is not the central focus of child protective services, and so program and divisional administrators could participate with less oversight and involvement from the overarching bureaucratic structure.

In this connection, we would like to propose that a project in its early exploratory phases is more likely to benefit by being located in a peripheral unit of the agency than by being located in a core operational setting. However, the adoption and dissemination phases will require that the project is later experienced and adopted by organizational units that are central in the agency.

CONCLUSION·

The perspective of interorganizational exchange is very useful for understanding an IR project that is conducted between a university and a social agency. There are several sources of potential conflict. To reiterate a few, there is the conflict between the university's knowledge development mission and the agency's service development perspective. There is also potential conflict over adoption and/or adaptation of project results that impinge on agency prerogatives. Further, there may be resource conflicts, conflicts over control of the project, dissemination of results, and conflicts that emerge from shifts in the continuity in agency or university commitment to and definition of the project, and so forth.

Each organization has its own interests, which the interorganizational exchange must somehow serve. Recall that we are defining success in terms of developing valid and useful practices, procedures, structures, or techniques, which are also adopted by the organization and can be disseminated to other relevant sites. The interorganizational exchange which fosters this outcome must acknowledge and contend with these potential conflicts of interest. In our analysis and experience (which has seen both successful and less than successful outcomes), the compatibility of motivations to enter the exchange, the interdependence of the parties as seen in a balanced power-dependence relationship which fosters trust, and the deliberate attention to linkages at all appropriate levels, are important prerequisites for successful intervention development.

REFERENCES

Astley, W. Graham and Paramjit S. Sachdeva. 1984. Structural sources of intraorganizational power: A theoretical synthesis. *Academy of Management Review,* 9(1), 104-113.

Benson, J. Kenneth. 1975. The interorganizational network as a political economy. *Administrative Science Quarterly, 2,* 229-249.

Cook, Karen. 1977. Exchange and power in network of interorganizational relations. *Sociological Quarterly, 18,* 62-82.

Levinthal, D. A. and M. Fichman. 1988. Dynamics of interorganizational attachments: Auditor-client relationships. *Administrative Science Quarterly, 33*(3), 345-369.

Oliver, Christine. 1990. Determinants of interorganizational relationships: Integration and future directions. *Academy of Management Review, 15*(2), 241-265.

Pennings, J. M. 1981. Strategically interdependent organizations. In *Handbook of Organizational Design,* edited by P. Nystrom and W. H. Starbuck. London: Oxford University Press, 433-455.

Pfeffer, Jeffrey and Gerald R. Salancik. 1978. *The External Control of Organizations: A Resource Dependence Perspective.* New York: Harper & Row.

Rich, Robert F. 1981. *Social Science Information and Public Policy Making.* San Francisco: Jossey-Bass.

Rogers, David L., David A. Wheatten, and Associates. 1982. *Interorganizational Coordination: Theory, Research and Implementation.* Iowa State University Press.

Rothman, J. (1980). *Using Research in Organizations.* Beverly Hills: Sage.

Rothman, J. 1987a. Case Management Action Guidelines: A Synthesis of Social Research. Center for Child and Family Policy Studies, School of Social Welfare, University of California, Los Angeles and Los Angeles County Department of Mental Health.

Rothman, J. 1987b. A Model of Case Management: Systematizing Case Management Intervention. Center for Child and Family Policy Studies, School of Social Welfare, University of California, Los Angeles and Los Angeles County Department of Mental Health.

Rothman, J. 1988a. An Empirically Based Model of Case Management: Results of a Field Study. Center for Child and Family Policy Studies, School of Social

Welfare, University of California, Los Angeles and Los Angeles County Department of Mental Health.

Rothman, J. 1988b. Guidelines for Dissemination and Training: Case Management Model. Center for Child and Family Policy Studies, School of Social Welfare, University of California, Los Angeles and Los Angeles County Department of Mental Health.

Rothman, J. and T. David. 1985. Status Offenders in Los Angeles County: Focus on Runaway and Homeless Youth–A Study and Policy Recommendations. School of Social Welfare, Bush Program in Child and Family Policy, University of California, Los Angeles, in Collaboration with Department of Children's Services, Los Angeles.

Rothman, J., W. Furman, and J. Weber. 1988 Aiding Runaway and Homeless Youth: Evaluation of a Community-Based Approach–The Runaway Adolescent Pilot Project. Center for Child and Family Policy Studies, School of Social Welfare, University of California, Los Angeles.

Rothman, J., W. Furman, J. Weber, D. Ayer, and D. Kaznelson. 1987. An Interim Evaluation of the Runaway Adolescent Pilot Program. Center for Child and Family Policy Studies, School of Social Welfare, University of California, Los Angeles.

Schneiderman, L., W. Furman, P. Lachenbruch, E. Fielder, M. Welch, and I. Chow. 1987. GAIN Participant Needs Assessment, Report Two, A Profile of Recipients of Aid to Families with Dependent Children in Los Angeles County Based on Sample Data from Both an In-Person Survey and the Los Angeles County Integrated Benefits Payment System. Center for Child and Family Policy Studies, School of Social Welfare, University of California, Los Angeles.

Thomas, Edwin, 1985. *Designing Interventions for the Helping Professions*. Beverly Hills, CA: Sage.

Van De Ven, A. and D. L. Ferry, 1980. *Measuring and Assessing Organizations*. New York: Wiley.

Warren, Roland, Stephen Rose, and Ann Bergunder. 1974. *The Structure of Urban Reform*. Lexington, MA: D. C. Heath.

Weick, K. 1976. Educational organizations as loosely coupled systems. *Administrative Science Quarterly*, *21*, 1-19.

Weiss, Carol H. 1980. *Social Science Research and Decision Making*. New York: Columbia University Press.

DISSEMINATION

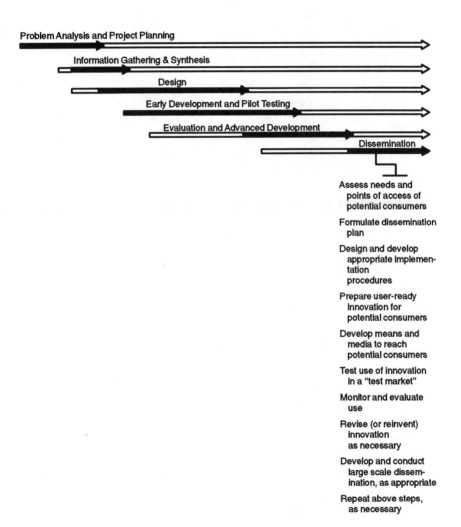

Problem Analysis and Project Planning

Information Gathering & Synthesis

Design

Early Development and Pilot Testing

Evaluation and Advanced Development

Dissemination

Assess needs and
points of access of
potential consumers

Formulate dissemination
plan

Design and develop
appropriate implemen-
tation
procedures

Prepare user-ready
innovation for
potential consumers

Develop means and
media to reach
potential consumers

Test use of innovation
in a "test market"

Monitor and evaluate
use

Revise (or reinvent)
innovation
as necessary

Develop and conduct
large scale dissem-
ination, as appropriate

Repeat above steps,
as necessary

Chapter 14

Skill Training Modules– A Strategy for Dissemination and Utilization of a Rehabilitation Innovation

Patrick W. Corrigan
Sally J. MacKain
Robert Paul Liberman

The best laid plans of mice and men
oft times are for nought.

–Shakespeare

Behavior therapists have produced many empirically valid treatment strategies for psychiatric disorders, including anxiety (Beck, Emery, and Greenberg 1985), depression (Beck et al. 1979; Rehm 1981), alcoholism (Marlatt and Gordon 1985; Sobell and Sobell 1988), mental retardation (Favell and Phillips 1986), and schizophrenia (Bellack 1984; Liberman 1990), as well as for treatment of marital and family problems (Baucom and Epstein 1989; Jacobson and Gurman 1986). In fact, behavior therapy has been shown to be more effective than other therapies in treatment of simple phobias, agoraphobia, panic, obsessive-compulsive disorder, schizophrenia, sexual dysfunctions, tobacco dependence, eating disorders, conduct disorders, and some psychosomatic conditions (Liberman and Bedell 1989; Liberman and Mueser 1989). Despite this success, behavioral interventions are not universally embraced.

317

In this chapter we will be discussing a particular behavioral intervention, skills training modules that were developed in the course of a long-term intervention research undertaking. We will start by indicating barriers to disseminating such practice–relevant products of intervention research.

BARRIERS TO IMPLEMENTING INNOVATIONS IN TREATMENT TECHNOLOGY

Barriers to the clinical dissemination and implementation of validated behavioral treatments derive from three sources: interventions themselves, institutional constraints, and therapist limitations (Backer, Liberman, and Kuehnel 1986; Corrigan, Kwartarini, and Pramana 1992). The recognition by scientists and practitioners alike of various barriers within treatment settings can germinate strategies that facilitate the implementation of new and improved clinical interventions. The types of barriers are summarized in Table 1.

INNOVATION-RELATED BARRIERS

More than ten journals are currently dedicated to reporting research on behavioral treatment strategies. Unfortunately, a tremendous gap exists between published and validated behavioral treatment methods and their use by most clinicians (Backer, Liberman, and Kuehnel 1986). The split between scientists and practitioners presents serious obstacles to the implementation of the clinical products of research in everyday treatment settings (Barlow 1981; Garfield and Kurtz 1976).

The rigorous methods and conservative inferences that guide clinical research do not readily yield meaningful clinical products. Evidence of statistical significance is typically a prerequisite for the publication of treatment research. However, investigators and clinicians alike recognize that statistical significance may have little correspondence with clinical significance (Barlow 1981). Treatments that produce greater scores on research measures may not show a concomitant improvement in patients' quality of life. More-

TABLE 1. Barriers to the dissemination and implementation of validated behavioral treatments.

LIMITATIONS INHERENT IN BEHAVIORAL PROGRAMS

1. Cultural specificity of the program.
2. Hawthorne effect from research demonstrations of behavior therapy.
3. Behavioral programs may be irrelevant to important treatment populations.
4. Complex behavioral programs are difficult to reproduce in the real world.
5. Behavioral programs often require ongoing measurement and quality assurance that are noxious to staff.
6. Behavioral therapy may be foreign to traditional office-based one-on-one psychotherapy.
7. Greater staff and budgetary resources are often required by behavioral programs than typical programs.
8. The problem of compromise.
9. Research significance is not clinical significance.

INSTITUTIONAL CONSTRAINTS

1. Little administrative or collegial support.
2. Bureaucratic red tape.
3. Insufficient ongoing supervision and quality assurance.
4. Transient staffing and program planning patterns.
5. Stressful job environment inhibiting implementation of most therapies.
6. Legislative or adminstrative barriers set up by independent governing bodies.
7. Incompetent staff members.
8. Heterogeneity of patients and inadequate staff/patient ratios.

PRACTITIONER BARRIERS

1. Many practitioners are unaware of the empirical validity of behavioral interventions.
2. Perception of behavior therapy as inflexible and hostile.
3. Unfamiliarity of practitioners with learning theory.
4. Reliance on medical model that obviates acceptance of behavior therapy.
5. Perceived lack of control of programmatic decisions.
6. Mistrust of implementing innovative programs.

over, clinical research summarizes the effects of treatment on the "hypothetical average" subject. There may be little correspondence between treatment effects on the "average" patient and real effects on the "everyday" patient who walks through the practitioner's door (Barlow and Hersen 1984).

Even if results of model research programs are translated into clinically relevant methods, innovative programs may not have the same impact in customary clinical settings where most community- or hospital-based patients are treated (Bachrach 1980, 1981). Frequently, "Hawthorne Effects" yield improved patient performance solely because participants bask in the research limelight. Reproducing a model program outside the luster of this limelight or without the enthusiastic leadership of a committed academic often results in more modest outcomes (Liberman 1983). Moreover, subjects recruited for participation in model programs are thoroughly screened using stringent selection criteria. The resultant homogeneous class may define a "unique culture" with therapeutic expectations and patterns of compliance that do not easily transfer to other patient populations (Bachrach 1980, 1986; Shepherd 1984). For example, few existing treatment programs can be generalized to address the complex needs of the mentally ill homeless or the dually diagnosed substance abusing mentally ill.

Differences in resources available to innovative treatment programs versus most community or hospital settings can impede implementation as well. Research programs are funded by grants which frequently provide large sums of money to support well-trained staffs and to provide necessary equipment, supplies, and subject fees that offer incentives for patient participation. In addition, research protocols attract students and postdoctoral fellows who are willing to provide services with youthful enthusiasm in exchange for training and research experience. Conversely, many hospital and community treatment programs report insufficient funds to provide satisfactory basic care, much less the funds and staffing levels required to meet the standards and criteria for fidelity to innovative programs (Repucci and Saunders 1974; Slama and Bannerman 1983). Transfer of innovative technologies to customary clinical settings with budgetary constraints requires strategies that can be implemented by existing professional and paraprofessional staff and that do not require expenditures for additional personnel and operating resources (Paul and Lentz 1977).

Research programs with precise measures and state-of-the-art technology frequently result in complex treatment protocols that are not readily assimilated by the practitioner community as a whole

(Backer, Liberman, and Kuehnel 1986). For example, many behavioral treatment techniques are foreign to the staff of programs that provide traditional one-on-one psychotherapy. Hence, traditional therapists do not readily adopt these treatments. Moreover, the demands of complex or novel therapies frequently exceed the clinical skills of ordinary practitioners. As a result, tracking the fidelity of the delivery of clinical innovations often requires unwieldy systems of quality assurance (Yeaton and Sechrest 1981).

Differences among model programs and everyday treatment may require compromise between treatment prescriptions and "real-world" demands (Liberman 1979; Repucci 1973; Repucci and Saunders 1974); hence, innovative technology must be flexible. However, clinical investigators who dedicate large amounts of resources and energy to designing and testing an innovation are frequently unwilling to modify their treatment protocols to fit with the idiosyncratic needs of specific milieus. Implementation of new programs that appear foreign to line level clinicians can be facilitated by independent consultants who help both innovators and yeoman staff mold new treatments to serve the needs of the specific treatment setting. For example, innovators from the Camarillo-UCLA Clinical Research Center for Schizophrenia and Psychiatric Rehabilitation have travelled to many institutional and community settings to introduce their psychoeducational treatment packages for schizophrenia and mold skill training modules to meet the specific needs of diverse staff and clientele.

INSTITUTIONAL CONSTRAINTS

Introducing innovative programs into existing treatment organizations requires targeting "two populations" for acceptance and use of the innovation: patients, for whom the treatment was developed, and change agents, responsible for carrying out the intervention (Repucci and Saunders 1974). Borrowing terminology from commercial enterprises, mental health innovators must "market" and "sell" their treatment programs to overcome institutional inertia and resistance. To motivate clinicians to change their treatment approaches and gain competence and comfort in using innovations may require control over rewards that affect staff behavior. Rewards include merit raises, bonuses, performance appraisals, job promotions, and public recognition for good work. Informal reinforcers exist in most institutions and practice settings as well; collegial approval, improved morale and self-esteem, and abundant interest and acknowledgement from supervisors are examples of consequences that can be harnessed to affect professional performance (Cullari and Ferguson 1981; Liberman 1979).

Researchers respond to a different set of reinforcers than line level practitioners; for example, investigators tend to value publications, scientific presentations, and promotion via advanced degrees or academic rank. Hence, outside innovators may not be cognizant of or sensitive to reinforcers valued by clinicians. Even when innovators actively seek to implement their new interventions, they are rarely in a position to control institutional or agency reinforcers. Program administrators must assume responsibility for implementing new programs (Greenblatt 1983), and hence must manipulate organizational contingencies so that novel interventions are carried out correctly. For example, behavior therapies often require highly specific competencies (e.g., employing learning principles such as positive reinforcement and collecting behavioral data) that need to be built into rewritten job descriptions. Ironically, the behavior of most administrators and supervisors is controlled by the same informal reinforcers that influence their staff. Supervisors need and seek approval and collegial support from others as well. If key administrators are unwilling to "rock the boat" and risk "flak" and disapproval from their peers and supervisors, they may initiate new programs halfheartedly, or may not maintain the consistent supervision required for program success.

Nursing staff in one psychiatric hospital reported that attempts to implement innovative behavior therapy programs failed without administrative or collegial support (Emerson and Emerson 1987). In another hospital, the head nurse of a psychiatric unit was found to be instrumental in changing the professional services of her staff through direct modeling of new treatment methods (Wallace et al. 1973). Hence, implementation of new treatment strategies require the allegiance of administrative parties. Even when administrators are supportive of change, red tape and stratified personnel levels characteristic of institutions may bog down the implementation of new interventions (Repucci and Saunders 1974; Tharp and Wetzel 1969). Layers of bureaucracy obfuscate clear lines of responsibility, thereby inhibiting innovation. Similarly, rigid administrative directives stifle initiative and inhibit personnel from supporting new programs (Paul and Lentz 1977; Liberman et al. 1975).

Frequently, decisions made by administrative officials within an institution are controlled by external pressures. Public treatment centers answer to independent governing bodies which not only administer budgetary concerns, but occasionally legislate treatment options. For example, use of seclusion, restraints, and contingent punishment has been tightly regulated in most states (Wexler 1984). In three examples of successful innovations for the treatment of autistic, retarded, and schizophrenic individuals, conflict between the values and goals of the clinical innovator and program director on the one hand, and the administrators or board of directors on the other, led to either the closure of the program or the departure of the innovator (Ball, Jarvis, and Pease 1983; Barber, Barber, and Clark 1983; Graziano 1969).

Patient treatment is also influenced by broader community and public concerns (Repucci and Saunders 1974). For example, the plight of the homeless mentally ill has sparked reinstitutionalization movements throughout the United States, thereby redirecting funds from community to inpatient settings (Wasow 1986). In addition to balancing institutional politics, professionals seeking to introduce innovations require a thorough understanding of political agendas and power struggles (Liberman 1979; Greenblatt 1983).

PRACTITIONER BARRIERS

Direct care staff, often with minimal professional preparation, spend the most time with psychiatric patients and are charged with implementing most treatments in community and institutional settings (Iwata et al. 1976; Reid and Whitman 1983). Hence, factors that impede the adoption of new treatments by line level clinicians greatly diminish the efficacy of innovations. For example, nursing level care staff in psychiatric institutions are comfortable with and overtrained for treating patients through use of medication. Expectations that they utilize psychosocial or behavioral techniques may clash with their professional role identity. In addition, there are few behavioral techniques that can match the "user-friendliness" of dispensing medications. In California, the curriculum for training licensed psychiatric technicians includes hundreds of hours of training in medication delivery but only eight hours in behavior therapy.

Some practitioners continue to deny the efficacy of behavioral treatment. Staff who closely identify with psychodynamic or medical models less readily understand the benefits of behavioral treatment (Backer, Liberman, and Kuehnel 1986). They may perceive environmental models of behavior change as threatening existing custodial or biological therapies on their unit. Similarly, many practitioners are ignorant of the principles that underlie behavior therapy (Emerson and Emerson 1987; Repucci and Saunders 1974). Learning theory has precise jargon which can sound foreign to uninitiated practitioners. As a result, specific terms may produce diverse connotations. For example, Repucci and Saunders (1974) listed the inaccuracies in treatment staff definitions of "time out": "an undesignated time period of sitting quietly," "a quiet period plus time-off during weekend visits home," "one hour of sitting and doing nothing, or calming down and then talking about the reason for time-out" (653). Frequently, differences in therapeutic language lead "naive" practitioners to judge behavior therapy as cruel or mechanistic. Some therapists perceive behaviorists as rigid, and their language inflexible.

The practice of mental health can be a demanding and difficult task with front-line staff most vulnerable to daily pressures, assaults, and injuries (Carmel and Hunter 1989). Witnessing or being victim of frequent patient violence was highly associated with job stress (Lion and Reid 1983; Lion, Snyder, and Merrill 1981; Madden, Lion, and Penna 1976; Klass, Growe, and Strizich 1977; Moos 1974). Work-related stress may impede faithful implementation of new strategies. For example, psychiatric technicians reported lack of control over their work settings as a major source of anxiety at work (Browner et al. 1987). Specific problems included psychologists developing treatment plans that were inconsistent with technicians' perceptions of patient skills, psychiatrists changing medication orders regardless of staff observations of patient behavior, supervisors scheduling work-hours without input from affected technicians, and administrators ordering inordinate amounts of paperwork to be completed. Frequent staff turnover resulting from job dissatisfaction prevents consistent implementation of programs. Staff with low morale may be poorly motivated or have little competence to faithfully carry out innovations (Repucci 1977).

Researchers have identified several ineffectual staff practices. Some clinicians have exhibited inaccurate use of psychoeducational training procedures with patients (Repp, Barton, and Brulle 1981; Storzbach 1989), while other studies have shown that staff have few quality social interactions with patients (Dailey et al. 1974). Completion of clinical duties has been further impeded by frequent, non-job related activities during scheduled work hours (Burg, Reid, and Lattimore 1979). This evidence shows that staff stressors must be diminished so that patient care remains at quality levels.

Attendants or nursing assistants who have worked in the mental health "trenches" for many years prior to the introduction of an innovative treatment may mistrust the new technology and the innovator introducing the technology (Repucci 1977). Entry of an "expert," who has been given an administrative mandate to promote change, may heighten staff concerns that they have little control over program development and direction. If innovators at the port of entry are viewed as outsiders, ignorant of existing program cultures, limits, and procedures, they may not be accorded credibility by line level staff and therefore will not be able to instigate change in the program (Levine 1973; Sarason et al. 1966).

OVERCOMING BARRIERS TO ADOPTION OF CLINICAL INNOVATIONS THROUGH DISSEMINATION OF MODULAR BEHAVIOR THERAPY PROGRAMS

Behavioral modules provide many benefits that circumvent barriers to the implementation of innovative programs. The combination of skill training and problem-solving approaches inherent in behavior therapy modules avoids the cultural specificity for which model programs have been criticized. Rather than teaching behaviors that are mainly appropriate for specific groups and locales, modules teach a range of behaviors from which individuals can select culturally meaningful skills. The flexibility inherent in problem solving allows individuals to adjust these skills vis-à-vis situational parameters. For example, when a patient discovers that the negotiation skills learned in medication management have limited impact on a new psychiatrist, the patient can brainstorm alternative approaches.

Behavioral modules also circumvent many institutional constraints to dissemination. Trainers' skills necessary to conduct modules are easy to learn and do not require a college education or extensive background in behavior therapy or psychopathology. The ward staff of most institutions and paraprofessionals in community support programs can acquire these skills after brief introductory training and are able to perform the skills at competent levels with minimal supervision. Hence, agencies and institutions do not need to spend large sums of money to hire specially educated staff. While obtaining the module requires purchasing manuals, learning materials, videotapes, and hardware like a video camera and recorder, these comprise a one-time, cost-efficient expenditure.

Behavioral modules have high face-validity that improves the likelihood that front-line staff will accept and implement the technology. Modules are not steeped in esoteric learning theory or pedantic jargon. Rather, they are presented within an educational framework in which staff assume the role of teachers and clients assume the role of students who learn instrumental and interpersonal skills that resolve social problems (Schade, Corrigan, and Liberman 1990). Hence, staff more readily understand the intent of modules as well as the means by which the change technology helps participants accomplish their goals.

Modules define a curriculum of discrete interpersonal, cognitive, coping, or self-care skills that are presented in structured, classroom-like settings. Highly specific curricula are consistent with the emphasis in behavior therapy on development of adaptive skills through educational technology (Curran and Monti 1982). Through psychoeducational strategies, staff can teach patients to replace behavioral deficits with appropriate responses, thereby assisting them in acquiring the skills to cope with interpersonal demands and stressors. Skills training has a prophylactic quality to it as well; acquisition of skills arms individuals with a repertoire of responses which help them to cope with future life problems. Implementation of most modules requires one or two practitioners who lead groups of up to twelve participants.

Modules comprise specific *micro-skills* which are taught to participants, and *trainer skills,* which clinicians use to facilitate skill acquisition. Some examples of micro-skill curricula are summarized in Table 2. From lists like these, practitioners choose modules that meet the unique needs of their patient population. Assignment to a specific module depends on individualized assessment of each patient's functioning and deficits. Hence, chronic schizophrenics with deteriorated functioning may be assigned to basic hygiene and conversation skills training while a higher functioning individual whose symptoms are under control may be assigned to a module on dating and friendship skills. Moreover, the form or process of training can be tailored to the learning capacity of the patient; more frequent prompting, modeling, and reinforcement can be effective with lower-functioning individuals while less structure and more initiative in goal setting and treatment are more effective with higher-functioning individuals.

Therapists who utilize skill modules assume a role similar to that of a coach, teacher, or trainer and call upon several trainer skills that can be applied in a stepwise fashion (Young 1982). First, module participants are instructed on the behavioral components to be taught in that day's session. Instruction highlights the benefits of incorporating these skills into their behavioral repertoire. Targeted skills are then modeled for the participants in prearranged vignettes (Perry and Furukawa 1986). The best models are high-status peers of the participants who struggle with mastering the skill, rather than performing the behavior at a flawless level (Bandura 1969). The range and efficiency of modeled vignettes can be greatly enhanced using videotapes produced for training purposes.

After participants have observed the modeled skill, they are provided opportunities to rehearse the skill in well-organized role plays. During the rehearsal, trainers provide prompts to direct the participant through troublesome interactions and feedback to guide subsequent performance. Rather than criticizing inaccurate performance, and thereby discouraging patients from subsequent learning, good feedback reinforces approximations to the targeted skill. Videotaping the rehearsal provides the added learning experiences

TABLE 2. Behavior therapy modules.

Teaching Family Model: A comprehensive intervention program for behavior disordered children that includes operant contingencies and communication skills (Phillips, Phillips, Fixsen, and Wolf 1974).

Couples Communication Skills: Teach couples to identify patterns that hinder communication and learn listening, assertion, and problem-solving skills (Gottman et al. 1976).

Conversation: Review basic conversational skills including eye contact, body language, and appropriate discussion topics (Gambrill and Richey 1985).

Medication Management: Teach patients with severe mental illness about the therapeutic and side effects of medication, means by which these effects can be tracked, and negotiation skills so that patients can collaborate with their psychiatrist regarding medication changes (Eckman, Liberman, Phipps, and Blair 1990).

Relapse Prevention: Patients who abuse alcohol or street drugs learn to identify situations in which relapse is likely to occur and to make a coping plan to be ready when these situations are encountered (Marlatt andd Gordon 1985).

Assertion Skills: The range of assertion skills are reviewed including saying no, making a complaint, and expressing a positive feeling (Lange and Jakubowski 1976).

Relaxation: Several exercises that foster relaxation are discussed including progressive muscle relaxation, deep breathing, and relaxing self-statements (Walker 1975).

Thinking Straight: Patients are taught to identify irrational statements that result in extreme emotions, to challange these beliefs, and to produce counters that will diminish the impact of similar future beliefs (McMullin and Casey 1975).

Job Finding Skills: Patients who have difficulty finding appropriate employment learn to search want ads, prepare a résumé, and interview with a prospective employer (Jacobs et al. 1984).

Basic Hygiene Skills: This module includes grooming (e.g., showering, brushing teeth, shaving, feminine hygiene) and clothes maintenance (washing and ironing clothes, hanging them up, mending rips, replacing buttons) (Spiegler and Agigian 1977).

Helper Skills: This module teaches counselors and other helpers various listening skills (Priestly and McGuire 1983).

Child Discipline: Parents learn nonaggressive disciplining techniques including response cost and time out (Silberman and Wheelan 1980).

Imagery: The module teaches participants to improve their control over imagination (Lazarus 1984).

of benefiting from video feedback as well as the special reinforcing qualities of seeing oneself on TV. At the end of each session, homework assignments are developed in which participants are instructed to practice the day's skill in some personally meaningful setting.

Each module generally has a Trainer's Manual which spells out the plan by which skills are trained and applied in the module. Manuals can be so specific as to provide text which prescribes instructions that trainers read to participants (e.g., questions to lead the discussion about the modeled vignette, dialogue for the rehearsal, and lists of problems that may impede subsequent skill use). At the other extreme, less specific manuals may provide only broad learning goals from which trainers must create the tasks for participants to accomplish these goals. In addition, some manuals come with instruments to assess a participant's level of competency before beginning training (which also permits clinicians to identify behavioral deficits), and after training to determine whether skills have been acquired. Trainees who have not demonstrated competence are encouraged to repeat the module. Each skill area of a module can be assessed for competence so that repetition can be limited to those skill areas in which mastery was not demonstrated.

DISTRIBUTION OF BEHAVIOR THERAPY MODULES

While behavioral modules avoid many barriers to implementation of treatment, the manner in which new strategies are introduced to institutions and their clinical practitioners affects the likelihood of acceptance and implementation. Glaser and his colleagues (1983) outlined five strategies that facilitate implementation as innovators introduce a new program into treatment settings.

1. *Staff more readily accept innovations if they are able to observe a demonstration of the intervention. A live role play or videotaped demonstration with patients facilitates this goal.* Training workshops offered as part of a dissemination project, "Adoption of Innovations in Mental Health," (AIMH) introduced and demonstrated Social and Independent Living Skills modules designed for rehabilitating persons with serious mental illness (Wallace et al. 1990). These demonstrations

were particularly effective when the host agency or institution selected their own patients to participate. Frequently, the target group of practitioners selected one or two "difficult" patients in an effort to challenge the innovator/trainer and to put the innovation to the test. Practitioners often reported being surprised when their more "resistant" patients willingly and even enthusiastically participated in the structured role play and question and answer components of the demonstration. Seeing their own patients enjoy the innovative activity led many staff members to become invested in the intervention.

2. *Innovators should clearly communicate the relevance of the technique to the resolution of problems in the treatment setting. The team that presents the new method should survey influential staff members regarding difficult clinical issues prior to presenting the innovation to the attending staff as a whole.* For example, staff at many facilities that received training in the use of the skills training modules in the AIMH project were under pressure to provide more patient contact hours and hence were anxious to learn techniques that would be easy to use in a group context. A number of practitioners worked with difficult patients and welcomed the highly structured format of the modules, seeing it as a means of coping with or even circumventing motivation and behavior problems. Other staff members were already conducting groups, but were eager for new ideas and procedures for working with patients and for documenting progress.

3. *The relative advantage of implementing new interventions in place of or through existing programs should be highlighted, especially in terms of difficult patient issues.* Therefore, innovators must know current methods used by staff with patients, as well as staff views regarding limits to these methods. In discussing these limits, innovators must avoid criticizing existing treatment protocols and thereby alienating staff. Instead, innovators must be empathic to treatment problems and be perceived as team players who offer alternative procedures that may be helpful.

4. *Staff more readily accept innovations that are easily understood. The prepackaged and highly prescribed nature of mod-*

ules facilitates this goal. However, innovators should be aware that the modules may be implemented by persons of a wide range of educational levels and must key their introductory discussions appropriately. In the AIMH project, audiences in attendance at introductory training workshops often comprised mental health care professionals with a variety of backgrounds and expertise. At some facilities, psychiatrists, psychologists, mental health administrators, nurses, recreation therapists, psychiatric technicians, and board and care home operators attended the same presentation, so trainers had to tailor terminology and level of complexity of the material to meet the diverse needs and goals of the audience. For example, the term "prodromal symptoms" might be used for medical audiences when introducing a module designed to teach symptom self-management, while "warning signs" would be sufficient for other audiences. While appropriate terminology is important in establishing credibility, presenters should avoid unnecessary jargon, which can instantly alienate the most dedicated line level staff.

5. *Implementation is facilitated when innovations can be "phased in" with evidence of incremental success along the way. Seasoned staff are wary of ambitious programs that seek to rewrite existing positions and practices. Behavior therapists can gradually train line level staff to implement discrete modules, rather than initiate wholesale implementation of a large scale treatment program.* For example, in the introduction of the skills training modules at facilities affiliated with the AIMH project, staff were typically trained to use the Medication Management Module (Liberman 1986) first and to implement it on a small scale as one portion of an entire program. Because the other modules are implemented using the same procedures, staff could observe the success of the first module and easily introduce others, gradually incorporating them into existing treatment practices.

These insights suggest that new innovations must be sensitively marketed to treatment staff (Fisher 1983). Findings from preliminary work with administrators and influential practitioners, along with the principles and training skills within each module, need to be communicated to staff *in person.* Interpersonal modes of communicating clinical innovations to potential practitioners far outweigh using the print media to convey information (Fairweather, Sanders, and Tornatzky 1974; Roberts and Larsen 1971). An action-oriented change agent who serves as a conveyor of knowledge about clinical innovation and assists potential users in adoption has been demonstrated to be the most viable model available (Larsen, Norris, and Knoll 1976).

In addition to selling the program to line level staff, administrators of treatment programs need to be convinced of its efficacy as well. For example, administrators who support the use of behavioral modules are more likely to allocate monetary and staff resources to this end. Moreover, administrators may become "champions" of the modules and motivate clinicians to sustain their involvement after the initial excitement and novelty of the intervention has waned.

EVALUATION OF MODULAR PROGRAMS

The Social and Independent Living Skills Modules

An innovative method of teaching skills for independent living has been developed for persons with disabling and chronic mental disorders at the UCLA Department of Psychiatry, Brentwood Veterans Affairs Medical Center, and Camarillo State Hospital. The Social and Independent Living Skills series, or "SILS modules" comprise a highly structured, prescriptive set of teaching tools. The SILS modules have been validated in controlled research (Liberman, Mueser, and Wallace 1986; Wallace and Liberman 1985; Wirshing et al. 1990) and have been field tested extensively at state hospitals, residential treatment facilities, and community mental health centers around the country (MacKain and Wallace 1989; Wallace et al. 1990).

Social and Independent Living Skills modules currently available or in various stages of development include Recreation for Leisure, Medication Self-Management, Symptom Self-Management, Grooming and Personal Hygiene, Job-Finding, Interpersonal Problem Solving, Money Management, Basic Conversation Skills, and Dating and Friendship. Each SILS module consists of a trainer's manual, patient workbooks, and a videotape that models the skills to be learned. The modules are professionally produced and thus are high quality and "user friendly."

SILS modules are used in training individuals, families, or groups consisting of from 1 to 15 patients, depending on the number and competency of trainers and the needs of the particular setting. Optimally, training should be conducted at a minimum of twice a week, in one-hour sessions. Given this schedule, approximately four months are needed to complete a module with a group of about ten participants.

The modules are divided into constituent skill areas as shown in Figure 1. Each skill area is taught using seven learning activities reviewed in Table 3. Each learning activity builds on information learned in previous steps and takes into consideration the cognitive deficits and need for acquiring problem-solving skills characteristic of people with serious mental illness. The first three activities focus on motivation and skill acquisition, the fourth and fifth teach the individual how to solve problems in the use of the skills, and the last two help the individual to generalize skills to settings outside the module group.

EVALUATION OF THE MEDICATION MANAGEMENT MODULES

Therapist-training activities that facilitate implementation of the Medication Management Module were tested in a national dissemination project (Eckman et al. 1990). Sites were solicited by telephone and mailings, in which the respective responsibilities of the project staff and participating field-test sites were discussed. Twenty-eight sites from around the country participated, representing inpatient and partial hospitalization programs in public and private psychiatric hospitals, community mental health centers, and residential care facilities. Trainers represented a wide range of dis-

FIGURE 1. Each module consists of skill areas related to the training objectives. The components of the skill area in the Medication Management Module, "Negotiating Medication Issues with Health Care Providers," include specific interpersonal behaviors that are the focus of training.

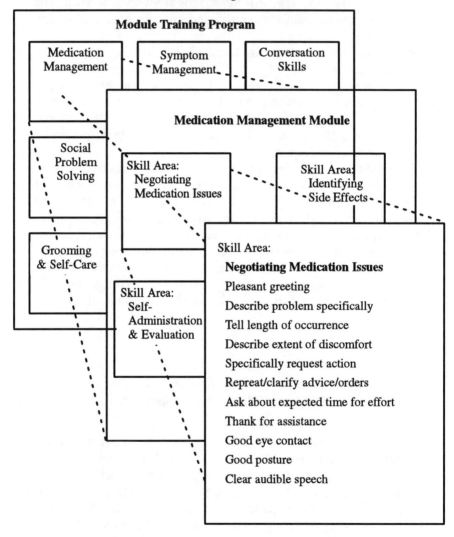

TABLE 3. The SILS modules learning activities.

1. Introduction to Skill Area:

The trainer sets the goals for the module and defines key terms. For example, in the Medication Management Module, introduction to Skill Area 1 includes a discussion of why medications are prescribed and what the benefits of medications are.

2. Videotape Questions and Answers:

Videotaped actors model a set of target behaviors succcessfully. The trainer pauses the tape periodically to ask the group members specified questions in order to increase patient involvement and to assess comprehension. For example, the videotape for the Medication Management Module shows a nurse discussing the therapeutic and side effects of medications with two patients.

3. Roleplay:

Patients are provided the opportunity to practice the skills they have recently viewed on the video, and to learn effective communication skills. During a roleplay in Medication Management, the patient pretends he/she is a nurse and explains the effects of antipsychotic drugs to a peer.

4. Resource Management:

Participants learn to identify and obtain resources essential to the skill being learned. For example, money and transportation are needed to get a prescription filled.

5. Outcome Problems:

Patients learn a 7-step method for solving problems that may arise when trying to use the skill. Problem situations in Medication Management include being offered an alcoholic beverage at a party and losing your medication.

6. Invivo Exercises:

Particpants practice newly learned skills in situations outside the training environment; the trainer accompanies the patient to provide moral support, prompts, and feedback. An example of an in vivo exercise includes completing the Medication Self-Assessment Rating Sheet.

7. Homework:

Patients perform the skill in "real life" situations without trainer support. For example, patients are asked to call a nearby emergency room and ask for the name of the person who handles psychiatric emergencies.

ciplines including psychiatry, psychology, social work, nursing, occupational therapy, and mental health workers.

The project team evaluated two modes of dissemination: the first fourteen sites that agreed to participate in the study were assigned to a *training plus consultation* condition while the second fourteen sites received *consultation* alone. The two-day training workshop began with a general overview to the skills training approach of the Medication Management Module. Therapist-trainees then observed a demonstration group in which expert therapists conducted a two-hour Medication Management session with volunteer patients. The remainder of the training consisted of structured practice and exercises under the guidance of experienced trainers, at the end of which all participants satisfactorily demonstrated the Module procedures. Clinicians in the *consultation only* condition learned about Module procedures from viewing a brief, introductory videotape and reading a detailed guide; no direct training was provided. Expert telephone consultation was available to all settings throughout the study.

Results showed that clinicians in both dissemination conditions showed significant increases in scores on a test measuring knowledge of module content and procedures. In addition, trainers in both conditions showed high fidelity in performing module skills while being observed during a sample module. However, participants who received the supervised training showed better performance scores than clinicians in the *consultation only* group. These results suggested that face-to-face training with modeling and guided practice augments trainer fidelity. However, even without structured training, therapists were able to follow the module procedures with a satisfactory degree of precision.

ADOPTION OF MODULES
FOR PSYCHIATRIC REHABILITATION

The Behavior Analysis and Modification Project (BAM) conducted over a five-year period at the Oxnard (California) Mental Health Center, led to the development and empirical validation of behavior therapy modules similar to those developed in the SILS project (Liberman and Bryan 1977; Liberman, King, and DeRisi

1976). Six of these modules were selected to be disseminated to Community Mental Health Centers (CMHC) across the United States via a learning activity training seminar (Liberman et al. 1982). To be included in the dissemination project, CMHCs had to demonstrate administrative and staff support for training; 40 centers met this criteria. The training program comprised two steps: (1) initial training aimed at familiarizing CMHC staff with the modules, led by "external experts" from the BAM Project; and (2) more extended training by "peer tutors."

During initial on-site training, action-oriented procedures that paralleled the module learning activities were used to help trainee-therapists acquire clinical skills. Upon completion of the initial training, six staff members were selected at each site as peer tutors to conduct the extended, inservice training. The extended training was outlined in detailed training guides provided by BAM innovators and mailed to each CMHC over the subsequent six weeks. On-site, peer tutors were not required to be experts in their content areas, but rather served to keep the inservice training sessions on task and to facilitate active rehearsal of trainee skills during the session.

Although the intervention program was carried out in forty CMHCs, complete data were collected from only the last eighteen centers visited (Liberman et al. 1982). From this group, 562 staff members completed the preintervention evaluation battery and attended the initial two-day, on-site training and program orientation. A 60-item multiple-choice test was given to participants before and after the 14-week period of training, measuring comprehension of basic behavioral principles and clinical application of these principles. Results showed that trainees who participated in the on-site workshop and in in-service training for a minimum of four modules showed a significant increase in conceptual mastery after training. Perhaps the most robust measure of the implementation of the BAM innovations is the extent to which the modular treatment procedures were put into practice by therapist-trainees. Of CMHCs that participated in the training program, 67 percent reported using one or more modules in a programmatic manner one year later. The vast majority of CMHCs reported continued use of modules by staff members in both individual and group therapies.

To learn even more about the process by which innovations are adopted by practitioners, "Adoption of Innovations in Mental Health," the aforementioned project sponsored by the California Department of Mental Health, studied "the life of a module" at various treatment facilities. The Medication Self-Management, Recreation for Leisure, and Symptom Self-Management Modules were distributed to mental health facilities around the country. In a preliminary investigation, 455 mental health facilities that had received the Medication Management Module were surveyed by mail regarding their use of the module (Blair and Wallace 1989). Of the 455 questionnaires mailed, 126 or 28 percent were returned within 18 months of having received the module; the limited response rate suggests that conclusions must be drawn tentatively. These sites received no professional orientation or training in the use of the Module; it was simply given to the site by a pharmaceutical company sales representative.

Therapists at 77 of the 126 sites (61 percent) reported continued use of the Module more than one year after receiving it. At 44 sites (35 percent), therapists were planning to use it but various administrative and logistical obstacles prevented immediate application. Staff at 4 sites (3 percent) stated that they would not be using the module; and one site rejected the Module after one trial. The vast majority of surveyed therapists (93 percent) had no prior exposure or specific training in use of the Module. Even without training, staff at all 77 sites where the Module was in use responded that it was easy to follow. Clinicians at 74 of these sites (96 percent) where the module was in use said participants gained as much or more from the Module than expected, and staff at all but one facility said that they would recommend the Module to other mental health professionals. Most facilities (80 percent) reported that trainers adapted the Module to meet specific needs of their patients and omitted some of the exercises.

To evaluate more completely the efficacy of the SILS modules when delivered by line level staff in a diversity of mental health settings, project staff telephoned or contacted by mail a variety of mental health facilities in California that were interested in using the SILS modules. Over a period of three years, staff at fourteen different sites and seventeen different programs within the sites received between eight and 24 hours of training by project team members. Staff trainees received approximately two hours of overview and demonstration of the modules, and then participated in a minimum of six hours of guided practice with the seven learning activities. After the training, staff at the facilities were then followed via periodic telephone contact and on-site consultation. Sixteen of the 17 programs also agreed to participate in the research relating to staff fidelity in delivering the modules and the effects of the modules on patients' acquisition of skills and knowledge.

Despite the small number of sites and programs involved in the project, certain trends among the programs were evident and worthy of discussion and future exploration. A description of project facilities is provided in Table 4. One of the state hospitals and the correctional facility had two and three inpatient programs, respectively, within the facility. These programs operated under somewhat differing circumstances and administrative structures. Therefore, rather than consider each facility or site as a single unit, programs within a site were treated as "subjects" of study.

Although over 350 staff members at the various facilities received training, only 39 actually conducted, or attempted to conduct, a module. The backgrounds of the trainers are listed in Table 5. The Trainer's Manuals were intended to be structured and specific such that virtually anyone, regardless of background or special

TABLE 4. Psychiatric facilities and programs participating in the study, "Adoption of Innovations in Mental Health."

Facility Sites		Distinct Programs	
State Hospitals	2	Inpatient	3
Correctional Facility	1	Inpatient	3
Residential Care	7	Residential	7
Day Treatment Centers	2	Day Treatment	2
Outpatient Clinics	2	Outpatient	2
Totals	14		17

TABLE 5. Job titles of trainers leading SILS modules in AIMH study.

Title	Number
Psychologist	5
Social Worker	4
Registered Nurse	2
Recreational and Occupational Therapist	5
Marriage/Family/Child Counselor	2
Psychiatric Technician (high school graduate)	4
Corrections Officer	10
Residential Facility Owner/Operator or Staff	7
Total	39

training, who enjoyed working with the mentally ill and who was willing and able to follow written instructions, would be able to lead a module effectively.

Up to 40 percent of the module sessions at the various programs were assessed for the fidelity with which trainers adhered to the prescribed learning activities. The fidelity instrument enabled the researchers to assess how closely trainers followed the module structure, and to evaluate how patients' learning of module skills and concepts thus might be affected. The observational instrument can also be used by supervisors or by other staff concerned with quality assurance to evaluate therapists' teaching techniques and style.

A program was considered to have "adopted" a module if one or more modules had been conducted in full, and if someone in that program expressed an intent to continue to conduct a module. Programs that did not conduct a module, after having received training, or that decided not to continue to offer a module or modules, were defined as "non-adopting" sites. A closer look at these adopting and non-adopting programs may provide clues to the characteristics that aid or impede the adoption of mental health innovations.

Of the 17 programs that received training and participated in the follow-up evaluation, ten had adopted at least one module, and were either teaching additional modules or continued to teach the same module to subsequent groups of patients. All ten of the adopting programs stated that they intended to offer module groups as part of their regular "menu" of treatment services. Based on interviews and questionnaires, a descriptive list of factors related to the adoption of the modules is provided in Table 6. The factors are cross-referenced to the taxonomy of barriers to innovation presented earlier in this chapter.

For the majority of the programs, the successful adoption of the SILS modules related to facilitative factors within the organization; for example, the presence of a local staff "champion" who was influential in using the modules, and/or on a mandate passed down from program administration. Other programs lacking an influential "champion," or administrative mandate, were successful primarily because of the extraordinary commitment of the trainer. As an example of the enthusiasm of these select, few trainers, patients who completed their modules were presented with a graduation ceremony, complete with a party and certificates. These trainers often operated in relative isolation, occasionally with a coleader, but with little peer or supervisory support or recognition.

Of the seven non-adopting sites, two never offered SILS groups, and the other five conducted all or part of a module, but discontinued their use after several months. None of these programs had current plans to conduct a module in the future. These non-adopting programs were similar to their adopting counterparts in terms of size, setting, and trainer qualifications. However, there were clear differences in the amount of external support trainers received. The trainers in the non-adopting sites were frequently in conflict with program administration and experienced more frustration. Trainers at these sites also worked independently, without coleaders, thereby adding to the "burnout" factor so common in the mental health field. Funding sources associated with these programs also tended to be precarious, compared to resources that were available to adopting programs, which were limited, but fairly predictable.

The patients in groups in which trainers followed the module as written–that is, completed 80 percent of prescribed trainers' behaviors on the fidelity measure–learned more than those in groups

TABLE 6. Characteristics of mental health programs adopting and not adopting the SILS modules.

"Adopting" Programs

No.	Type of Program	Setting	Reasons for Adoption	Taxonomy
2	Chronic inpatients	State hospital	Trainer, administrative commitment	Institutional and Practitioner
2	Acute inpatients	State prison	Administrative mandate, Administrative "champion"	Institutional
1	Transitional inpatient	State prison	Administrative mandate, Administrative "champion"	Institutional
2	Residential community	Small <25 beds	Owner/operator conducts module groups	Practitioner
1	Residential/ educational	Large 50 beds	Administrative mandate, but staff turnover jeopardizes continued implementation	Institutional
1	Day Treatment	County CMHC	Trainer commitment	Practitioner
1	Outpatient	County CMHC	Trainer commitment, Administrative "champion"	Institutional and Practitioner

"Non-Adopting" Programs

No.	Type of Program	Setting	Reasons for Nonadoption	Taxonomy
1	Inpatient	State hospital	Staff turnover, no mandate, coordinator, or champion	Institutional

No.	Type of Program	Setting	Reasons for Nonadoption	Taxonomy
2	Residential	Small <12 beds	(1) Cut in funding, never offered module (1) owner/ operator conducted group, but did not follow manual and lost interest	Institutional and Practitioner
2	Residential	Large >50 beds	(1) Trainer ill, had conflicts with administration, quit job (1) Administration thought module was not "worth the time it took"	Institutional and Practitioner
1	Outpatient	County CMHC	Funding cuts, no staff volunteered or were assigned to lead a group	Institutional
1	Day Treatment	County MHC	Funding cuts, county mental health reorganization	Institutional

where the trainer deviated from the basic structure. Patients whose trainers extracted various exercises from a module (for example, used the videotape only and deleted all other exercises) gained little if any information and skills from their experience. Also, trainers who skipped large portions of the module tended to be less likely to continue to use the module in subsequent groups. On the other hand, when interviewed, trainers who followed the module as written tended to express more satisfaction regarding the quality of the group, believed that patients gained from the material, and were more likely to continue to use the modules.

Because the number of programs investigated was so small, each program was treated as a case study, and analyses were primarily descriptive. To understand the process by which an institution adopts or rejects an innovative treatment, contextual and sequential information is required. Although case studies have been criticized on the basis of their lack of objectivity, reliance on retrospective reports, and lack of controls, these criticisms are frequently misguided (Runyan 1982, 1983; Bem 1983) and overlook the unique value of the case study approach (Strauss and Hafez 1981).

The cases of two residential treatment facilities–one that adopted the modules (Facility A) and one that did not (Facility B)–can illuminate the manner in which various impediments can affect the implementation of an innovation such as skills training modules. Two staff members from each of these two board-and-care facilities attended a two-day training seminar on how to use the Medication Management Module at their local community mental health center (CMHC). The two board-and-care homes had received supplemental funds from the state to provide additional psychosocial treatment for their residents. The facilities were within five miles of each other, were a conglomerate of individual apartments, and were served by the same CMHC, which provided all psychiatric treatment for their residents other than the modules. At both sites, residents were expected to keep their own bedrooms neat and clean, but meals were prepared for them. On the average, residents of these homes had a total of eight months previous hospitalization and were 33 years old. The vast majority had current diagnoses of schizophrenia.

Facility A served 12 residents and employed four people. The same woman who owned the care home also served as its chief administrator and conducted the modules herself. Her activity director and manager co-led the group of 11 participants. Although neither the group leader nor the coleader had prior experience leading groups, they approached the task with enthusiasm, if not a bit of apprehension. At the initiation of training, the activity director said, "I know the guys need this Medication Management Module but I'm a little uneasy because I've never led a group like this before." The trainers requested that project staff visit weekly for a period of time to provide them with support and guidance. They followed the modules as written, with a fidelity rate of more than 90 percent. Attendance by residents was nearly 100 percent. Patients who completed the Medication Management Module in the facility almost doubled their scores of knowledge about antipsychotic medication; scores remained improved at a one-year follow-up.

At the close of the first Module, the group in Facility A celebrated with a pizza party, where each participant was awarded a certificate of completion. The owner/trainer eagerly requested assistance from the project team in adding a second module to her facility. She stated, "The guys are all asking what they get to do next. We have the two meeting times each week set aside to do the modules, and I can't imagine not spending that time doing a skills training group with them." She subsequently conducted three additional modules: Recreation for Leisure, Grooming and Self-Care, and Symptom Self-Management.

Facility B hired a staff member to do recreational activities and skills training with the Modules for the 30 residents of this facility. An experimental test of the Module was attempted with patients randomly assigned either to an experimental group that would receive the Module or to a waiting-list control group. Ten residents were randomly selected to begin the Medication Management Module within several weeks of the staff training, while another ten were administered the Module-related assessment measures but waited to receive the Module.

Although the care home administrative director attended the initial training at the CMHC, she did not attend the Module groups. The newly hired staff person conducted the Medication Management Module alone, although the activity director observed several of the final sessions. The trainer appeared to be self-confident, although she had never conducted a structured group before. During each visit by project staff, the trainer complained that she did not agree with some of the Module content, such as a problem-solving exercise that related to avoidance of illicit drugs. "I don't think this is very realistic," she explained, and skipped the exercise. She followed the Module with 70 percent fidelity, based on observation of 35 percent of her sessions. Nevertheless, the Module was well received by patients as reflected by her comment:

I was surprised that during the break, when we have refreshments, the group members made positive remarks about the module. It was Social Security payday, but everybody was here except for one person. I couldn't believe it–usually you can't get anybody to show up for anything on payday!

Despite the positive reception she and the Module received from participants, the trainer felt isolated from and unappreciated by her program management. The administrator believed that "too little was gained for the amount of time and energy that went into it." Although scores on knowledge and skills almost tripled for patients attending the module–while scores for the control group remained the same–the administrator decided not to continue the module, and the wait-list control group never received the training. The trainer explained, "Since the funds are so tight, they want me to spend treatment time with the really low-functioning residents, and we don't even want to try to do the Modules with them." Offers by the project team to help conduct a group with lower-functioning residents were politely rejected, the Modules were discontinued, and no follow-up testing was completed. Soon after the Module was finished, the trainer left her position with the facility.

The six other non-adopting facilities shared a number of characteristics exemplified by Facility B. At these sites, program reorganization or reprioritization, as well as the departure of key staff, were factors associated with the decision not to implement the Module or to discontinue it. Five of the seven trainers at non-adopting sites left the facility before implementing the Module, while it was being conducted, or shortly after its completion. Their departure was most often attributable to financial constraints that affected programming and staffing, and to the lack of financial and professional support of administration and coworkers.

Although these trainers did not adopt the Module, all but one trainer in both adopting and non-adopting facilities stated that the Module would benefit their patients. The exception was a trainer who believed the Module might actually harm patients because of the active and directive training techniques. This trainer discontinued the Module after one of his patients was rehospitalized. The trainer subsequently pursued employment as a recreational counselor elsewhere.

Trainers at adopting sites, as illustrated by Facility A, more often had coleaders or colleagues who were involved with and supportive of the modules; therefore, these trainers felt less isolated. Adopting facilities had an overarching treatment philosophy that was in harmony with the goals and structured format of the modules, and most enjoyed financial and program stability.

SUMMARY

Behavioral modules are a user-friendly product of intervention research and facilitate implementation of effective treatment innovations. The predesigned curricula with videos and trainer manuals make adoption and utilization of the technology relatively easy. The psychoeducational principles underlying modular approaches help to obviate many staff barriers to implementation since they are both user friendly and cost effective. However, while the requisite trainer skills defined by a module are easy to acquire and clearly improve patients' clinically relevant behaviors, innovators must still incorporate dissemination strategies that will promote adoption and utilization by practitioners.

Strategies that facilitate the dissemination process include: (1) face-to-face introduction of the innovation with "live" demonstration of the skills to clinical staff; (2) clear evidence of administrative leadership that provides the resources and staff mandate to schedule and implement modules: and (3) a respected practitioner who serves as a "champion" of the innovation and who encourages colleagues to incorporate the module curricula and constituent trainer skills into daily treatment plans. The combination of behavior therapy modules and effective dissemination strategies should increase the utilization of behavior therapy in many mental health facilities containing needy and underserved patient populations.

REFERENCES

Bachrach, L. L. 1980. Overview: Model programs for chronic mental patients. *American Journal of Psychiatry, 137,* 1023-1031.

Bachrach, L. L. 1981. Discussion: The role of model programs in the care of chronic mental patients. In *Chronic Mental Patients: Treatment Programs, Systems,* edited by J. A. Talbott. New York: Human Sciences.

Bachrach, L. L. 1986. Dimensions of disability in the chronic mentally ill. *Hospital and Community Psychiatry, 37*, 981-982.

Backer, T. E., R. P. Liberman, and T. G. Kuehnel. 1986. Dissemination and adoption of innovative psychosocial interventions. *Journal of Consulting and Clinical Psychology, 54*, 111-118.

Ball, T., R. M. Jarvis, and S. S. Pease. 1983. Interinstitutional misadventures in a training program for parents of retarded children. *Analysis and Intervention in Developmental Disabilities, 3*, 239-248.

Bandura, A. 1969. *Principles of Behavior Modification.* New York: Holt, Rinehart, and Winston.

Barber, K., M. Barber, and H. B. Clark. 1983. Establishing a community-oriented group home and ensuring its survival: A case study of failure. *Analysis and Intervention in Developmental Disabilities, 3*, 227-238.

Barlow, D. H. 1981. On the relation of clinical research to clinical practice: Current issues, new directions. *Journal of Consulting and Clinical Psychology, 49*, 147-155.

Barlow, D. H. and M. Hersen. 1984. *Single Case Experimental Designs: Strategies for Studying Behavior Change* (2nd edition). New York: Pergamon.

Baucom, D. H. and W. Epstein. 1989. *Cognitive-behavioral Marital Therapy.* New York: Brunner-Mazel.

Beck, A. T., G. Emery, and R. Greenberg. 1985. *Anxiety Disorders and Phobias: A Cognitive Perspective.* New York: Basic Books.

Beck, A. T., A. J. Rush, B. F. Shaw, and G. Emery. 1979. *Cognitive Therapy of Depression.* New York: Guilford.

Bellack, A. S. (ed.) 1984. *Schizophrenia: Treatment, Management, and Rehabilitation.* New York: Grune & Stratton.

Bem, D. J. 1983. Toward a response style theory of persons in situations. In *Nebraska Symposium on Motivation, 1982–Personality: Current Theory and Research, 30*, edited by R. A. Dienstbier and M. M. Page. Lincoln: University of Nebraska Press, 211-221.

Blair, K. and C. Wallace. 1989. Evaluation of the dissemination of the medication management module. Unpublished report available from Camarillo/UCLA Clinical Research Center, P.O. Box 6022, Camarillo, CA 93011-6022.

Browner, C. H., K. A. Ellis, T. Ford, J. Silsby, J. Tampoya, and C. Yee. 1987. Stress, social support, and health of psychiatric technicians in a state facility. *Mental Retardation, 25*, 31-37.

Burg, M. M., D. H. Reid, and J. Lattimore. 1979. Use of a self-recording and supervision program to change institutional staff behavior. *Journal of Applied Behavior Analysis, 12*, 363-375.

Carmel, H. and M. Hunter. 1989. Staff injuries from inpatient violence. *Hospital and Community Psychiatry, 40*, 41-46.

Corrigan, P. W., W. Y. Kwartarini, and W. Pramana. 1992. Barriers to the implementation of behavior therapy. *Behavior Modification, 16*, 132-144.

Cullari, S. and D. G. Ferguson. 1981. Individual behavior change: Problems with programming in institutions for mentally retarded persons. *Mental Retardation, 19,* 267-270.

Curran, J. P. and P. Monti. (eds.) 1982. *Social Skills Training: A Practical Handbook for Assessment and Treatment.* New York: Guilford.

Dailey, W. F., G. J. Allen, J. M. Chinsky, and S. W. Veit. 1974. Attendant behavior and attitudes toward institutionalized retarded children. *American Journal of Mental Deficiency, 78,* 586-591.

Eckman, T. A., R. P. Liberman, C. C. Phipps, and K. Blair. 1990. Teaching medication self-management to chronic schizophrenics. *Journal of Clinical Psychopharmacology.*

Emerson, E. and C. Emerson. 1987. Barriers to the effective implementation of habilitative behavioral programs in an institutional setting. *Mental Retardation, 25,* 101-106.

Fairweather, G. W., D. H. Sanders, and L. G. Tornatzky. 1974. *Creating Change in Mental Health Organizations.* New York: Pergamon.

Favell, J. E. and J. E. Phillips. 1986. Behavior therapy in residential programs for retarded persons. In *Behavior Analysis and Therapy in Residential Programs,* edited by F. J. Fuoco and W. P. Christian. New York: Van Nostrand, Reinhold, 260-279.

Fisher, D. 1983. The going gets tough when we descend from the ivory tower. *Analysis and Intervention in Developmental Disabilities, 3,* 249-256.

Gambrill, E. and L. Richey. 1985. *Taking Charge of Your Social Life.* Belmont, CA: Wadsworth.

Garfield, S. L. and R. Kurtz. 1976. Clinical psychologists in the 1970's. *American Psychologist, 31,* 1-9.

Glaser, E. M., H. H. Abelson, and K. N. Garrison. 1983. *Putting Knowledge to Use.* San Francisco: Jossey-Bass.

Gottman, J., C. Notarius, J. Gonso, and H. Markman. 1976. *A Couple's Guide to Communication.* Champaign, IL: Research Press.

Graziano, A. M. 1969. Clinical innovation and the mental health power structure. *American Psychologist, 24,* 10-18.

Greenblatt, M. 1983. Some principles guiding institutional change. *Analysis and Intervention in Developmental Disabilities, 3,* 257-259.

Iwata, B. A., J. S. Bailey, K. M. Brown, T. J. Foshee, and M. A. Alpern. 1976. A performance based lottery to improve residential care and training by institutional staff. *Journal of Applied Behavior Analysis. 9,* 417-431.

Jacobs, H. E., S. Kardashian, P. K. Kreinbring, R. Ponder, and A. R. Simpson. 1984. A skills-oriented model facilitating employment among psychiatrically disabled persons. *Rehabilitation Counseling Bulletin, 28,* 87-96.

Jacobson, N. S. and A. S. Gurman. 1986. *Clinical Handbook of Marital Therapy.* New York: Guilford.

Klass, D. G., A. Growe, and M. Strizich. 1977. Ward treatment milieu and post hospital functioning. *Archives of General Psychiatry, 34,* 1047-1052.

Lange, A. J. and P. Jakubowski. 1976. *Responsible Assertive Behavior: Cognitive/ Behavioral Procedures for Trainers.* Champaign, IL: Research Press.

Larsen, J., E. L. Norris, and J. Knoll. 1976. *Consultation and its Outcome: Community Mental Health Centers*. Palo Alto, CA: American Institutes for Research.

Lazarus, A. A. 1984. *In the Mind's Eye*. New York: Guilford.

Levine, M. 1973. Problems of entry in light of some postulates of practice in community psychology. In *The Helping Professions in the World of Action*, edited by I. I. Goldenberg. Lexington, MA: Heath.

Liberman, R. P. 1979. Social and political challenges to the development of behavioral programs in organizations. In *Trends in Behavior Therapy*, edited by P. O. Sjoden, W. S. Dockens, and S. Bates. New York: Academic Press.

Liberman, R. P. 1983. Special issue on sociopolitics of behavioral programs in institutions and community agencies. *Analysis and Intervention in Developmental Disabilities, 3*, 131-259.

Liberman, R. P. 1986. *Medication Management Module*. Camarillo, CA: UCLA Clinical Research Center.

Liberman, R. P. (ed.) 1990. *Handbook of Psychiatric Rehabilitation*. Elmsford, New York: Pergamon.

Liberman, R. P., T. Ball, L. Siddach, C. J. Wallace, L. Guyette, P. Magaro, and W. DiScipio. 1975. Behavior therapy in state hospitals. In *Future Role of the State Hospital*, edited by J. Zusman and E. Bertsche. Lexington, MA: D. C. Heath & Co, 157-189.

Liberman, R. P. and J. R. Bedell. 1989. Behavior therapy. In *Comprehensive Textbook of Psychiatry (Fifth edition)*, edited by H. Kaplan and B. Sadosck. Baltimore: Williams & Wilkins.

Liberman, R. P. and E. Bryan. 1977. Behavior therapy in a community mental health center. *American Journal of Psychiatry, 134*, 401-406.

Liberman, R. P., T. Eckman, T. Kuehner, J. Rosenstein, and J. Kuehnel. 1982. Dissemination of new behavior therapy programs to community mental health centers. *American Journal of Psychiatry, 139*, 224-226.

Liberman, R. P., L. W. King, and W. J. DeRisi. 1976. Behavior analysis and modification in community mental health. In *Handbook of Behavior Therapy and Modification*, edited by H. Leitenberg. Englewood Cliffs, NJ: Prentice-Hall, 101-171.

Liberman, R. P. and K. T. Mueser. 1989. Schizophrenia. In *Comprehensive Textbook of Psychiatry (Fifth edition)*, edited by H. Kaplan and B. Sadock. Baltimore: Williams & Wilkins.

Liberman, R. P., K. T. Mueser, and C. J. Wallace. 1986. Social skills training for schizophrenic individuals at risk for relapse. *American Journal of Psychiatry, 143*, 523-526.

Lion, J. R. and W. H. Reid. 1983. *Assaults within Psychiatric Facilities*. New York: Grune & Stratton.

Lion, J. R., W. Snyder, and G. L. Merrill. 1981. Underreporting of assaults on staff in a state hospital. *Hospital and Community Psychiatry, 32*, 497-498.

MacKain, S. J. and C. J. Wallace. 1989. *Adoptions of Innovations in Mental Health*. Unpublished report available from Camarillo/UCLA Clinical Research Center, P.O. Box 6022, Camarillo, CA 93011-6022.

Madden, D. J., J. R. Lion, and M. W. Penna. 1976. Assaults on psychiatrists by patients. *American Journal of Psychiatry, 133*, 422-425.

Marlatt, G. A. and J. R. Gordon. (eds.) 1985. *Relapse Prevention.* New York: Guilford.

McMullin, R. and B. Casey. 1975. *Talk Sense to Yourself: A Guide to Cognitive Restructuring Therapy.* Lakewood, CO: Counseling Research Institute.

Moos, R. H. 1974. *Evaluating Treatment Environments: A Social Ecological Approach.* New York: John Wiley.

Paul, G. L. and R. J. Lentz. 1977. *Psychosocial Treatment of Chronic Mental Patients: Milieu vs. Social Learning Programs.* Cambridge: Harvard University Press.

Perry, M. A. and M. J. Furukawa. 1986. Modeling methods. In *Helping People Change (Third edition),* edited by F. H. Kanfer and A. P. Goldstein. New York: Pergamon.

Phillips, E. L., E. A. Phillips, D. L. Fixsen, and M. M. Wolf. 1974. *The Teaching-Family Handbook.* Lawrence, KS: Bureau of Child Research.

Priestly, P. and J. McGuire. 1983. *Learning to Help: Basic Skills Exercises.* London: Tavistock Publication.

Rehm, L. P. (ed.) 1981. *Behavior Therapy for Depression: Present Status and Future Directions.* New York: Academic.

Reid, D. H. and T. L. Whitman. 1983. Behavioral staff management in institutions: A critical review of effectiveness and acceptability. *Analysis and Intervention in Developmental Disabilities, 3,* 131-150.

Repp, A. C., L. E. Barton, and A. R. Brulle. 1981. Correspondence between effectiveness and staff use of instructions for severely retarded persons. *Applied Research in Mental Retardation, 2,* 237-245.

Repucci, N. D. 1973. The social psychology of institutional change: General principles for intervention. *American Journal of Community Psychology, 1,* 330-341.

Repucci, N. D. 1977. Implementation issues for the behavior modifier as institutional change agent. *Behavior Therapy, 8,* 594-605.

Repucci, N. D. and J. T. Saunders. 1974. Social psychology of behavior modification: Problems of implementation in natural settings. *American Psychologist, 29,* 649-660.

Roberts, A. O. H. and J. K. Larsen. 1971. *Effective Use of Mental Health Research Information.* Palo Alto, CA: American Institutes for Research.

Runyan, W. M. 1982. In defense of the case study method. *American Journal of Orthopsychiatry, 52,* 440-446.

Runyan, W. M. 1983. Idiographic goals and methods in the study of lives. *Journal of Personality, 51,* 413-437.

Sarason, S. B., M. Levine, I. I. Goldenberg, D. K. Cherlin, and E. M. Bennett. 1966. *Psychology in Community Settings.* New York: Wiley.

Schade, M. L., P. W. Corrigan, and R. P. Liberman. 1990. Prescriptive rehabilitation for severely disabled psychiatric patients. *New Directions in Mental Health Services, 45,* 3-17.

Shepherd, G. 1984. *Institutional Care and Rehabilitation*. London: Longman.

Silberman, M. L. and S. A. Wheelan. 1980. *How to Discipline Without Feeling Guilty: Assertive Relationships with Children*. Champaign, IL: Research Press.

Slama, K. M. and D. J. Bannerman. 1983. Implementing and maintaining a behavioral treatment system in an institutional setting. *Analysis and Intervention in Developmental Disabilities, 3*, 171-192.

Sobell, L. C. and M. B. Sobell. 1988. Behavioral assessment and treatment planning with alcohol and substance abuse: A review with emphasis on clinical application. *Clinical Psychology Review, 8*, 19-54.

Spiegler, M. D. and H. Agigian. 1977. *Community Training Center: An Educational-Behavioral-Social Systems Model for Rehabilitating Psychiatric Patients*. New York: Bruner-Mazel.

Storzbach, D. 1989. *The Use of a Staff Self-Monitoring Procedure for Improving the Fidelity of Behavioral Programming on a Behavioral Research Unit*. Unpublished Master's Thesis: California Lutheran University, Thousand Oaks, CA.

Strauss, J. S. and H. Hafez. 1981. Clinical questions and "real" research. *American Journal of Psychiatry, 138*, 1592-1597.

Tharp, R. and R. Wetzel. 1969. *Behavior Modification in the Natural Environment*. New York: Academic.

Walker, C. F. 1975. *Learn to Relax: 13 Ways to Reduce Tension*. Englewood Cliffs. NJ: Prentice Hall.

Wallace, C. J., J. R. Davis, R. P. Liberman, and V. Baker. 1973. Modeling and staff behavior. *Journal of Consulting and Clinical Psychology, 41*, 422-425.

Wallace, C. J. and R. P. Liberman. 1985. Social skills training for patients with schizophrenia: A controlled clinical trial. *Psychiatry Research, 15*, 239-247.

Wallace, C. J., R. P. Liberman, S. MacKain, G. Blackwell, and T. Eckman. 1990. Modules for training social and independent living skills: Application and impact. Submitted to *Archives of General Psychiatry*.

Wasow, M. 1986. The need for asylum for the chronically mentally ill. *Schizophrenia Bulletin, 12*, 162-167.

Wexler, D. B. 1984. Legal aspects of seclusion and restraint. In *The Psychiatric Uses of Seclusion and Restraint*, edited by K. Tardiff. Washington, DC: American Psychiatric Press.

Wirshing, W., T. A. Eckman, R. P. Liberman, and S. M. Marder. 1990. Management of risk of relapse through skills training of chronic schizophrenics. In *Advances in Schizophrenia Research*, edited by C. Tamminga and S. C. Schulz. New York: Raven Press.

Yeaton, W. H. and L. Sechrest. 1981. Critical dimensions in the choice and maintenance of successful treatments: Strength, integrity, and effectiveness. *Journal of Consulting and Clinical Psychology, 49*, 156-167.

Young, W. T. 1982. Structured learning therapy: Problem-solving skills training and socialization skills training. In *Multimodal Handbook for a Mental Hospital: Designing Specific Treatments for Specific Problems*, New York: Springer.

Chapter 15

Disseminating Intervention Research in Academic Settings– A View from Social Work

Ronald H. Rooney

Research instruction in social work education and professional education generally has focused on increasing skills in the critical consumption of studies to inform practice and in conducting research in practice settings. While this focus assists in applying known technologies and assessing knowledge about well-studied problems, the approach does not prepare students to deal with emerging areas of practice, including the development of new intervention technologies. Thomas has proposed Intervention Research (IR) as the single most appropriate model of research for social professions, as it assists in the development of technology for addressing social problems (Thomas 1978). However, the utilization of IR in academic settings has not been studied, and critics claim that the paradigm contains barriers which inhibit widespread utilization. In this chapter I discuss several barriers and suggest a three-tiered approach for enhancing IR dissemination in academic settings such that increasingly sophisticated models and increasingly skilled model developers are produced (Rooney 1990). The methodology of intervention research has itself been formulated through a process of design and development, thus it too represents a product whose dissemination is appropriate and necessary.

BARRIERS TO THE DISSEMINATION OF INTERVENTION RESEARCH

As in other social professions, a gap between research and practice has plagued social work throughout its history (Blythe and

Briar 1985). IR provides one promising solution for this problem through its guidance in the design, product testing, evaluation, and dissemination of innovative solutions to practice problems (Rothman 1989; Thomas 1989). The primary product of IR is empirically based service approaches in the form of service manuals and program designs with knowledge development about practice as a by-product (Reid 1987a). Hence, IR assists in the provision of practical guidance for practitioners, while focusing researchers on relevant practice problems. IR further promotes the integration of practice and research through training in the role of model developer.

The promise of the IR approach for addressing the research-practice gap is largely unstudied in academic settings. Further, critics suggest that the paradigm contains inherent barriers and disincentives to utilization. These barriers can be described as *forbidding complexity* and *lack of academic rewards*.

Forbidding Complexity

Rino Patti suggests that the comprehensive nature of the design, development, and testing processes in IR precludes widespread adoption in practice settings facing short policy and funding cycles. For example, agencies feel pressure to demonstrate results on innovative programs in annual funding cycles which may short-circuit the time required to complete all the phases of IR. Rather than disseminating an aggregated approach involving all the phases, Patti recommends the development of disaggregated steps which better fit agency constraints (Patti 1981, 1989). For example, the knowledge retrieval steps could be used in compact form to inform program development and pilot studies may need to be conducted and completed within a single year for funding purposes.

Lack of Academic Rewards

Jeanne Giovannoni suggests that since knowledge development continues to be the main basis in academia for promotion and tenure, IR researchers are advised to include knowledge development products as well as practice and program manuals in their career planning (Giovannoni 1989). For example, research reports published in refereed journals assessing the effectiveness of models developed in addition to the development and dissemination of practice models are advised for junior faculty needing to satisfy conventional requirements for scholarship.

These criticisms can be addressed in the light of knowledge developed inside and outside IR about effective dissemination and utilization. Within IR, Thomas proposes that innovations will be successfully disseminated and utilized to the degree that they are behavior guiding, codified, simple, flexible, modular, inexpensive, and designed for usability from the outset (Thomas 1989; Paine, Bellamy, and Wilcox 1984; Rogers and Shoemaker 1971).

These criteria support research dissemination reports suggesting that those research methods which are readily encompassable and applied at low cost are likely to be adopted (Blythe and Briar 1985; Fischer 1981). Specifically, the use of rapid assessment scales, single organism designs, and the study of critical incidents have made research more accessible to students and practitioners (Levitt and Reid 1981; Edleson 1985; Davis and Reid 1988).

IR dissemination has, however, emphasized multiple phases and advanced models which might be described as *programs of model development* (Figure 1). For example, Thomas has published several studies which document the elaboration of a practice model for intervening with the spouses of alcohol abusers, and Rothman has published studies of the utilization of program development guidelines (Thomas and Santa 1982; Rothman, Teresa, and Erlich 1978; Reid 1987b). These models represent a level of model development to which many model developers aspire. They involve procedures that make them appear neither simple nor modular for aspiring model developers. While such programs of model development may be appropriate goals for model developers who can conduct extensive field tests, presenting them as the primary model for initiates may produce the same ambivalence that those students learning experimental design often have to the Solomon Four Group design. While that design is intellectually attractive in its comprehensive approach to addressing problems of reliability and validity, the requirement of random assignment to four groups makes dissemination of the design impractical in most practice settings.

Programs involving full-scale model development might be bet-

FIGURE 1

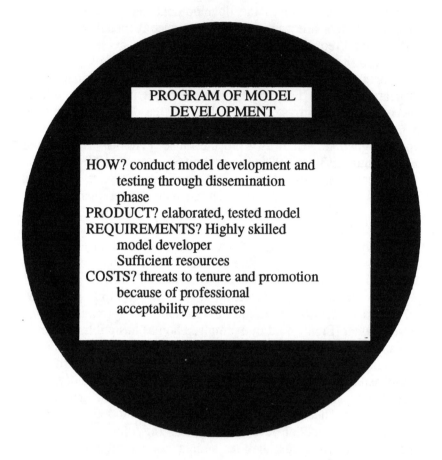

PROGRAM OF MODEL
DEVELOPMENT

HOW? conduct model development and
    testing through dissemination
    phase
PRODUCT? elaborated, tested model
REQUIREMENTS? Highly skilled
    model developer
    Sufficient resources
COSTS? threats to tenure and promotion
    because of professional
    acceptability pressures

ter presented as examples of the potential of the paradigm when the
model developer is highly skilled, and has adequate resources, institutional support, and time. Such programs can be presented as
somewhat unique products of IR specialists. There is, however,
room for many other IR practitioners who use the paradigm more
selectively to work on particular problems at particular times, while
conducting other research using other methodologies.

Based on these conclusions, an association might be hypothe-
sized between increased IR utilization and the extent to which it is

disseminated in modular fashion. A correlated human product is the IR researcher.

In this chapter I describe efforts to promote utilization and acceptance of IR by students through a three-tiered approach, modular in nature, in an academic setting. The first tier comprises the presentation of IR modules in introductory research courses and practice courses; the second tier constitutes a doctoral course in intervention research, and the third tier represents IR dissertations. The activities involved in each tier are delineated and the potential costs and benefits of each are assessed. This three-tiered approach produces increasingly sophisticated models and increasingly skilled model developers (Figure 2).

FIRST TIER: USE OF IR AS MODULES IN RESEARCH AND PRACTICE COURSES

IR in modular form may be introduced to a variety of potential users. Students in introductory research courses represent one such group of potential users. Such courses frequently have a goal of enhancing informed consumption of research studies, and students in such courses are often called upon to select a problem of interest and analyze a certain number of studies, assess their adequacy, and provide implications for practice. However, students frequently select a problem that has not been well researched and they abandon the problem when few studies that are specifically focused on their chosen subject are found. If they do continue with the problem, their newly developed analytic skills mainly permit them to pick apart the few available studies. Too often, their learning becomes an exercise in critiquing the validity of studies, rather than focusing on the utilization of suggestive but partially flawed studies (Hanrahan and Reid 1984). An unintended consequence may be continued reliance on practice wisdom because the research is "too flawed."

While there is value in learning how to assess the reliability and validity of well-designed studies, the message that research is not useful with less well-studied problems is dysfunctional in applied fields. IR can be presented as a useful approach at an early stage of inquiry where a problem with important consequences but lacking adequate solution has been identified. Instead of dismissing the

FIGURE 2

TIER 1: Presentation of modules to research classes, concentration courses. Instruction in analysis, design phases. Learn how to develop summary generalizations and practice guidelines

PRODUCTS: orientation to IR paradigm
    preliminary model guidelines
    preliminary model guideline developers

ADVANTAGES: low cost, widespread orientation
DISADVANTAGES: evaluation phases not included

TIER 2: Presentation of IR course. Includes instruction in evaluation and dissemination.
PRODUCTS: preliminary untested models: "models in waiting"
    some preliminary tested models
    preliminary model developers

ADVANTAGES: more elaborate models
DISADVANTAGES: requires course development
    often lacks testing or only has had pilot
    study

TIER 3: Support of IR dissertators

PRODUCTS: models which have undergone main field tests
    model developers

ADVANTAGES: prepares way for being able to develop programs of model development
DISADVANTAGES: requires some preparation and orientation of committee members

problem or devastating the few available studies, initial steps from the IR paradigm can be presented. Following this route, students are taught to define the problem, to describe the benefits of dealing with the problem and the costs of ignoring it, and to engage in a broader scope of knowledge retrieval (Thomas 1984; Rothman 1980).

IR can help students consider potential information sources that are broader in scope through expanding the original conceptualization of the problem. Guidelines from IR about fruitful potential areas of inquiry, such as law, technology, ethics, and developments in parallel fields (Thomas 1984: 108-109), can be shared. Bounds are set around the search process to make the task feasible within the constraints of the course quarter or semester timeline. Students can then learn how to search the literature with advanced bibliographic sources such as computerized social and psychological databases.

A major contribution of IR at this stage is the development of summary generalizations, which push the student to find the forest in the trees, and to assess the adequacy of those generalizations analytically. A second major contribution is the translation of these summary generalizations into practice guidelines.

I have used this first tier of dissemination in introductory research courses at the University of Minnesota and University of Wisconsin, as well as in other elective and curriculum concentration courses that involve literature reviews for practice relevance. The IR phases of analysis, retrieval, and design of intervention guidelines are introduced to all students in contexts where knowledge about adequate solutions is not in an advanced state (Thomas 1984; Rothman 1980).

Additionally, some students pursue an IR option in completion of a course paper. For those who carry out the IR option, preliminary model guidelines are developed based on a review of the literature. The human product of this approach is the preliminary guideline developer. Skills acquired by the guideline developer can lead to model testing in additional course work and independent studies. The process can also serve as a model for how graduates can rapidly educate themselves about a new problem or practice area (Rooney 1980).

Student preliminary model developers engaged in this process at first often felt overwhelmed with the complexity of the task and wondered if model development was better performed by theorists (Marsh 1983). When the steps of problem definition, identification of relevant resources, and development of summary generalizations and practice guidelines were broken down with concrete examples, including those developed by other students, many proceeded successfully with the task. Production of preliminary model guidelines was typically a source of great satisfaction. They were, however, admonished not to overestimate the value of their guidelines without testing (Mullen 1978). Nonetheless, it was indicated to them that the development of empirically derived practice guidelines is an improvement over practice ideas lacking any empirical backing (Reid 1977).

SECOND TIER:
THE DEVELOPMENT OF A COURSE IN IR

Subsequently, a doctoral course in IR was developed that emphasizes evaluation and diffusion phases in addition to analysis and design. This doctoral course has now been offered three times and several MSW students have also selected it as an elective.

This IR course has now produced 20 preliminary untested models. For example, a student was concerned with the fact that victim offender reconciliation programs for property crimes are frequently successful, but programs often operate far below capacity because there are often more offenders than victims willing to participate. The student combined knowledge about reconciliation programs with ethical principles of self-determination and research on ethical persuasion to develop a stepwise procedure for soliciting the involvement of victims (Bae 1988). Research on interpersonal influence suggests that liked, respected, trusted sources are more influential in changing attitudes than persons lacking those characteristics (Feld and Radin 1982). Since victims now received a letter introducing the program from reconciliation program staff who might be presumed to be in favor of participation, the first step in the proposed intervention was to prepare such a letter to be sent out by the judge who had heard their case, on court letterhead. Research on influence further suggested that persons not already inclined to the viewpoint of the influence source are more persuaded by two-sided arguments which begin with the position now held by the person (Feld and Radin 1982). Following this generalization, victims who did not respond to the letter would be telephoned by program staff with a persuasive appeal which acknowledged their reservations and presented advantages and disadvantages of program participation in an even-handed fashion. Previous research had indicated that victims who do not volunteer cite as reasons that their loss was slight, that they are unsure that the program will help perpetrators, and that they have concerns about their own safety in such interaction. These potential reasons would be assessed with each victim in a two-sided argument about the costs and benefits of project participation. Victims who did not respond to this appeal would be sent a follow-up letter respecting their decision and leaving an address should they reconsider.

Practice models were also developed at larger system levels. For example, one student, who was also an administrator for a national chemical dependency treatment program, developed a model for national dissemination through regional site managers of information about the problems of the elderly with alcoholism (Gilmore 1988).

In addition, many international students have developed practice models which adapt Western technologies to non-Western settings (Haj-Yahia 1988). For example, a student from India developed a model for organizing the homeless in India to build their own housing (Chandy 1988).

These "models in waiting" are more fully formed than the preliminary guidelines produced by the module approach. While these models may cohere conceptually and are empirically based, they lack field testing. Consequently, they are only partial applications of IR and may include elements which in fact do not work in actual practice settings.

This disadvantage of preliminary untested models can be corrected if students go on to conduct pilot field testing. As this requires more time than the quarter in which the preliminary model is developed, I have worked with two MSW students through independent studies to conduct pilot tests. Wanless developed a caseload management method which allowed her to make decisions about intensity of service and permitted an active rather than reactive approach to caseload decisions (Rooney and Wanless 1985). The student-researcher implemented the model with her own caseload for nine months and, guided by her decision-making model, was able to open and close twice as many cases as other practitioners in her adult service unit. Macy-Lewis developed and implemented an adaptation of the Task-Centered approach for a group of single parents (Macy-Lewis 1985). A six-week pilot group intervention was conducted with six single parents. Parents identified target problems such as feeling irritable with their children and the lack of involvement with other single parents. Tasks were developed in the group for each member to try in the home environment. Five of the six single parents reported that the group was good to very successful in addressing their concerns. These preliminary tested models were realized at relatively low cost. Students were able to complete them in field or work settings and received course credit for the independent study. Published articles were an additional by-product of each study.

In addition to "models in waiting" and preliminary tested models, an important result of the IR course has been the academic preparation of prelimary model developers who are positioned to move ahead to model testing or development of preliminary models on other problems.

THIRD TIER: SUPPORT OF IR DISSERTATIONS

Two graduates of the doctoral course in IR at the University of Minnesota have now pursued IR dissertations. Dissertations can produce models which have undergone advanced field tests and so help train more advanced model developers (Reid 1978, 1979). Bonnie used IR to develop and test a group intervention program to assist children grieving the loss by death of a parent or sibling. Summary generalizations indicated that many bereaved children struggle to understand that everyone dies; death is final and irreversible. Further, bereaved children frequently have difficulty expressing verbally about the loss and coping with resulting changes in family systems and roles. Following a pilot study, a six-week group intervention was conducted with nine bereaved children while a control group of 12 bereaved children did not receive the intervention. The intervention included a series of structured exercises related to the analysis of a film about a child's experience of loss by death. The children learned to identify beliefs about death, emotions experienced, and changes occurring to the child in the film. The children were then helped to explore these issues related to their own loss by identifying emotions they had experienced, coming to terms with the facts and details of the death, and exploring changes in their roles and family system. While improvement in depression scores as measured by the Children's Depression Inventory (Kovacs 1983) was similar for both the intervention and control groups, clinical symptomatology as measured by the Child Behavior Checklist (Achenbach and Brown 1988) decreased to 44 percent of the members of the intervention group over the course of the intervention and increased to 100 percent for the control group (Bonnie 1989).

Chou has recently completed an intervention research study to develop, implement, and assess a family intervention program designed to assist the parents of developmentally disabled children in Taiwan. This model is based on research which suggests that parents and siblings frequently have physical, psychological, and financial difficulties as a result of having a disabled child. These difficulties are frequently compounded in Taiwan by shame influenced by beliefs that the disability was caused by sin of the parents or their ancestors. Consequently, North American intervention models which emphasize group interventions to provide alternative explanations for the cause of the disability and empowerment of the caregivers through expansion of support networks were modified by developing a family intervention approach to occur in the family's home setting based on the Family Problem Solving approach (Reid 1985). The intervention included exploration of problems as perceived by family members, presentation of alternative explanations about the cause of disability, and increasing social support resources for caregivers (Chou 1992).

The costs for doctoral students in conducting IR dissertations have been relatively modest. Bonnie was able to secure permission to conduct his study at an agency without substantial cost. Chou received an innovative research grant from the University of Minnesota to support her dissertation study in Taiwan. Faculty involvement has been similar to that in other dissertation committees, with the exception that more time was devoted to educating other committee members about the purposes, products, and means of evaluation of IR dissertations. As committee members were unaccustomed to the emphasis on intervention development and pilot testing, the education effort included sharing articles and presenting a student-faculty colloquium about IR. While developed models require more field testing prior to broader dissemination, a key personnel product is the more advanced model developer.

SUMMARY AND DISCUSSION

This paper has presented three tiers of educational activity for increasing usage of IR by students in an academic setting. Presentation of IR in modules taught in research and practice courses orients a large number of potential users and stimulates some to develop preliminary model guidelines. Use of IR in full course format produces preliminary untested "models in waiting" in many cases, preliminary tested models in others, and preliminary model developers. Finally, the dissertation tier produces models which have undergone a main field test as well as well-prepared model developers.

This three-tiered approach is suggested as a way of disaggregating the IR process such that potential users can assimilate chunks which are appropriate to their level of knowledge, interest, and skill. The approach also suggests indicators that could be used to assess the dissemination of IR in academic settings. At the first tier, the extent to which IR modules are utilized in research and other courses could be tracked through a national survey. At the second, the number of courses specific to IR could be monitored. The number and type of models produced through those courses could also be tracked, as well as the extent of model testing that they have undergone. Finally, at the third tier, the number of dissertations produced based in IR could be measured. Additional criteria might include tabulating the number of articles, manuals, and other products that are generated.

Additional issues have been raised professionally about use of IR by faculty member researchers. While it is beyond the scope of this chapter to address these issues in detail, usage could be enhanced by presenting workshops on how to teach IR in modular or course form at annual meetings of professional associations, arranging special conferences in which IR model developers could make presentations and develop a network, and arranging interest group meetings at national conferences. Such interest groups could share practical information on securing grant support for IR research, and on how to prepare interim project reports and knowledge products for publication to assist in quests for tenure and promotion.

Dissemination of IR in modular form at both student and faculty levels should assist in enhancing the potential of IR as one of the most appropriate paradigms for research in the human service fields.

REFERENCES

Achenbach, T., and J. Brown. 1988. *Bibliography of Published Studies Using the Child Behavior Checklist and Related Materials.* Burlington, VT: University of Vermont.

Bae, Im Ho. 1988. Model for the enhancement of participation by victims in Victim-Offender Reconciliation Programs. Unpublished paper. School of Social Work, University of Minnesota.

Blythe, Betty J. and Scott Briar. 1985. Developing empirically based models of practice. *Social Work.* 30, 483-488.

Bonnie, Ed. 1989. Impact of death on latency aged children: Formulation of a clinical intervention. Doctoral dissertation. School of Social Work, University of Minnesota.

Chandy, Joseph. 1988. Model for development of housing for the homeless in India. Unpublished paper. School of Social Work, University of Minnesota.

Chou, Yueh Ching. 1992. Development and testing of a model for assisting families who care for a child with developmental disabilities in Taiwan. Doctoral dissertation. Minneapolis, Minnesota: School of Social Work, University of Minnesota.

Davis, Inger P. and William J. Reid. 1988. Event analysis in clinical practice and process research. *Social Casework.* 69 (May), 298-306.

Edleson, Jeffrey L. 1985. Rapid-assessment instruments for evaluating practice with children and youth. *Journal of Social Service Research.* 8,3, 17-31.

Feld, Sheila and Norma Radin. 1982. *Social Psychology for Social Work and the Mental Health Professions.* New York: Columbia University Press.

Fischer, Joel. 1981. The social work revolution. *Social Work, 26* (3), 199-207.

Giovannoni, Jeanne. 1989. Commentary-intervention research: What's distinctive. Conference on Intervention Research: Research for Practice, UCLA, Los Angeles. March 19-21, 1989.

Gilmore, Kathy. 1988. Facilitating alcoholism education for the elderly. Unpublished paper. School of Social Work, University of Minnesota.

Haj-Yahia, Mohammed. 1988. Contracting model for working with the families of nonvoluntary mentally ill clients in Israel. Unpublished paper. School of Social Work, University of Minnesota.

Hanrahan, Patricia and William J. Reid. 1984. Choosing effective interventions. *Social Service Review,* 58, 244-258.

Kovacs, M. 1983. *The Children's Depression Inventory: A Self-Rated Depression Scale for School-Aged Youngsters.* Unpublished manuscript. Pittsburgh, PA: University of Pittsburgh.

Levitt, John L. and William J. Reid. 1981. Rapid assessment instruments for practice. *Social Work Research & Abstracts,* 17, 13-19.

Macy-Lewis, Jane A. 1985. Single-parent groups. In *Task-Centered Practice with Families and Groups,* edited by Anne E. Fortune. New York: Springer, 92-100.

Marsh, Jeanne C. 1983. Research and innovation in social work practice. Avoiding the headless machine. *Social Service Review,* 57, 582-598.

Mullen, Edward J. 1978. The construction of personal models for effective practice. A method for utilizing research findings to guide social interventions. *Journal of Social Service Research.* 2, 1, 45-63.

Patti, Rino J. 1981. The prospects for social R&D: An essay review. *Social Work Research and Abstracts.* 17, 2, 38-44.

Patti, Rino J. 1989. Commentary–Organizational aspects of intervention research. Conference on Intervention Research: Research for Practice, UCLA, Los Angeles. March 19-21, 1989.

Paine, S. C., G. T. Bellamy, and B. L. Wilcox. (eds.) 1984. *Human Services that Work: From Innovation to Standard Practice.* Baltimore: Paul H. Brookes, 269-277.

Reid, William J. 1977. Social work for social problems. *Social Work,* 23, 374-382.

Reid, William J. 1978. Some Reflections of the Practice Doctorate, *Social Service Review,* 51, 449-455.

Reid, William J. 1979. The model development dissertation, *Journal of Social Service Research,* 3, 2, 215-225.

Reid, William J. 1985. *Family Problem Solving.* New York, Columbia University Press.

Reid, William J. 1987a. Evaluating an intervention in developmental research. *Journal of Social Service Research.* 11, 1, 17-37.

Reid, William J. 1987b. Research in social work. *Encyclopedia of Social Work,* 18th edition, Silver Spring, Maryland: National Association of Social Workers, 477-487. See page 480.

Rogers, E. M. and F. F. Shoemaker. 1971. *Communication of Innovations: A Cross-Cultural Approach.* New York: The Free Press.

Rooney, Ronald H. 1980. Training the generalist who can specialize or the specialist who can do more than one thing. CSWE APM, Los Angeles, April 1980.

Rooney, Ronald H. 1990. Increasing use of intervention research by social work students. Paper presented as part of Intervention Research Network Panel at the Annual Program Meeting, Council on Social Work Education, March 6, 1990, Reno, Nevada.

Rooney, Ronald H. and Marsha Wanless. 1985. A model for caseload management based on task-centered casework, 187-199. In *Task-Centered Practice with Families and Groups,* edited by Anne Fortune. 92-100. New York: Springer Publishing Company.

Rothman, Jack. 1980. *Social R&D: Research and Development in the Human Services.* Englewood Cliffs, NJ: Prentice-Hall.

Rothman, Jack. 1989. Intervention research: Application to runaway and homeless youth. *Social Work Research and Abstracts,* 25, (March), 13-18.

Rothman, Jack, Joseph G. Teresa, and John L. Erlich. 1978. *Fostering Participation and Promoting Innovation.* Itasca, IL: F. E. Peacock.

Thomas, Edwin J. 1978. Mousetraps, developmental research and social work education. *Social Service Review,* 51, 468-483.

Thomas, Edwin J. 1984. *Designing Interventions for the Helping Professions.* Beverly Hills, CA: Sage.

Thomas, Edwin J. 1989. Advances in developmental research. *Social Service Review,* 63, (December), 578-597.

Thomas, Edwin J. and Catherine A. Santa. 1982. Unilateral family therapy for alcohol abuse: A working conception. *American Journal of Family Therapy.* 10, 49-58.

Chapter 16

Afterword–
Competencies for Intervention Research

Edwin J. Thomas
Jack Rothman

The methods of intervention research build upon the traditions of diverse available research and practice modalities. Some of these make a direct contribution to intervention research and may be utilized in existing form. Others need to be modified or reconceptualized for intervention research purposes. A unique character of the intervention research paradigm is the integration and configuring of these established methodologies. To meet these research requirements, the tasks of intervention research call for special combinations of competencies. Which configuration is most appropriate depends upon the tasks to be addressed in the research and the particular facet of intervention research to which the tasks are most closely related.

A wide range of competencies presently appear to be relevant to carrying out the tasks of intervention research. These include (a) knowledge of social science theory and research, (b) knowledge of the specific intervention problem area of the research, (c) general knowledge of human service problems and practice methods, (d) methods of knowledge utilization, (e) D&D methods, and (f) selected special capabilities. Further details and examples of each area of competence are provided in Table 1.

Two types of competence are essential for all aspects of intervention research. One is familiarity with conventional social science theory and research methods applicable to the intervention research area. The other is familiarity with the specific intervention problem area of the research, an applied focus that distinguishes intervention

369

TABLE 1. Areas of competence suggested for the facets of intervention research.

Areas of Competence	Facets of intervention research		
	Knowledge Development (KD)	Knowledge Utilization (KU)	Design and Development (D&D)
Social science theory and methods (social/behavioral theory in the area of the research; and social/behavior science research methods including problem formulation; research strategies, such as case studies, surveys, or experiments; data-gathering procedures, such as questionnaires, interviews, and observation schedules; and analysis procedures, such as coding, scaling, and statistical methods).	Essential	Essential	Essential
Knowledge of the specific intervention problem area of the research (e.g., substance abuse, poverty, domestic violence, crime, delinquency, marital problems, parent-child problems, school difficulties, health behavior).	Essential	Essential	Essential
General knowledge of human service problems and practice methods.	Desirable	Highly Desirable	Highly Desirable
Methods of knowledge utilization (e.g., procedures of information retrieval and review, synthesis, and application; meta-analysis; knowledge dissemination and planned change).		Essential	Essential
D&D methods (e.g., the paradigm of intervention research; D&D methods relating to intervention design, development, evaluation, and dissemination; concepts of D&D, such as developmental validity; and D&D techniques, such as developmental testing, proceduralization, developmental logs and task analysis).		Desirable	Essential

	Facets of intervention research		
Areas of Competence	Knowledge Development (KD)	Knowledge Utilization (KU)	Design and Development (D&D)
Special capabilities (e.g., organizational, administrative, interactional and interorganizational skills; ability to analyze and apply one's own experience; ability to think through and to solve practical problems systematically; ability to observe and obtain data accurately; ability to adhere to new intervention procedures yet be able to appraise their adequacy; dependability and reliability; strong dedication to the developmental mission).			Essential/ Highly Desirable

research from the basic research conducted in the disciplines, which may have no applied relevance.

The different areas of competence are grouped somewhat differently for each of the facets of intervention research. To conduct KD, the essential competencies, of course, are knowledge of social science theory and research and knowledge of the specific intervention problem area of the research. General knowledge of human service problems and practice methods would also be desirable.

Turning to the KU facet, the methods of knowledge utilization would clearly be central. Knowledge of the specific intervention problem area of the research would also be essential as would familiarity with the social science theory and research being drawn on. General knowledge of human service problems and practice methods and the methodology of intervention D&D would again also be desirable.

D&D requires the broadest range of competencies. As indicated in the right-hand column of Table 1, all areas of competence are identified as essential or highly desirable. Foremost, of course, is familiarity with D&D methods, the methodology that has been the main thrust of the approach presented in this book. A number of special capabilities were also identified as essential or highly desirable for D&D, examples of which have been given in the table. While the other areas of intervention research also clearly call for special capabilities, some of these that appear particularly relevant to the successful completion of tasks requiring design and development may not be as obvious and, hence, have been underscored here.

Looking at the D&D competencies further as they relate to the diverse requirements of D&D, a summarizing comprehensive repertoire may embrace the following:

1. Mastery of theoretical and conceptual background knowledge concerning human service problems, social science disciplines, and research methodologies.

2. Ability to identify, define and conceptualize major social and behavioral problems, treatment methods and unresolved issues for intervention modalities.

3. Ability to identify relevant sources of knowledge and information for problem solution (e.g., empirical research, related practice and technology, social innovation), and to retrieve, assess, order, and synthesize their contributions for application purposes.

4. Ability to design innovative intervention strategies and techniques derived from the diverse sources of knowledge and information. This requires familiarity with social science and related data, with treatment and related technology, and a capacity to relate one to the other in new and potentially productive ways. It necessitates knowledge of the methodology of intervention design.

5. Ability to engage in development processes, that is, to operationalize appropriate intervention procedures, to submit them to pilot and developmental testing, to revise and proceduralize them as appropriate and to come up with innovative, field tested interventions.

6. Ability to employ multiple methodologies in development and evaluation—needs assessments; quantitative and qualitative approaches; basic research methods; single-case experimental designs; group- and quasi-experimental designs; measurement

instruments and practice related recording procedures; developmental practice and methods of proceduralization; diverse techniques, such as those of human service practice (e.g., treatment planning), task analysis and flowcharting; and selected aspects of program evaluation now employed for assessing, modifying and developing interventions in a phased D&D sequence.

7. Ability to work cooperatively in practice settings, to gain the support of practitioners and other agency actors, and to handle the politics of field research generally and of outcome evaluation in particular.

8. Ability to communicate research results differentially both to the scientific community and to the community of professional practitioners and administrators.

The skills required by intervention researchers in D&D are thus broad and varied. Fortunately, since projects are generally conducted on a team basis in an organizational setting, skills can be distributed among several different individuals and do not need to be concentrated in a single person.

Systematic training for the different competencies is a requisite for advancing this work. Training encompassing the competencies outlined in this discussion and reflected in this book is a vital necessity for expanding effective human service technology. We do not minimize the complexity implied in mounting such training or of the work that still needs to be done on the methods of intervention research. However, as conceptual and methodological progress in intervention research is achieved, the need for appropriate training becomes more salient and a critical focal point for further attention.

APPENDIXES:
ILLUSTRATIVE PRACTICE TOOLS–
DESIGN AND DEVELOPMENT
PRODUCTS OF INTERVENTION
RESEARCH

Appendix A

Fostering Participation
and Promoting Innovation–
Handbook for Human Service
Professionals

Jack Rothman
Joseph G. Teresa
John L. Erlich

INTRODUCTION

Mental health professionals realize that they cannot serve families and individuals in a vacuum. In an increasingly còmplex and interdependent environment, family services must consider social conditions that strain family life, and community forces that aid family unity and strength.

A group of mental health specialists meeting at Boston University stated the matter squarely:

> Increasingly, the mental health professions are delivering services to the community–not just responding to the onset of

The research that produced this procedural practice guide is described in Jack Rothman, John L. Erlich, and Joseph G. Teresa *Promoting Innovation and Change in Organizations and Communities: A Planning Manual*. New York: John Wiley and Sons, 1976. Also in Jack Rothman, Joseph G. Teresa, and John L. Erlich, *Developing Effective Strategies of Social Intervention: A Research and Development Methodology*. PB-272454 TR-1-RD, National Technical Information Service, Springfield, VA, 1977. Issued originally by F. E. Peacock Publishers, Itasca, Illinois, 1978. Out of Print. Reprinted by permission of F. E. Peacock Publishers.

pathology. A broad spectrum of professional activity is emerging, generally characterized as community mental health. It involves active participation in community affairs on the part of mental health personnel, preventive intervention at the community level, and collaboration with responsible laymen in reducing community tensions. Consultant services are being offered to the institutions of the community and new methods are being developed for working with and through other professional groups in support of mental health. The community itself is being taught to collaborate in creating health-giving environments.

Gerald Caplan and Henry Grunebaum, leading community mental health theorists, point out the centrality of family integration here:

> Intervention should support the integrity of the family in its own home and should prevent its fragmentation.

A wide range of programs has been developed within this broadened framework of service. For example:

- Family and Child Advocacy Programs (social legislation, child advocacy councils)
- Family life education (shifting family roles, discipline, understanding feelings)
- Consultation to primary care-giving institutions (such as schools and community centers)
- Special services to high risk populations (minorities, preschoolers, the mentally retarded, the aging)
- Mobilizing community resources to assist families (coordination, general health care)
- Halfway houses and community placement (preparing patients for transition back into home and community)
- Support of natural, informal care-giving systems (neighborhood groups, opinion leaders)
- Outreach and decentralized services (hotlines, crisis intervention)

• Encouraging meaningful community participation and problem solving by families (social action, creative use of leisure).

Purpose of this Handbook

The above initiatives require skills and strategies that are not often found in standard clinical and casework practice. A deficit in such skills has thwarted many well-intentioned mental health and family service professionals.

This handbook will offer you two fundamental sets of skills: fostering participation in your agency (clients, staff members) or in the community (residents public officials, other agencies) through the principle of *relevant benefits* (rewarding desired behavior); promoting a new service or program in your agency or community through the principle of *partialization* (starting with a small group and spreading to a larger one).

These intervention strategies are basic for gaining the involvement of key parties such as clients, colleagues, or community agencies, and for setting up innovative programs, such as outreach or advocacy. In addition to expressing commonsensical ideas, the principles are consistent with experience in systems intervention. As will be shown, they are supported by basic research. Among the many tools in the professional's kit, these two may be drawn upon frequently.

Practical Advice Derived from Research

This handbook was developed over a six-year period at The University of Michigan, through a research grant by the National Institute of Mental Health. The intervention principles ("Action Guidelines") resulted from an exhaustive search of the social science research literature. They were field tested and made operational by human service professionals in a variety of agencies (community mental health, family service, schools, courts, planning councils, etc.). Based on the field experience a working manual was composed, refined, and streamlined to produce this handbook. In the problems and actions described, we will concentrate on the experience in community mental health and family service settings, although examples from other agency situations will be introduced when useful.

How to Use the Handbook

Different readers may use the handbook in different ways. Some users may be able to employ the Action Guidelines with full autonomy within their existing assignments, for example, increasing the extent of client or community participation in a regular family life education program. In other cases, where a totally new program, such as family advocacy or a community residence, is the aim, the cooperation or approval of agency colleagues, administrators, or the board may be necessary.

This handbook is not meant to be a conventional textbook. Rather, the concepts will best be understood through an attempt to apply them.

Each chapter contains a "Getting Started" section. Here we pose a series of questions to help you through the planning phase. An "Initial Log" form (in two parts) is provided for noting your preliminary thoughts. The emphasis is on specifying realistic and short-term goals and clear means to reach them. Examples from the field study may aid in filling out the form.

Feel free to read the chapters in alternate order, to "skip around" as you read, and to write your own notes in the margins. Later, a second reading should help to solidify your understanding. On implementing either (or both) of the Action Guidelines, the manual should be returned to as a periodic reference.

Limitations and Capabilities

This handbook is not a technical blueprint. It offers a general strategic direction to achieve an objective which you define. You cannot expect to proceed step by step in cookbook fashion, as in baking a pie. Sensitivity, judgment, creativity, and moral choice on the part of the user are essential.

Furthermore, the handbook is not intended as an all-inclusive diagnostic and problem-solving tool. It must be supplemented by other approaches and materials. For the purposes of systems diagnosis, a variety of supplementary sources may be tapped. See the bibliography for some especially helpful references.

The handbook is designed to be of use to a variety of direct service practitioners (social workers, psychologists, psychiatrists, psychiatric nurses), as well as administrative and supervisory personnel in mental health and family service agencies. In this text the "practitioner" is understood to be the user of the guideline, regardless of his agency position.

Our experience with a wide range of professionals suggests that this material can be used successfully. If you apply the guidelines with care, your "unattainable" objectives may well come within reach.

FOSTERING PARTICIPATION

Introduction to the Problem

The promotion of positive mental health is closely connected to active and meaningful *participation*. Clients must be motivated to participate in programs, such as family life education or drop-in centers. The open support of fellow staff members can enhance agency work in outreach or family advocacy services. The involvement of volunteers can expand community placement programs or crisis walk-in centers. The cooperation of additional community agencies may be vital for mobilizing appropriate resources and for engaging in preventive efforts, such as pre-care and community education.

The value of participation in the mental health field is evident. There remains, however, the vital question of how to get people to attend, join up, speak out, work on a committee, or lend support.

A school social worker faced this kind of practical problem:

> The mothers' program began in October and ultimately involved nine mothers–seven tutoring and two helping with the materials center. In April, the teacher in charge of the program sought my assistance. Two mothers had recently dropped out of the program, and only three mothers were attending their general meetings.

Conclusions of Research

Findings of recent research on participation (see the bibliography) can be summarized in this generalization:

> The amount of voluntary participation in an organization depends on the benefits gained from participation, and the degree to which the benefits are shown to result directly from participation.

The Action Guideline

The concept of benefit provision suggests the following Action Guideline:

> To foster participation in organizations, programs, or task groups, practitioners should provide or increase relevant benefits.

The term "participation" in the guideline should be interpreted in a broad sense. The term is meant to include not only the recruitment of new members, but also changes in the patterns of existing members' participation. For example, an individual who had merely attended an activity might shoulder responsibilities or become an officer.

Many professionals intuitively use benefits as a tool in their work, and the guideline may seem an obvious statement. However, we are trying to make this common approach more explicit and more systematic so that it may have a greater impact on participation in programs and services. Though derived from an independent literature source, the guideline is related to certain learning theory or behavior modification concepts, as we will discuss shortly.

Types of Benefits

Benefits may be described as either *instrumental* or *expressive*. Instrumental benefits provide material, tangible, task-oriented returns, such as getting an increased welfare allotment or new equipment for the agency. Expressive benefits are intangible and psychological in character, such as increased friendships, personal satisfaction, or pride. Further distinctions may be made within the two categories.

1. *Instrumental benefits* may be:
   a. *material*–obtaining a loan or grant, securing needed information or authorization, etc.
   b. *anticipatory*–setting up an action structure, or obtaining a verbal commitment as a partial achievement toward the material gain.
2. *Expressive benefits* may be:
   a. *interpersonal*–making new friends, having an enjoyable social experience, etc.
   b. *symbolic*–receiving an award which represents public approval or recognition of an individual's participatory activities, being mentioned in a newspaper article, etc.

In practice, these approaches are often used in combination; sometimes one is given special emphasis and supplemented by others.

Illustrations of Benefits from Practice

Here are descriptions of how professionals used the four different types of relevant benefits with different groups:

(1) Instrumental Benefits: Material

Our community mental health program in the housing project was floundering. I had been working with a few residents in the project to develop a self-help group. When our efforts faltered, I decided to use the guideline with the goal of increasing participation in group meetings.

We elected to increase benefits by resolving specific problems for each family; for example, getting free roach spray from the manager (he usually charged residents), getting a toilet repaired, obtaining special educational attention for certain children, and transporting families to the dentist. At the same time we saw the families individually and informally, and decreased the number of group meetings from weekly to biweekly to "on call." In a sense, elimination of unnecessary meetings was another reward. On a group level, when tenants ran into rent disagreements with the management, we set up contacts with Legal Aid.

Eventually we called the group together, and then personally visited those who did not come suggesting that we could not continue to help them unless they attended the group sessions! It worked. By providing concrete benefits and by making them depend upon participation, the group began to function again.

(2) Instrumental Benefits: Anticipatory

I used this guideline to help organize the Black Student Union at the junior high school. The kids had come to me for help because of my role as program director at the local community center.

We called a meeting in which the students identified the areas for union concern, and set up appropriate committees supervised by my staff. The organization devised plans for a Black History Week. This effort enabled the student union to develop a program with a large number of black students participating.

This satisfying action structure achieved, the group proceeded to establish broader goals and 1 was able to withdraw my staff.

(3) Expressive Benefits: Interpersonal

By employing the guideline, I was able to increase participation in our district-wide organization of secondary students. Meeting with their steering committee, I suggested that the group might enjoy a weekend "retreat." When the school agreed to cover part of the expenses, I proceeded to plan the excursion. The event was a definite success: the students interacted socially and looked forward to meeting one another again.

The eventual effect was that our regular attendance nearly doubled, and previously inactive members became more vital participants.

(4) Expressive Benefits: Symbolic

As a school-community agent, I desired to increase community participation in the school and to improve services to children through volunteer help. Special classes were decided upon according to the interests of the students and volunteers. These included: arts and crafts, cooking, crochet, dramatics, modern dance, and sewing.

The participation guideline gave continuity to the program. I provided recognition for the volunteers by working toward a presentation of activity "products" at the end of the program, offering service awards, and providing publicity. I requested that a regular PTO meeting be rescheduled for the final presentation, in order to reach a large number of community people. The program met with great success: the volunteers and students both wanted to repeat it for another six-week session.

The Pattern of Implementation

We have found that one general pattern was followed in all the cases in our field tests. This pattern consists of five steps:

1. goal determination
2. selection of benefits to be used
3. initial contact with potential participants
4. follow-up contact with potential participants
5. delivery of benefits, or operation of the event

We will consider each of these steps in turn.

(1) Goal Determination

The first step is to select the goal of participation. In our experience, the guideline was used to form new groups or to maintain or increase participation in existing groups. Here are illustrations of these objectives, as stated by participants in the field study:

> My goal is to increase the number of participants in the Mental Health Association's annual chapter leadership workshop.

> My goal is to get the Welfare Rights Organization groups in the area to participate in securing an Early Preventive Screening, Diagnosis, and Treatment program for their local communities.

My goal is to maintain the current level of participation in the mothers' tutoring program in the school, and to increase the number who attend the group meetings.

(2) Selection of Relevant Benefits

The selection of relevant benefits for increasing participation is apparently a two-stage process. First, the practitioner must identify the benefits available; second, the benefits must be matched to the target population. (If the practitioner has access to ample resources, it may be possible to reverse the order of these steps.)

In our experience, the majority of the practitioners who used the participation guideline provided multiple benefits. Most chose a combination of instrumental and expressive benefits, frequently combining material and interpersonal rewards.

(3) Initial Contact with Potential Participants

The method used for the initial contact varied according to the nature of the target system. The major difference in approach lay in the ease with which the potential membership could be identified and located, and in the degree to which the practitioner was in day-to-day contact with that membership. The types of initial contacts varied, ranging from direct personal conversations and telephone discussions, to flyers, mailings, and notices in the newspapers.

(4) Follow-Up Contact with Potential Participants

Practitioners in our study tended to use a different medium for the recontact than was used for the initial contact. When the potential membership was individually identifiable, the contact and follow-up were usually by formal letter or memo in alternation with an informal conversation, either face to face or by telephone. When the potential membership was diffusive or broadly defined, practitioners tended to use a different form of mass media for the recontact stage than they had used for the initial contact. The value of newspapers, radio, or television in supplementing handbills and posters should be considered. Note that a variation in the follow-up medium is not a necessity; it is simply a common practice.

(5) Delivery of Benefits

The actual delivery of the promised benefits is particularly important. When the benefits are in the form of a social event, the practitioner should oversee the proper operation of the event.

Several professionals in our study developed contingency plans, so that if one benefit turned out to be unavailable, another could be substituted. If the benefits were interpersonal, the worker had to expend more energy during an event. Other types of benefits, particularly material, required greater effort prior to an event. Generally speaking, the less control workers had over the delivery of the rewards, the more active the workers were, often using multiple and contingency approaches.

Ideas from Behavior Modification

Readers may have recognized this reward (or reinforcement) principle as an element of behavior modification. Although behaviorist concepts have not been generally directed to systems intervention, a few ideas and terms are relevant to community and organizational work. While the concepts may be familiar to some readers, their application to social systems will be new. We believe that these behaviorist ideas can be used without any coercion to foster voluntary participation.

Behavior Specification: It is essential that the user specify the exact nature of the behavior to be changed. In the case of participation, we may be attempting to increase:

1. *rate:* the frequency with which an individual attends meetings, programs, etc.
2. *form:* the type or quality of participation, that is, attendance, committee chairmanship, making financial or other material contributions, speaking up at meetings, etc.
3. *duration:* the extent of participation over a period of time
4. *variability:* the stability or regularity of participation

The assumption is that different types of benefits may be effective in encouraging different aspects of participation behavior.

Positive Reinforcement: This refers to benefits contingent upon the performance of some desired behavior. The clinician or caseworker has certain direct reinforcers available in relationships with clients. These include approval, attention, and affection. In a group or community context, these rewards may be offered to one individual through other individuals. In classroom situations the following positive reinforcements have been suggested; information regarding performance ("Your answer is correct"); material rewards (good grades, refreshments); and opportunity to encourage in preferred behaviors (personal selection of preferred study subjects). In human service community work the agency's resources offer varied reinforcement possibilities, as do those external community resources with which the agency has operating ties. The trick is to locate these, recognize their reward potentials and make them available.

Contracting: There has been increasing use of this concept in settings such as schools and community mental health programs. A practitioner might come to an agreement about a level of participation, which, if followed for a designated time, could result in a desired outcome. For example, contracting was used in the issuance of a certificate to leaders who completed the six-week volunteer service session in the school-community example cited earlier.

Shaping: This involves a series of sequential goals leading up to a long-range objective. In an organizational context, one might speak of "interim goals." As a hypothetical example, a community worker wants a woman to take on an appointive office; the worker starts by asking her to attend a committee, then later asks her to chair a committee, and finally to hold an office.

Group Contingencies: Benefits may be offered to groups as well as to individuals. The United Fund offers a great number of social and symbolic rewards to volunteers who achieve their goals, often using graphs and charts to dramatize the group objective. A committee or organization might set certain goals or standards for participation, and foster group satisfactions for successful attainment.

Problems of Executing the Guideline Strategy

Our field staff encountered some difficulties implementing the guideline, and they made a variety of suggestions.

First of all, they pointed out that the benefits selected must have real significance for the target group. One worker stated:

> I had to be sure that the benefits were really viewed as worthy by the group members. Without this, the whole thing would have failed.

Another noted that:

> The benefits must be perceived as important by participants. The benefits could be potential as well as actual.

The need for interim, short-range benefits to sustain motivation was also stressed.

> I often feel that a long-range goal is achievable but a group may not be able to keep that goal in sight–or even to agree with it at that stage of the game.

> Because of existing power relationships in society, low income persons lack the clout to make rapid gains or to resolve their pressing problems. This means that their participation must be sustained while they struggle with those problems. The structuring of participation to provide expressive experiences and immediate social gratification permits this. Those of us who are highly issue oriented tend to forget or neglect that. We dare not!

Many workers highlighted the difficulties of choosing appropriate benefits.

> Since instrumental or expressive rewards vary by individual and by situation, the determination of rewards was a problem. Also, it was not within my power to assure delivery of all the benefits which might have reinforced participation.

Guaranteeing the benefits was the most difficult aspect of this approach.

I think that a practitioner who promises only expressive benefits, without any instrumental rewards, is fighting an uphill battle.

Getting Started

(1) Think of some existing family-related problem in your agency situation that could be aided through increased or improved participation (by clients, other agencies, staff members, etc.). A glance at the listing of programs on page 3 in the introduction may suggest some options.

(2) Specify the nature of participation behavior that you will be dealing with in your intervention and the direction in which you would like to change it. For example, will you be dealing with:

recruitment

retention or maintenance

increasing the rate of participation

changing the form of participation

(attendance, membership, committee participation, volunteer work, officership, contributions)

stabilizing or varying the pattern of participation

(3) Try to select relevant benefits which are both attractive to target groups and available for you to deliver. What types of benefits would be effective in stimulating the desired participation? consider:

Instrumental:

material

anticipatory

Expressive:

interpersonal

symbolic

Consider multiple rewards. Get to know your group. Observe them; ask them about their likes; ask other experienced professionals. What types of benefits are available to you? Consider such sources as:

your personal relations

agency resources and good will (the board, volunteers)

agency links with external resources

the group itself

(4) Decide whether some special reinforcement technique may be applied, such as:

shaping

contracting

group contingency

Don't let these get in your way, however. Use them only if they are applicable and potentially useful in your situation.

(5) Consider ways of making benefits known and available to the relevant target group.

(6) Carry out the guideline. Don't forget follow-up contact.

(7) Try to assess the results of your work. Specify real indicators of change in participation. These may include such factors as:

change in specific number of persons at meetings

changes in number and/or percentage of dropouts from programs

increase or decrease in the number of individuals who collaborate by taking responsibility

Initial Log Form–Part I

As a further step toward getting started, we suggest now that you write down your tentative thoughts regarding implementation of the guideline. The Initial Log is a tool for organizing your thinking. It has proved valuable to the professionals taking part in our field tests. Following the Log form are illustrations of key sections that they completed.

INITIAL LOG

1. Date of preparation: _____

2. In relation to the guideline, what is your proximate goal (i.e., type or amount of participation)? Be as specific as possible. The goal should be moderate and short-range: something that can be accomplished in a five- to twelve-week period.

3. Describe the circumstances (conditions, assignments, events, requests, etc.) which led you to use this guideline to achieve your proximate goal.

4. Look back at the intervention guideline. How would you begin to define each element of the guideline in your immediate situation? (How might you operationalize these components?)

    (a) What is your proximate participation goal?
        Indicate *current* level of participation: _____

        Indicate *intended* level of participation: _____

        Within what time period: _____

    (b) What benefits will you offer?
        Instrumental
            material: _____
            anticipatory: _____
        Expressive
            interpersonal: _____
            symbolic: _____

5. How will you deliver these benefits? (Are they available to you? Do you control their use or can you obtain a measure of control? Have you contingency benefits available?)

6. List the major steps you anticipate taking in order to use this guideline.

_____

_____

_____

_____

_____

_____

SAMPLE INITIAL LOG ENTRIES

I. Example of a Community Mental Health Program in a Public Housing Project (Family Agency)

A. *Goal Statement* (Log item 2)
My goal is to increase tenant participation in our biweekly group meetings on "Y" Court in the Public Housing Project from five families to ten families.

B. *Operationalization of the Guideline Elements* (Log item 4)
Increase participation in organizations, programs, or task groups:
Increase tenant participation in our group meetings on "Y" Court in the Public Housing Project.

Provide (or increase) appropriate benefits:
I will try to do this by seeing that specific problems of each attending family are resolved. These might include: repairing faulty plumbing; obtaining free roach spray; serving as an advocate for children having school difficulty, and so forth.

II. Example of a Black Student Union in a Junior High School

A. *Goal Statement* (Log item 2)
My goal is to set up a black student organization which will be responsive to the needs of black students and will not be controlled by the school administration.

B. *Operationalization of the Guideline Elements* (Log item 4)
Increase participation in organizations, programs, or task groups:
Boost the average monthly committee attendance of black students from fifteen to twenty-five.

Provide (or increase) appropriate benefits:
I will try to do this by having a committee of black students organize a Black History Week program. This should encourage participation in the student organization and its committees.

Practical Advice Derived from the Field Study

The personal resources of the practitioner are his most effective tools. These include: selecting appropriate benefits, announcing them, motivating people, and delivering both interpersonal and material rewards.

It is advisable to choose a goal and a strategy that are consistent with (or which can be enhanced by) your experience and position in the agency. Choose a goal about which you have conviction and enthusiasm.

With regard to your agency situation, seek a goal that will fit in with your other assignments, and attempt to gain whatever support you can from fellow staff members and agency administrators. Try to locate suitable physical facilities, or plan a program that fits the available facilities.

Choose a program that will be of specific interest to clients, or work hard at developing their interests. It helps if you choose a group of clients who are receptive to your agency and the program; attempt to build this kind of receptivity as you proceed.

Try to clarify your personal goals and assignments in the agency, so that you are free to concentrate on this task without heavy pressure from other demands or without the neglect of other assignments. Lack of staff and resources may impede you; selection of a feasible objective is an important strategic consideration.

Several field workers warned that the intervention cannot be carried out in a mechanical, ritualistic manner. The art of practice has to shape the science of any intervention strategy. This involves the practitioner's attitudes, interpersonal skills, sense of timing, etc. As two of them advised us:

> There is a need to develop trust and a decent relationship with client groups. This takes time and demonstrated proof that you can deliver.

> There is the consideration of the personal qualities of members, as well as the level of enthusiasm conveyed by the practitioners.

More specific observations were offered:

> I found little difficulty in using this guideline. The only problem was self-imposed: a limited time in which to develop the offered benefits.

> One difficulty was my lack of information about the community I was working in. Insufficient time forced me to form a group before I had adequate community information.

> Do not burden the staff or clientele by trying to solve the problem in one day.

> The phone conversations proved to be crucial to the success of this guideline. Through these personal contacts, we were able to respond to the needs and concerns of those to whom we spoke.

> I ran into the usual organizational interferences. Too many complicated chains of communication hindered the application of a simple idea.

Realize also that clients and community people will have other activities that compete for their time and interests. The benefits you offer must be strong enough to gain their attention and capture their motivation. Clients and residents may lack knowledge of the organization or may not possess certain skills for adequate participation. You may need to make up these deficits as you continue.

Initial Log Form–Part II

As a final planning aid, you should consider the key community groups and individuals that may support your efforts. You should also think about the factors which will affect your progress. We have provided checklists of common *facilitating factors*, those which will assist you to carry out the guideline, and typical *limiting factors*, those which may inhibit your success. As an aid to planning, we have listed conditions which were frequently singled out by practitioners in the field study. Check any factors that apply to your own situation.

What key community groups, if any, will you probably involve?

Group   Reason for contact

_____   _____

_____   _____

_____   _____

_____   _____

_____   _____

What key individuals, if any, will you probably involve?

Individuals   Title and/or affiliation   Reason for contact

_____   _____   _____

_____   _____   _____

_____   _____   _____

_____   _____   _____

_____   _____   _____

_____   _____   _____

PERSONAL FACTORS

Facilitating

☐ Good personal relationships with staff.

☐ Good personal relationships with clients.

☐ Personal commitment to the agency.

☐ Personal commitment to the program.

☐ Personal commitment to the guideline.

☐ Personal knowledge of the community.

☐ Peronal knowledge of the programs.

☐ Personal knowledge of the relevant ideology (and theory).

☐ Personal gain (promotion, job title, etc.).

☐ Prior experience.

☐ Self-confidence.

☐ Other:_____

_____

Limiting

☐ Personal knowledge of clients.

☐ Personal position or role.

☐ Personal loss (demotion, job title, etc.).

☐ Impatience.

☐ Other:_____

_____

AGENCY FACTORS

Facilitating	*Limiting*
☐ Affiliated organizational support or involvement.	☐ Unclear or shifting goals, programs, or assignments.
☐ Board support or involvement.	☐ Hindering structure of the organization.
☐ Administration support or involvement.	☐ Negative agency attitudes toward the clients or community.
☐ Supervisor support or involvement.	☐ Practitioner-organization conflict.
☐ Supervisor disinterest.	☐ Lack of staff or training.
☐ Practitioner assignments are consistent with effort.	☐ Lack of funds, facilities, or other resources.
☐ Physical facilities aid the effort.	☐ Lack of support of supervisor.
☐ Other: _____	☐ Lack of support of staff.
	☐ Other: _____

CLIENT FACTORS

Facilitating

☐ Client disinterst or dissatisfaction with the agency or program, leading to a desire for change.

☐ Other: _____

Limiting

☐ Client disinterest or dissatisfaction with the agency or its activities.

☐ Client specifically disinterested in your program.

☐ Client lack of knowledge about the organization, its purpose, programs, or activities.

☐ Clients interfere with organization activities.

☐ Pressure from clients.

☐ Dissension among clients.

☐ Other:_____

COMMUNITY FACTORS

Facilitating

☐ Community receptivity to your organization or program.

☐ Support of (influential) community groups for your organization or program.

☐ External influences making the community support your organization or program.

☐ Community support of the practitioner.

☐ Other: _____

Limiting

☐ Community residents lack necessary knowledge or skills.

☐ Community residents interfere with organization activities.

☐ Other activities compete for the time and interest of residents.

☐ Community lacks funds needed to support your organization or program.

☐ Other: _____

PROMOTING AN INNOVATION

Introduction to the Problem

The mental health field is dedicated to new ways of serving individuals, strengthening families, and creating more humane communities. Innovation is a distinguishing mark of the field. Mental health professionals are constantly faced with the challenge of producing new programs, new services, new attitudes in the organizations and communities they serve.

An innovation may be any new programs service, or idea, the target of which is a social group or population. The professional may deal with an innovation that is entirely new, or one that is already established elsewhere and is new only to the particular location or context.

Professionals are often overwhelmed when attempting to introduce innovations. The task may seem too large or the time available too restrictive. A youth guidance worker described her innovation and its obstacles as follows:

> I had been working with pregnant girls who attended our community center. As a member of the School-Age Parent Program Committee, I discovered that the girls were having a very limited educational experience in the public schools. Many had given up hoping for any kind of future after high school. They needed help in planning for themselves, and they needed special skills to carry out their ambitions.

> I became convinced that a more substantial guidance program was necessary. But I took no specific steps because: (1) I knew that I would have to face administrative resistance from the secondary education bureaucracy; and (2) a great deal of my own time would be required.

Perhaps you have faced similar problems in your own practice. The innovation guideline is directed to such difficulties.

Conclusions of Research

From a number of studies on the diffusion of innovations (see the bibliography), we have drawn this generalization:

Innovations which can be tried on a partial basis are more likely to succeed than innovations which require total adoption without a preliminary trial.

This concept, termed "partialization," stresses the advantage of displaying an innovation in a preliminary small-scale demonstration. The innovation is more likely to be adopted by a general target group if they can first witness its successful performance in a smaller segment of that group.

There are many examples of this approach to the mental health field. Specialized programs for community care givers (such as clergymen) are often begun on a small scale. The same is true for the use of paraprofessionals: a start is made in one program area, say home treatment, with the hope that it will spread to other areas. Drop-in programs for recently released patients are usually begun on a trial basis. Most of the services designed to be alternatives to institutionalization have followed this pattern.

A detailed illustration of the concept is provided by a study of how the "new math" joined the curriculum of schools in Allegheny County, Pennsylvania. A group of five superintendents who had close association with one another introduced the new approach in 1959. As a result of their example and their contacts with other superintendents, another ten schools adopted the new math in 1960. Still another twelve schools were added in 1961; and by the end of 1963, thirty-eight schools were employing this altogether different method of teaching mathematics. This snowball effect can be found in the spreading of many innovations.

Proximate Goals

Related to the principle of partialization is the vital concept of *proximate goals*. These are moderate, tangible objectives that can be attained in the short term. In the new math illustration, a partial target group of five superintendents initiated the innovation. A proximate general target system of ten additional schools accepted this method in the next year. Those fifteen can be considered a new partial target group, as the basis for reaching the next proximate stage. (Visualize a rippling effect resulting from throwing a pebble into a pond.) Some targets may be of small enough scale to be considered proximates.

The Action Guideline

The idea of partialization suggests the following Action Guideline:

> To promote an innovation in a general target system, first develop the innovation in a limited portion of the target system.

The guideline directs the practitioner to single out a limited or "partial target" group with which to begin. This provides an initial leverage on what might otherwise be an overwhelming task.

This stepping-stone procedure is particularly useful with the following considerations:

- The innovation should be reasonably legitimate and non-controversial. (Otherwise a more political power strategy may be necessary.)
- The innovation should be a process which is not easily reversible once begun.
- Scale is important: you may have little information about the value or cost of a large-scale implementation; or the cost of a large-scale effort may be high, while the limited demonstration may be relatively inexpensive.
- A large-scale application might alert and mobilize the opposition, but a small-scale one would not.
- If the larger population has little or no receptivity to the innovation, confronting them all at once may be self-defeating.

Depending on the innovation and how it is apt to be transmitted, either of two basic partial groups may be recommended:

(1) Similar Values. Communication may be facilitated when the general and partial target groups possess similarities of outlook, social status, or education. If the innovation will be spread by word of mouth or individual contacts, there may be more comfort and trust among people who are similar, and messages are more likely to be transmitted accurately.

(2) Opinion Leaders. New ideas often enter a system through higher status, more sophisticated opinion leaders. These individuals are distinguished by their greater education, media exposure, higher contact with the change agent, and openness to innovative ideas. These characteristics may be sought in a partial target population, particularly one using mass communications as the medium of transmittal.

The selection of an appropriate partial target system is crucial. The partial system chosen should improve the innovation's chances for success. As an example, an organizer in a welfare workers' union wanted to introduce a plan for bringing the union's programs to the individual building level. He considered several factors in choosing an initial target building:

> I was able to employ the following elements in selecting a target subpopulation:
>
> Geographical location
>
> History of organizational activity (how long the people had been relating to each other organizationally)
>
> Leadership (both actual and potential) within the partial target population
>
> Skill and experience within the target population

The following chart illustrates four innovation promotions, demonstrating how practitioners have applied the ideas of a general target system and a partial target system. The chart also indicates the mechanisms by which the transfer was made from the smaller to the larger target system. Such transfer mechanisms ordinarily involve a board of directors, a policy committee, or an agency unit with responsibility for decisions on program matters.

SETTING:	INNOVATION:	GENERAL TARGET:
A community mental health center in a semi-rural county.	Stimulate local unions to accept the function of community care givers for their members.	All 200 local unions in the county.
Traditional settlement house serving a largely black population.	Introducing an intensive educational focus into a program that had been essentially recreational.	Entire school age membership of the settlement house.
A regional planning council serving several counties.	Have the planning council gain responsibility for advising HUD on housing applications from all regional municipalities.	All 30 municipalities in the region.
A social welfare employees union in a metropolitan community.	Decentralize program implementation through building level unit committees.	All 25 building level units in the union: the total membership.

PROXIMATE (short-run) TARGET:	PARTIAL TARGET:	TRANSFER MECHANISM:
Fifty unions from around the county.	A limited number of union members and leaders participated in a workshop on community care giving–including ten unions.	The county-wide (all-inclusive) AFL-CIO Labor Education Committee voted sponsorship of a follow-up workshop to be offered to all county locals.
The same as general target.	A group of 20 teen members were involved in two educational counseling sessions.	Board of directors voted an allocation for hiring an educational director to serve the membership.
12 municipalities with whom practitioners have had positive previous contact.	With HUD approval, reviewed and assessed trial applications from four municipalities.	HUD approved review procedure for all municipality applications.
Six units in a contiguous area.	Shop stewards at a single building location were involved successfully in union program implementation functions.	The union executive board instituted a policy of building level program implementation.

Patterns of Implementation

Two basic patterns have been observed in the actual application of the guideline. (Other refinements will be discussed later.) The first pattern, a "Direct Flow" model, works as follows:

PRACTITIONERS → PARTIAL TARGET →
PROXIMATE TARGET

Here the action flows from the practitioner to the partial target system to the proximate target system. This pattern is typical of the agricultural extension approach in which a farmer is motivated by the worker to use a new seed. He is successful, his neighbors see the results, and they plant the same seed. In the direct flow model, the proximate target population accepts the innovation directly.

The second pattern is a "Decision-Making Unit" model:

PRACTITIONER → PARTIAL TARGET →
DECISION-MAKING UNIT → PROXIMATE TARGET

In this pattern, the action moves from the practitioner to the partial target system to a relevant decision-making unit (such as a board of directors or policy committee), and only then to the proximate target system. This process typically is used in organizational situations. In the decision-making unit arrangement, a transfer mechanism authorizes the passage from the smaller to the larger group.

There are many variations on this model. Sometimes the practitioner needs initial approval from a supervisor. In some cases there are two decision-making units involved. Some practitioners arrange to have the decision makers experience the demonstration directly, as in holding a conference for board members at which a new technique is employed.

Examples from the Field Test

Our field staff followed both of the basic patterns. The direct flow model was illustrated by the president of a social workers' union who wished to set up a training program for his executive board. He desired to teach them a new method in which case examples and the sharing of personal experiences would be used to deal with grievances more effectively. He obtained approval from the board to begin the process.

I then selected four board members to participate on the committee. They each agreed to present a case example for the meeting.

I chaired the committee meeting, suggested the rationale for the model to be used, and assumed responsibility for following up on specific tasks. The committee decided to conduct the training session before the board, following the format of the committee meeting. Individual contacts were made to publicize the event. The model was used at the training session, and the response was very favorable. The board had directly seen and experienced what I was trying to get across.

The proximate target system, the executive board, participated in the training session with positive evaluative comments: "We were able to share problems in a new way"; "It was helpful to know that other people had some of the same problems."

The key suggestion at the training session was that the next target system could be the general membership, with the same model being applied.

The decision-making unit pattern was followed by family service worker, who was attempting to develop the concept of outreach services. She believed the agency should work directly with clients in a low-income housing project, rather than expecting them (or middle-class substitutes) to come to the agency office. The problem was to convince the agency board to provide this type of service, and to persuade the housing manager to accept it within the project.

My use of the guideline involved a small group of residents living on a court in a low-cost housing project. We were able to convince the Housing Authority that social intervention could make a difference in the social problems of the housing project–that we could reduce the social causes for eviction. We selected one court (five families) out of the entire project as a demonstration. We set up a time limit for evaluative purposes; we promised progress reports at specific intervals; and we met with the residents regularly, and sometimes "dropped in" as well. This plan was submitted in writing to the board along with my periodic progress reports.

The plan worked almost too well; it was constantly referred to in agency board meetings. The outreach idea was new here, but it so impressed the board and the housing director, that it was accepted as a legitimate and appropriate agency program. The results with the residents were not as spectacular, but did constitute a beginning, and we gradually expanded to other courts.

In practice, the majority of cases require a formal decision-making unit to foster or legitimate the spread of the innovation. This is because many human service workers are organizationally based and require formal procedures to institute new programs.

Degrees of Effort

As we have seen (in the social work union training example), the partial target may do the actual "selling" to the broader target group, while the worker remains in the background.

In other instances, the worker may be highly energetic in the transfer. This was true in the example of the youth guidance worker quoted at the beginning. After demonstrating an intensive guidance program for unwed mothers within one high school, she worked hard to introduce the same format throughout the school system:

I now had to involve additional individuals and groups. I proceeded to develop a proposal and arrange for meetings with the following: my center's board of directors, the school-age parents advisory board, Episcopal officials, school administrators, teachers, and students.

After many meetings we were able to gain administrative approval and a verbal commitment for funding of the program.

"Product" Innovations vs. "Process" Innovations

Some professionals attempted to introduce a fairly concrete, detailed "product"; for example:

> The development of a policy statement calling for an increase in the number of psychiatric beds for children in the metropolitan area.

> The establishment of a poverty and social problems curriculum in six schools in the tri-county area.

> A rotating toy library for the use of six child care centers.

Others sought to establish a more fluid "process" of participation within the target population; for example

> A subcommittee or task force of the eight private agencies involved in institutional work with children, who will work cooperatively with three representatives of the public sector.

> Small groups of black and white students who will meet together in one junior high school.

Practitioner Confidence

As we have seen, some practitioners were certain of the validity and workability of the innovation; others were less confident and viewed the partial implementation as a feasibility study. A family service worker expressed this position:

> My innovation was a program designed to prove that services for mentally retarded adults could be delivered with volunteer help. Until that time, the agency had resisted using volunteers to any extent. Two small groups of adults were selected from community care homes. Other home operators asked that their residents be allowed to participate, and eventually we used our experience to write a proposal to the public school's adult education department, requesting a weekly socialization program for 200 mentally retarded adults. All of

this took detailed planning because we could not afford the failure of those first few programs.

We recruited and trained volunteers, we selected the initial group with care, and we tried to monitor everything constantly.

Our demonstration with a small portion of the target population allowed us to open the program to the larger target. If we had not limited the group initially, we would have had disaster: we had neither the volunteers, the space, the equipment, nor the know-how to handle a large group. In addition, we did not have the agency approval to proceed with this program.

Oversimplification: A Warning

We have spoken of exclusive categories– with or without a decision-making unit, automatic or guided diffusion, etc.–but the processes of social change are more complex than that. If we trace the steps of a practitioner in action, perhaps we can correct any tendency to oversimplification. Below, the director of a mental health association describes the steps he followed in getting the county mental health board (the proximate target) to endorse a policy statement calling for the provision of more psychiatric beds for emotionally disturbed children. The partial target was the Children and Youth Committee of the board.

> I first discussed the need for additional beds with several committee members and the committee staff person. These contacts were with people who were not resistive on doctrinaire grounds. They encouraged me to bring the issue to the full committee for general discussion.
>
> During the next two weeks, I again talked informally with several committee members. I also spent time with county mental health board staff, in an effort to help them understand the nature of the need and the more desirable options available. The key staff person agreed that it would be helpful for me to present basic information to the committee at its next meeting, and informed the committee chairman that I was going to prepare some helpful information.
>
> With staff assistance from my own agency, I researched

some of the issues related to inpatient care. It was possible to prepare materials that provided valid answers.

Prior to the actual committee meeting, I again discussed the matter informally with several key committee members. I shared the data I was collecting and asked them for their thoughts and suggestions, which I included in my presentation.

At the December 15th meeting I presented the information that had been collected. Surprisingly, there was general agreement about the validity of the data, and little support for the notion that there were alternatives to hospital care for the children in question. The time seemed right to suggest a formal policy statement. Although I had not prepared one, I decided to take advantage of the favorable tone that had developed. After some discussion, the policy statement was adopted.

The committee, through its chairman (a member of the fall board), made its recommendation to the County Mental Health Board at its late December meeting. The board adopted the policy statement and directed the committee to work for its implementation

Problems of Executing the Guideline Strategy

Several practitioners expressed support for the principle underlying the guideline. As two of them noted:

> There is a universality about the application of the principle of spreading an innovation from a small group of "converts" to a wider clientele. The guideline works because it reflects truth about the way people learn.

> I feel the guideline itself is sound. If meetings of black and white students are ever to becomes regular part of the curriculum in my school, the value and feasibility of the innovation will first have to be demonstrated with small group. It would be too risky to implement the approach on a large scale without any prior demonstration of its worth.

Other practitioners noted that the guideline is useful in long- and medium-range planning, because operational problems can be seen on a small scale before the innovation is attempted on a large scale. They also felt that the initial experience by a limited portion of the target system was helpful in determining the potential success of the innovation.

> You have an opportunity to work out problems of the innovation and to test its value before trying it on the total target system.

> It offers a test of the idea for the practitioner, as well as a strategy for gaining acceptance.

Our field staff commented on the selection of an appropriate partial target system.

> The most difficult thing is defining the appropriate "limited portion" of the target population.

> It is important to choose a partial target system that will carry the innovation to the intended target.

The experience of a health planner, who attempted to establish a preventive patient education program by working with a portion of the agency staff, illustrates some hazards involved in selecting the partial group:

> The partialization of the staff backfired in this situation. There was little experience of staff involvement in such work. Those in the partial group became extremely ego-involved; the others developed a "we-they" attitude as if they had no role whatever, even though they were needed to help carry out contacts. In this particular case, due to the inexperience and attitudes of the staff group, partialization did not work.

Two general recommendations regarding the selection of a partial target group can be drawn from the experience of the field test. First, the group should be so constituted as to expedite the success of the limited demonstration. That is, it should have some of the following characteristics:

- Receptiveness to the innovation
- General acceptance of change
- Good relations with the practitioner
- Good motivation
- Special qualifications such as education, skills, or experiences which would facilitate a successful demonstration

Second, the partial group should be respected by the general target population (or at least not be a deviant disapproved segment). There should be strong links and good means of communication between the partial and general targets. However, this second recommendation would not apply when one wanted to complete the total demonstration before diffusing, so as not to arouse a known opposition.

Getting Started

In attempting to use this guideline for the first time, you might follow a thought-action process as follows:

(1) Think of some new program, service, or activity that you have been planning to carry out, or that ties in with general tasks and objectives of your current position or assignment. A review of program listings on page two may be helpful.

(2) Attempt to set this down as a goal, one of moderate scope and of short-term duration; something that could be completed in a minimum of roughly five weeks, and a maximum of twelve weeks.

(3) Picture the general or total target system at which this innovation is directed. If the general group is very large, scale it down to a workable proximate target.

(4) Think about a partial segment of that target system, a limited subgroup: (a) who might relatively easily be involved in an immediate trial or demonstration of the innovation; (b) with whom there is high likelihood of success in an initial trial; and (c) whose success would likely have an impact on the larger target system, or on a relevant decision-making unit that could legitimate or authorize transfer of the innovation to the larger target system. Will it be possible to go from the partial to the proximate target in a short time? If not, you may want to further reduce your proximate target.

(5) Our review of patterns of implementation suggests that autho-

rization or legitimation is often needed early in the game in order to proceed. This might be obtained from a supervisor, an agency director, or from the agency board. Another priority may be contact with persons or organizations who can provide resources for the small scale demonstration, or who can offer access to the smaller target system. Make a list of those individuals, groups, or organizations whose acceptance needs to be gained.

(6) When you have worked the issue through to this point, begin to fill out the Initial Log. This is designed assist you in formulating (on paper) some early steps that you might take in starting to carry out this guideline.

Initial Log Form–Part I

The next step toward getting started involves recording your tentative thoughts on implementing the guideline. The Initial Log is a tool for organizing your thinking; it proved to be valuable to the practitioners in our field study. It is geared to help you think about your goal and ways of operationalizing the guideline.

Part II of the Log will cover key individual and community groups to involve, and facilitating and limiting factors in your situation.

Following the Log form you will find illustrations of key sections that were completed by project practitioners.

INITIAL LOG

1. Date of preparation: _____

2. What is your goal (i.e., the innovation) in using the guideline? Be as specific as possible. Keep a short-term time perspective (five to twelve weeks).

3. Describe the circumstances (conditions, assignments, events, requests, etc.) which led you to use this guideline to achieve the above goal.

4. Look back at the Action Guideline. How would you begin to define each element of the guideline in your immediate situation? (How might you operationalize these components?) Keep in mind the innovation goal stated in #2.

   (a) What is the general target system?

      The proximate target?

   (b) What is the specific partial target system?

   (c) What decision-making unit, if any, is involved? How will its members be encouraged to accept the innovation?

   (d) How will you foster diffusion (forms of linkage, communication, promotion, etc.) from the partial to the general target?

5. List the major steps you anticipate taking in employing this guideline.

_____

_____

_____

_____

_____

_____

SAMPLE INITIAL LOG ENTRIES

I. Example of Outreach Programs in a Housing Project

   A. *Goal Statement* (Log item 2)
   My goal is to establish outreach services for tenants in a housing project served by a traditional Family Service Agency. (A
   broader goal, beyond the application of the guideline in this
   instance, is related to the agency's desire to establish outreach
   services in the general community.)

   B. *Application of the Guideline Elements* (Log item 4)
   General Target System: All tenants of the housing project
   (twenty courts).
   In Proximate terms: Tenants in six courts.
   Partial Target System: One court of six families. This court
   will be selected at random because there is no basis for knowing which court offers the best potential.

II. Example of a Social Welfare Employees' Union

   A. *Goal Statement* (Log item 2)
   My goal is to establish a pattern of implementation of union
   programs at the building level through committees at each
   work location.

   B. *Application of the Guideline Elements* (Log item 4)
   General Target System: All twenty-five building units.
   In Proximate terms: Six units contiguous to one another and to
   the partial system.
   Partial Target System: One building-level committee structure
   where staff has already expressed an interest in our operation.

Practical Advice Derived from the Field Study

Some advice has been drawn from questionnaire analysis in our
field study. First of all, there are several ways in which you may use
personal resources, including:

1. develop and rely upon good relationships within the agency;
2. select a program to which you are committed and which is logically related to your position in the agency;
3. take advantage of your prior experience–select a program and setting in which your experience will be an asset.

In addition, you should consider fostering support for the program at all levels within the agency, particularly at the upper levels. If the program is consistent with your other assignments, this can serve to legitimize the activity and allow a concentration of energy.

Community support of your organization and yourself may be significant; build such support, or select groups to work with in which such support already exists. Client participation may be important. Their interest in, and receptivity to, the program is also a consideration. Select a program which interests clients, or work hard to develop such interest.

Limiting forces are most likely to appear within your own agency. Such agency limitations frequently stem from lack of clarity, so clarification of your goals, programs, and assignments may be a useful tactic. If internal lack of funds or staff is a problem, you must plan a program realistically within the means of the agency, or think of tapping external resources. To a lesser extent, the agency's structure may be an obstacle, or its lack of authority may be limiting. Both of these factors suggest strategic considerations in choosing a program.

The need to manage time and energy efficiently was frequently emphasized in the field study, as was the related factor of the need to select a feasible, moderate-sized proximate goal:

I had little time to implement the guideline.

One problem was having to be patient before things started happening. Constant assessment had to take place, along with an incredible amount of public relations.

The guideline is valid, but one should remember to think clearly and to limit the goal sufficiently.

I would not advise another person to work on as many communities as I have attempted. Responsibilities should be delegated to other leaders and organizations.

Within the client population and the larger community, the biggest limitations are likely to be competition from other activities, and lack of knowledge. This highlights the educational functions of the practitioner's job (interpretation, communication, public relations) and the need to formulate programs that are meaningful and interesting enough to compete with the many forces demanding the attention of clients and community people.

Initial Log Form–Part II

As a final planning aid, you should list the key community groups and individuals that are likely to support your efforts. You should also consider the factors which will affect your progress. We have provided checklists of common *facilitating* and *limiting* factors found in our field study. It will assist you to note any factors that apply to your own practice.

What key community groups, if any, will you probably involve?

Group   Reason for contact

_____   _____

_____   _____

_____   _____

_____   _____

_____   _____

What key individuals, if any, will you probably involve?

Individual   Title and/or affiliation   Reason for contact

_____   _____   _____

_____   _____   _____

_____   _____   _____

_____   _____   _____

_____   _____   _____

_____   _____   _____

PERSONAL FACTORS

Facilitating	*Limiting*
☐ Good personal relationship with administrator.	☐ Poor personal relationships with board (members).
☐ Good personal relationship with supervisor.	☐ Lack of personal knowledge of the community.
☐ Good personal relationships with staff.	☐ Poor personal reputation.
☐ Personal commitment to the agency.	☐ Personal loss (demotion, job title, etc.).
☐ Personal knowledge of clients.	☐ Overinvolvement.
☐ Personal position or role.	☐ Fatigue.
☐ Good personal reputation.	☐ Lack of time.
☐ Self-confidence.	☐ Other:_____
	_____
☐ Other: _____	
_____	

AGENCY FACTORS

Facilitating	*Limiting*
☐ External authority requires your organization to support your effort.	☐ Lack of power or authority of your organization.
☐ Affiliated organizational support.	☐ Unclear or shifting goals, programs, or assignments.
☐ Board involvement.	☐ Lack of agency knowledge of clients or community.
☐ Administration support or involvement.	☐ Lack of agency support, or hindering action of affiliated organizations.
☐ Administration disinterest.	☐ Lack of agency support, or hindering action of supervisor.
☐ Supervisor involvement.	☐ Other:_____
☐ Supervisor disinterest.	
☐ Physical facilities aid the effort.	
☐ Other: _____	

CLIENT FACTORS

Facilitating

☐ Voluntary client participation in your organization or program.

☐ Client participation in your organization or program through a legal or administrative ruling.

☐ Client is generally interested in your organization

☐ Client shows receptivity to your organization or program

☐ Other: _____
_____

Limiting

☐ Client shows a general negative response to your organization.

☐ Client is disinterested or dissatisfied with your organization or program.

☐ Client lack of knowledge of your organization, its purposes, programs, or activities.

☐ Other: _____
_____

COMMUNITY FACTORS

Facilitating

☐ Voluntary community participation in your organization.

☐ Community support of clients.

☐ Other: _____
_____

Limiting

☐ Community disinterest or dissatisfaction with your organization or program.

☐ Community lack of knowledge of your organization, its purposes, programs or activities.

☐ External influences make the community unsupportive of your organization or program.

☐ Community residents are specifically disinterested in your program.

☐ Other: _____
_____

AN AFTERWORD

While the guidelines have been derived from social science research, and field experience with them has given the authors confidence in their utility, they are not presented as a panacea or a routine prescription for solving all mental health problems. The reader will have to rely on personal judgment in the application:

Does this initiative fit my situation?

Am I comfortable with it organizationally? philosophically?

Does it seem as good or better than alternative approaches that come to mind?

The procedures incorporated in the handbook, particularly in the Getting Started sections, represent a general scheme for systematic problem solving. Through the repeated use of the Initial Log, this type of analytic planning for systems intervention can become automatic, perhaps with the use of a few informal notes.

This endeavor has not been an academic exercise: we have not attempted to produce a library dust collector. These strategies should be used to deal with real mental health problems and to strengthen family life. We offer a set of tools that must be employed with skill. There is no magic in the guidelines, no sources of strength beyond thoughtful application by committed professionals. And there is little value in the handbook unless that happens.

GLOSSARY

Definitions of Key Terms
As They Have Been Used in This Handbook

ACTION GUIDELINE–The basic strategy contained in the intervention principle.

BENEFITS–Rewards for desired behavior.

CONTRACTING–The agreement to provide a benefit for sustained participation.

DIFFUSION–The spreading of an innovation to larger populations.

EXPRESSIVE BENEFITS–Intangible, psychological rewards.

GROUP CONTINGENCY–Supplying benefits to a group which meets desired standards.

INNOVATION–Any program, technique, or activity perceived as new by an organization or population group.

INSTRUMENTAL BENEFITS–Material, tangible rewards.

OPINION LEADERS–Those individuals within a target group who are looked to for advice and guidance.

PARTIAL GROUP–An initial division of a larger population.

PARTIALIZATION–Division of a target system for the introduction of an innovation. Often involves the selection of a smaller group of opinion leaders from the total population.

PARTICIPATION–The act of taking part in a social activity.

POSITIVE REINFORCEMENT–The provision of benefits for the performance of desired behavior.

PROMOTION–(As in "promoting an innovation") The process of diffusing and insuring acceptance of an innovation.

PROXIMATE GOAL–A moderate, tangible objective that can be achieved within a short term.

REINFORCEMENT–See "Positive Reinforcement."

SHAPING–The establishment of a sequence of goals leading to a long-range objective.

TARGET SYSTEM–An organization or population group toward which an innovation is directed. (Also "target group" and "target")

TRANSFER MECHANISM–A means (often a decision-making unit) by which an innovation is spread from a smaller to a larger target system.

BIBLIOGRAPHY

Fostering Participation

Mulford, Lee, and Klonglan, Gerald E. "The Significance of Attitudes for Formal Voluntary Organizations: A Synthesis of Existing Research and Theory." Paper presented at a meeting of the American Sociological Association, Washington, DC, 1970.

Orum, Anthony. "Structural Sources of Negro Student Protest: Campus and Community." Paper presented at a meeting of the American Sociological Association, San Francisco, California, 1969.

Schneiderman, Leonard. "Value Orientation Preferences of Chronic Relief Recipients." *Social Work*, July 1966, pp. 58-67.

Seals, Alvin, and Malaja, Jiri. "A Study of Negro Voluntary Organizations in Lexington, Kentucky." *Phylon*, Spring 1964, pp. 27-31.

Warner, Keith W., and Henterman, William. "The Benefit-Participation Contingency in Voluntary Farm Organization." *Rural Sociology*, June 1967, pp. 133-153.

Weissman, Harold. "An Exploratory Study of a Neighborhood Council." PhD dissertation, Columbia University, 1966.

Promoting an Innovation

Arnt, Johan. "A Test of the Two Step Flow in Diffusion of a New Product." *Journalism Quarterly*, Vol. 45, 1968, pp. 457-465.

Becker, Marshall H. "Patterns of Interpersonal Influence and Sources of Information in the Diffusion of Two Public Health Innovations." Ann Arbor: University of Michigan, Public Health Practice Research Program, Report, 1968.

Coleman, James, et al. *Medical Innovation: A Diffusion Study*. New York: The Bobbs-Merrill Co. 1966.

Fliegel, Frederick C., and Kivlin, Joseph E. "Attributes of Innovations as Factors in Diffusion." *American Journal of Sociology*, Vol. 72, 1966, pp. 235-248.

Fliegel, Frederick C., and Kivlin, Joseph E. "Farm Practice Attributes and Adoption Rates." *Social Forces*, Vol. 40, 1962, pp. 364-370.

Havens, Eugene A., and Rogers, Everett M. "Adoption of Hybrid Corn: Profitability and the Interaction Effect." *Rural Sociology,* Vol. 26, 1961, pp. 409-414.

Hruschka, E., and Rheinwald, H. "The Effectiveness of German Pilot Farms." *Sociologia Ruralis,* Vol. 5, 1965, pp. 101-111.

Katz, Elihu, and Lazaisfeld, Paul F. *Personal Influence: The Part Played by People in the Flow of Mass Communications.* New York: The Free Press, 1955.

Kivlin, Joseph E., and Fliegel, Frederick C. "Differential Perceptions of Innovations and Rate of Adoption." *Rural Sociology.* Vol. 32, 1967, pp. 78-91.

Mansfield, Edwin. "Technical Change and the Rate of Imitation." *Econometrica,* Vol. 20, 1961, pp. 741-766.

Menzel, Herbert, and Katz, Elihu. "Social Relations and Innovation in the Medical Profession: The Epidemiology of a New Drug." *Public Opinion Quarterly,* Vol. 19, 1955, pp. 337-352.

Polgar, Stephen, et al. "Diffusion and Farming Advice: A Test of Some Current Notions." *Social Forces,* Vol. 41, 1963, pp. 104-111.

Rogers, Everett. *The Diffusion of Innovations.* New York: The Free Press, 1962.

Rogers, Everett, and Shoemaker, F. Floyd. *The Communication of Innovations.* New York: The Free Press, 1971.

Rogers, Everett, and Beal, George M. "Community Norms, Opinion Leaderships and Innovativeness among Truck Growers," Wooster: *Ohio Agricultural Experimental Station,* Research Bulletin, No. 912, 1962.

Rogers, Everett, and Svenning, Lynne. *Modernization among Peasants: The Impact of Communication.* New York: Holt, Rinehart & Winston, 1969.

Systems Analysis and Problem Diagnosis

Bennis, Warren G. *Changing Organizations.* New York: McGraw-Hill Book Co., 1966.

Cox, Fred, et al. *Strategies of Community Organization.* Itasca, Illinois: F. E. Peacock Publishers, 1974.

Etzioni, Amitai, ed. *Complex Organizations: A Sociological Reader.* New York: Holt, Rinehart & Winston, 1964.

Hasenfeld, Yeheskel, and English, Richard, eds. *Human Service Organizations.* Ann Arbor, Michigan: University of Michigan Press, 1974.

Kramer, Ralph, and Specht, Harry. *Readings in Community Organization Practice.* Englewood Cliffs, New Jersey: Prentice-Hall, 1969.

O. M. Collective. *The Organizer's Manual.* New York: Bantam Books, 1971.

Perlman, Robert, and Gurin, Arnold. *Community Organizations and Social Planning.* New York: John Wiley & Sons, 1972.

Rothman, Jack. *Organizing and Planning for Social Change: Action Principles from Social Science Research.* New York: Columbia University Press, 1974.

Zald, Mayer N., ed. *Social Welfare Institutions.* New York: John Wiley & Sons, 1965.

Appendix B

The Unilateral Treatment Program for Alcohol Abuse– Background, Selected Procedures, and Case Applications

Edwin J. Thomas

BACKGROUND

Unilateral family therapy (UFT) is intervention directed toward changing the behavior of an uncooperative family member through working with a cooperative member as mediator (Thomas and Santa 1982). As applied to the uncooperative alcohol abuser, cooperative, nonalcohol abusing spouses are assisted to influence their alcoholic partners to stop drinking, enter treatment, or both (Thomas 1989; Thomas, Santa, Bronson, and Oyserman 1987). Their alcohol abusing partners do not (and, at least initially, will not) participate in the treatment. This approach does not assume that the cooperative spouse is to blame for the difficulties. However, that spouse is viewed as a vital and potentially crucial point of leverage who may be the main or only rehabilitative influence accessible to the therapist.

The unilateral approach to family therapy has three foci of intervention. The *individual focus* emphasizes assisting the cooperative

The research reported here was supported in part by Grants 1 R01 AA04163-03 and 5 R01 AA04163-07 of the National Institute on Alcohol Abuse and Alcoholism, Edwin J. Thomas, Principal Investigator. I wish to acknowledge the contributions of Denise Bronson, Cathleen Santa, Joanne Yaffe, and Daphna Oyserman in the pilot phase of the research and of Richard D. Ager, Marianne Yoshioka, Kathryn Betts Adams and David Moxley in the evaluation phase.

family member with his or her coping (e.g., reducing stress and anxiety about the abuser's drinking and channeling the spouse's efforts toward specific ways to address the drinking problem). The *interactional focus* entails mediating changes in marital and family functioning (e.g., reducing marital discord through unilateral relationship enhancement, reducing nagging and other customary drinking control efforts and spouse enabling of the abuser's alcohol abuse). The *third-party focus* involves work with the spouse or other family members to bring about change in the uncooperative family member (e.g., inducing the alcohol abuser to seek treatment or other assistance, to stop drinking, or both). It is this combination of interventional foci along with working with one or a few cooperative family members in a rehabilitative capacity to reach an uncooperative family member that makes the unilateral approach a distinctive mode of therapy (for further details, see Thomas 1989; Thomas and Santa 1982).

The major emphasis of the treatment program is on assisting the spouse to become a positive rehabilitative influence with the resistant drinker. There are three main phases of treatment. The first involves *preparing the spouse to assume a positive rehabilitative role.* This phase involves (a) the treatment orientation; (b) monitoring of the abuser's alcohol consumption through the spouse; (c) alcohol education for the spouse; (d) unilateral relationship enhancement to reduce the level of conflict in the marital relationship and to increase the spouse's ability to influence the abuser; (e) reduction of the spouse's customary drinking control behavior; and (f) disenabling to reduce the ways in which the spouse has enabled the abuser to drink. The second phase consists of *conducting abuser-directed interventions to actively influence the alcohol abuser to enter treatment, stop drinking, or both.* Among the possible interventions in this phase are the spouse carrying out a programmed confrontation or programmed request with the abuser, use of agreements/contracts, providing sobriety support, follow-up interventions, such as spouse-invoked contingent consequences, and various supplementary interventions. The third area involves *maintaining spouse and abuser treatment gains.* Beneficial outcomes were reported in two studies of this treatment program, details of which are reported elsewhere (Thomas et al. 1987; Thomas, Yoshioka, Ager, and Adams 1993).

In selecting spouses and abusers most likely to benefit from this type of treatment, it has become clear that potential participants should also meet the same eligibility criteria as those employed in the research. Criteria for the spouse included recognition that the partner had a drinking problem, willingness to receive help to try to do something about that problem, and absence of a drinking problem. Criteria for the abuser included a drinking problem for which he or she was unwilling to receive treatment. Additional criteria for both partners were absence of domestic violence, no other problem of drug abuse, no history of severe emotional disorder, no immediate plans for marital dissolution, and no other concurrent professional counseling. While aspects of this treatment program might well apply to cases not meeting these criteria (e.g., abuse of other drugs in addition to alcohol), the use of confrontive interventions in cases in which these criteria are not met could increase the risk of failure and precipitate such adverse complications as domestic violence, martial estrangement, and self-destructive acts by the abuser.

Although space does not permit coverage here of details for the entire treatment program, selected procedures and applications for program components are included as illustrative D&D products. Other aspects of the unilateral approach and treatment program are to be found in Thomas (1989), Thomas and Ager (1992), and Thomas and Ager (in press).

SPOUSE-ORIENTED INTERVENTIONS

Spouse-oriented interventions, as indicated, are part of the spouse role induction and are directed toward preparing the spouse to assume a positive rehabilitative role. Two program components for these interventions are presented below: unilateral relationship enhancement and modification of the spouse's customary drinking control.

Unilateral Relationship Enhancement

Purpose

The purpose of unilateral relationship enhancement (URE)[1] is to improve the relationship between the marital partners and to increase the ability of the spouse to influence the abuser. Accordingly, the spouse is requested to carry out behaviors when the abuser is sober that the abuser would find enjoyable and that the spouse is willing and able to carry out. Enhancing behaviors of the spouse may be "pleasers," such as initiating sex or making special meals, or not engaging in "displeasers," such as being critical or leaving the bathroom in a mess.

Introduction

Clients are introduced to URE in their first or second treatment session, and a good portion of one or two sessions is spent setting up the initial program. It is best to begin with examples from the spouse's experience rather than with general explanations. For example, the therapist can introduce URE by indicating that it is common in marriages where there is an alcohol problem that the non-drinking spouse stops or decreases certain pleasing behaviors. The client may then be asked to think of any examples from her or his own marriage. Starting with these examples, the therapist moves in a stepwise fashion through the process of setting up and explaining the program.

Identifying Potential Enhancers

The client is then asked to think of behaviors she or he could engage in that would be pleasing to the alcohol-abusing spouse and that have either dropped to a low level or are no longer occurring in the marriage. If the client is having difficulty thinking of examples, it can also be helpful to consider other potentially pleasing behaviors that never took place frequently. The therapist may also show the client an illustrative list to help generate ideas. If a list is used, the therapist and client should first review the entire list to trigger ideas before evaluating each item suggested as a possibility.

Screening Behaviors

After identifying a preliminary list of enhancers, the therapist reviews the items on it with the client. Items are removed if they represent a behavior which the client cannot readily perform, if too much time or resources are required to change them, or if there are limited opportunities to perform the behaviors. Displeasers should be carefully screened to exclude complaints based on "real" problems (e.g., a leaking roof) that need to be solved *versus* complaints that are needlessly aversive to the abuser (e.g., nagging) and that can be reduced without adverse consequences. If there are legitimate, unresolved marital problems underlying the complaints, clients are asked to put these issues aside for a later time until progress can be made in attempting to address the alcohol problem.

Specification of Behaviors

Surviving items are then carefully specified, so that the therapist and client agree on the particular behavior to be carried out. Specification is necessary because there are typically alternative definitions and indicators of a given pleaser. Often a targeted displeaser can readily be turned into a pleaser. For example, "not going to bed at the same time" can become "going to bed at the same time," and be recorded as a positive.

It is also advisable to specify the particular circumstances in which the spouse should engage in each behavior. Occasions are best when the alcohol abuser is sober and most receptive, and when the client has adequate time and energy to carry out the behavior.

Assigning the Program

After the items have been screened and determined to be appropriate and feasible, the client is asked if she or he is willing to change the selected behaviors and, if so, to proceed to increase the pleasers and decrease the displeasers. Behaviors relating to all items, such as giving affection or engaging in sex or conversation, should be carried out when the client feels comfortable engaging in the behavior. The client is told that there are no quotas or expectations of maximum or minimum performance; rather, the objective is to do her or his best.

The therapist emphasizes that the program by itself is not intended to correct major marital problems or reduce the drinking, but is one of several components that help to prepare the marital relationship for later changes. The program can be described as an "investment" made now by the client to be realized later in beneficial changes that URE and the other aspects of the treatment may produce. It is explained that the goals of URE should not be revealed to the partner. The behaviors should be carried out without announcement or comment, thus allowing the URE actions to speak for themselves, and not to request or necessarily to anticipate a positive response from the drinker.

Baseline

The therapist takes a retrospective baseline for each targeted item by determining how often the client has engaged in the behavior in question during the month before entering treatment.[2] Information can generally be obtained more readily for the month by obtaining the data week-by-week, beginning with the most recent week. In obtaining the base rates, a method of measuring each behavior needs to be determined (e.g., frequency or duration, etc.).

Recording and Monitoring

The client is asked to record the behaviors engaged in and the therapist prepares or otherwise makes available a recording form for that purpose. The therapist writes the targeted behaviors on the recording form and instructs the client to note each time during the week when a selected behavior is carried out.

The program is then reviewed in the following weeks to determine whether and how well the client is carrying out and recording the behaviors, how the methods of measurement are working, and whether the enhancing behaviors continue to be appropriate.

For the most part, if appropriately selected, the enhancers selected for the program should be kept throughout the course of treatment, with no new behaviors added. However, the client may suggest new enhancers subsequently that are appropriate and these can be added to a general "special events" category. Alternatively, a new, more specific category may be considered. If so, the therapist and client should go through all the steps that were used to screen, choose and measure the original behavior before including the new item as a separate category.

Handling Resistance and Other Difficulties

Occasionally some clients are reluctant to carry out the program. One type of resistance to URE involves clients who say that they are already making efforts in all positive areas and avoiding all negative areas, and there is no room for improvement. Even so, the therapist can explore and often identify "extras" that might enhance the relationship. The therapist can also choose a less structured program with a client who is resistant to formalizing URE. This might consist of settling on some behaviors that the client agrees to work on but not monitor on the forms, or foregoing behavior selection altogether and informally monitoring the pre-existing relationship enhancement activities.

Another potential difficulty results from the client's anger toward the drinking marital partner. When this feeling is strong at the outset, the client may openly oppose doing anything to enhance the relationship. The client's willingness to perform the behaviors of URE is a necessary condition to initiating a program. It may be necessary to postpone further program development until such time as the client is willing.

Some abusers drink so heavily and consistently that there are few opportunities to enhance the relationship interpersonally when they are sober. In such circumstances, the client may choose times when there is both little or no alcohol in the abuser's system and no active drinking. Also, enhancers can be selected to include at least some that do not require interpersonal contact (e.g., buying special foods or doing other small favors).

Case Application

Mrs. D is a 60-year-old part-time secretary whose husband is a machine operator and a longtime heavy drinker unmotivated for treatment. In her second session, with the aid of the list of Illustrative Pleasers and Displeasers,[3] Mrs. D identified several items that eventually survived the screening and were selected for her URE program. In recent years she had not been initiating much in the way of physical affection with her husband and the other behaviors she chose as pleasers had stopped because of her anger about the drinking.

The therapist obtained a retrospective baseline from Mrs. D for each item, as shown in Table 1. Most of the pleasers were at a rate of 0 times per month prior to treatment and the two displeasers were carried out about once daily.

Mrs. D was cautioned not to expect responses from her husband, and not to anticipate a decrease in the drinking due to these efforts alone. She adopted a positive attitude about URE from the start. She began to carry out the behaviors right away and reported that her feelings towards the marriage improved, and there were a few positive reactions from Mr. D.

TABLE 1. Frequency of relationship enhancement behaviors before and during treatment for Mrs. D.

Areas of Behavior	Monthly Mean	
	Restrospective Baseline	Treatment Phase
Pleasers		
Going out alone with H	0	4.4
Initiating hugs, kisses, touching	0	13.6
Bringing coffee or a snack	0	2.5
Discussing future plans	0	6.7
"Special things": meals, gifts	1	5.1
Expressing affection/approval	3	4.0
Displeasers		
Critical or sarcastic remarks	30	7.1
Nagging about smoking or chores	35	3.5

Note. The mean for the retrospective baseline is the client's estimated frequency for the month before treatment began and, for the treatment phase, it is the monthly mean of the behaviors during 5.5 months of treatment.

The frequency with which Mrs. D engaged in the behaviors varied somewhat from week to week, but she continued URE activities and monitoring throughout the course of treatment. Her pleasers increased markedly and her displeasers decreased to levels well below her retrospective baseline (see Table 1). In particular, she began to show more affection (e.g., hugs, kisses) and reduced conflictual interactions such as nagging, criticism, and sarcasm. When she actively intervened later in the course of treatment, her husband agreed to stop drinking and did so. Although there were no doubt many factors contributing to this success, Mrs. D. performed the tasks of URE consistently as part of the preparation to help establish conditions in the marital system that would favor achieving change in her husband's drinking. For further details concerning this program, the reader is referred to Thomas, Adams, Yoshioka, and Ager (1990).

Modification of the Spouse's Customary Drinking Control

Purpose

The modification program to reduce spouse customary drinking control (DC)[4] is carried out to reduce the general aversiveness of drinking control efforts and to help make way for the spouse to assume a more positive rehabilitative role. Subsequently, an active intervention intended to influence the abuser to reduce drinking, enter treatment, or both is planned and implemented.

Introducing the Program and Identifying DC Behaviors

In an early session, the program is initiated by identifying the spouse's drinking control behaviors that might be potential targets of change. To facilitate the process of identifying potential targets of change, the Spouse Sobriety Influence Inventory (SSII) may be employed, which makes it possible to assess the frequency of 45 DC behaviors.[5] The therapist reviews the spouse's responses on this scale, which should be completed prior to treatment. Each item for which the spouse reports having engaged in the behavior occasionally or more over the past six months (i.e., which was given a score of three or more) is flagged as a potential target for change, and is listed on a separate piece of paper without any indication of its source.

If the Inventory is not used, the spouse is asked for examples of his/her past behaviors which were aimed at reducing or stopping the abuser's drinking. Useful opening questions are "How do you let the drinker know you dislike his/her drinking?" or "How have you tried to get him/her to stop drinking?" All spouse mentions of drinking control behaviors are listed on a separate piece of paper.

After the preliminary list of target behaviors has been identified, the therapist reviews them with the spouse to obtain examples of how the particular behavior is engaged in as well as abuser reactions.[6]

At this point the therapist orients the spouse further to the concept of drinking control by describing some of the dysfunctions associated with these behaviors. Drinking control is described as part of the spouse's "old sobriety influence system" which we hope to have put aside so that other, more appropriate ways of responding can be initiated. Instances of drinking control are thereafter referred to as the "old system," a convenient short-hand concept that is readily understood.

Screening Behaviors

The final list should be screened to eliminate behaviors not specifically related to drinking or its control (e.g., general complaints about the marriage or efforts to change it). In some instances, the drinking control behaviors of the spouse are intended to avert or reduce danger to the spouse or others occasioned by the drinking (e.g., the spouse refusing to let a child get into a car about to be driven by a drunken marital partner). When there is evident danger or other risks, control efforts related to these factors clearly should be excluded from the DC modification program.

Assigning the Program

Control behaviors that survive the screening should be specified and appropriate alternative responses identified. Once all behaviors have been screened, the spouse's willingness to reduce the frequency of the old drinking control efforts is sought. If the spouse is willing, the therapist selects several items (usually three) from the list of surviving items which the spouse and therapist believe are among the easiest to change. The spouse is asked to stop the chosen behavior as best as he/she can and to engage in alternative responses.

The spouse also is requested not to reveal the goals of the program to the drinker and to carry it out without any announcement. The spouse is cautioned against anticipating any positive response from the abuser and that the program, by itself, is not expected to bring about changes in the drinking. However, the program is described as having its own benefits for the spouse and as one of many changes that help to prepare the marital relationship for more active intervention to follow.

Monitoring

At the next session, the therapist reviews the behaviors chosen for reduction the week before, and any problems are addressed. If the spouse was able to reduce the frequency of the targeted behaviors sufficiently, additional behaviors are selected from the surviving items and are targeted for the upcoming week. If the spouse has been doing well in reducing the targeted behaviors, and is willing to take on others, additional selections are made each week until all behaviors on the list have been targeted for change.

Handling Difficulties and Special Problems

Although the DC modification program should remain more or less intact throughout the treatment period, it may be necessary to make adjustments, depending upon such factors as the number of areas of drinking control targeted, the rate of spouse progress, and program compliance.

In some instances, the spouse may report that she or he has already stopped engaging in all DC behavior. Rather than avoid doing anything further on DC, the therapist may wish to begin monitoring in an informal way the spouse's possible DC activities.

The spouse may resume control efforts or have mistakenly failed to recognize some of his or her actions as attempts to change the drinking. The therapist should be particularly attentive to indirect or non-verbal behavior that conveys disapproval of drinking so that such behaviors can be addressed and included in the program.

The spouse may be reluctant to stop engaging in DC, fearing that in so doing, there will be an increase in the partner's drinking. Spouses also may worry that by not criticizing the drinking, she or he will be condoning the drinking. The therapist can acknowledge that these concerns are understandable yet indicate that such control behaviors do not promote long-term recovery. Instead, they often cause marital conflict, and DC and its negative effects may interfere with planned abuser-directed interventions that will be conducted later.

The therapist also may need to help the spouse distinguish enabling from DC. Here it can be pointed out that, in contrast to DC, enabling typically involves promoting the drinking, for example, by serving drinks or buying alcohol for the drinker.

While successfully trying to reduce DC, some spouses will continue to be preoccupied with related cognitions, such as negative thoughts involving the drinking, or affect, such as anxiety or anger about the abuser's drinking. Some continuing indications of the cognitive and affective correlates of DC are common and are to be expected, at least to some extent, particularly in the early stages of DC modification. As the program continues, however, and there is more and more detachment of the spouse as evidenced by reductions in the overt behavioral aspects of DC, the cognitive and affective correlates likewise abate for most spouses.

However, in some cases spouses will persist in having intense negative thoughts or feelings about the drinking, despite successful reduction of the targeted DC behaviors. In such cases, it may be necessary to address detachment directly and more broadly to assist the spouse further to "back off," "let go" and achieve greater emotional distance from the drinking and its effects (e.g., Leite 1987).

Case Application

In their mid-sixties, Mrs. Y was employed part time out of the home and Mr. Y was retired. Mrs. Y reported that overall they both found their relationship to be rewarding and loving. A long-time heavy drinker, Mr. Y had slowly increased his drinking since his retirement several years earlier.

Mrs. Y had endorsed a total of 19 items on her pre-treatment scale. Review of these during the second session suggested that three of them were particularly problematic as they almost always resulted in the couple's arguing. These three were: expressing disapproval of the drinking (Item 2), asking the drinker before he goes out to drink less (Item 5), and trying to get the drinker to reduce his/her drinking while at a social function (Item 12). The therapist introduced the concept of drinking control as involving part of the "old sobriety influence system" and Mrs. Y readily agreed to try to refrain from engaging in the three behaviors. Weekly review of her progress indicated that she had discontinued the behaviors altogether.

At the tenth session, Mrs. Y expressed concern about continuing the program because she noted that Mr. Y was drinking more heavily since the program began and seemed to have more blackouts and other alcohol-related symptoms. The therapist reminded Mrs. Y that the purpose of the DC modification was not to reduce Mr. Y's drinking but to help set the tone for the programmed request that they were then planning. After brief discussion, Mrs. Y concluded that, in the meantime, she would continue with the program and allow Mr. Y to experience the full effects of his drinking.

The mean for the targeted DC behaviors was reduced from a pre-treatment level of 4.00 (indicating frequently) to 1.00 (rarely) at post-treatment. Concurrent with work on the DC modification, the therapist and Mrs. Y together planned a programmed request, an abuser-directed intervention deemed to be appropriate in her situation. In response to her carefully scripted and delivered request for him to enter treatment for his drinking, Mr. Y entered an outpatient program for his alcohol abuse. For further details, see Yoshioka, Thomas, and Ager (1992).

ABUSER-DIRECTED INTERVENTIONS

The purpose of abuser-directed interventions,[7] as indicated, is to induce the abuser to enter treatment for his or her alcohol abuse, to reduce drinking including abstinence, or both. Such interventions are undertaken only after sufficient progress has been made in the areas of spouse role induction.

Presented below are two important abuser-directed interventions: the programmed confrontation and programmed request. Both interventions involve systematic assessment, careful intervention planning, organization, implementation, and follow-up. Preconditions for carrying out a programmed confrontation include the spouse's recognition that other, less intrusive interventions are not more appropriate and the spouse's willingness to follow through with a strong contingent consequence if the action recommended for treatment for the abuser is not followed. For example, the spouse may be willing to separate, divorce, develop a separate life within the marriage, or alter domestic arrangements for household work if the recommendation is not followed. Conditions that need to be met to implement a programmed request include evidence of some readiness on the part of the abuser to respond favorably to the request and, in general, unwillingness of the spouse to make any significant alteration in behavior or situation if the abuser fails to comply with the request. The recommended steps in the development of either a programmed confrontation or a programmed request are presented in Table 2.

Two cases from the same crossover experimental dyad are briefly summarized. The first case of the dyad, which was assigned at random to receive immediate treatment, highlights the use of the programmed confrontation, and the second case, assigned to receive delayed treatment, illustrates the use of the programmed request. Each case indicates applications of the procedural steps given in Table 2.

Programmed Confrontation

Mr. and Mrs. X, a professional couple in their fifties, had been married for twelve years–the second marriage for both of them. Mrs. X had two children from her previous marriage; one child, an eleven-year-old, was still living at home. Mr. X, the alcohol abuser, had been a heavy drinker since before their marriage. He drank approximately 21 ounces of 80-proof spirits every evening.

TABLE 2. Selected steps in programmed confrontation and programmed request.*

1. Determination of suitability

2. Determination of feasibility

3. Preparation of spouse's script

    a. Declaration of affection

    b. Statement of concern about the abuser's drinking and its effects

    c. Specification of drinking level and severity

    d. Itemization of drinking-related incidents, problems, and their effects

    e. Specification of action recommendations (for example, to enter treatment)

    f. Specification of consequences if action not taken

4. Rehearsal of presentation

5. Staging of the confrontation

6. Postconfrontation planning

7. Conduct of the confrontation

8. Postconfrontation monitoring and follow-through

*Adapted with permission from Thomas, E. J. (1989), Unilateral family therapy to reach the uncooperative alcohol abuser. In B. A. Thyer (Ed.), *Behavioral Family Therapy*. Springfield, IL: Charles C Thomas.

Sessions 1-9 of the 34 weekly sessions were devoted to orientation, clinical assessment, and development and introduction of the spouse role-induction components. Preparation for work on the programmed confrontation occurred during sessions 10-17; the confrontation was provided in session 18. Sessions 19-34 focused on the development and maintenance of a "self-control" component for Mr. X. The steps of programmed confrontation in this case are summarized and illustrated below.

Determination of Suitability

Assessment disclosed that Mr. X was strong willed and stubbornly resistant to Mrs. X's efforts to bring about change in his drinking habits. Mrs. X believed that a very strong intervention was required to bring about any change and was dissatisfied with the marriage, given her husband's current level of drinking. She was seriously considering separation or divorce if Mr. X did not receive help for his drinking. The risk of violence was assessed to be low.

Determination of Feasibility

It was determined that Mrs. X was capable of making direct requests of Mr. X and of speaking to him about his alcohol use in a firm and calm manner. Further, if Mr. X refused treatment, Mrs. X was willing to follow through with contingent consequences, as indicated below.

Preparation of the Spouse's Script

Drawing from a list of instances of Mr. X's excessive drinking and their adverse consequences, four extreme and factual events, difficult to dispute, were selected for scripting. Several revisions of the script were required before the examples were made sufficiently specific to highlight the reality of the events without blame, guilt inducement, or use of language from the spouse's old influence system. Mrs. X was helped to draft a statement of her strong concern about her husband's drinking in the introduction. She indicated that she cared about him very much and she documented her husband's drinking behavior and alcohol consumption, on the basis of records she kept during the alcohol monitoring. A summary of the more general problems associated with the drinking and their effects was drafted next. The recommendation that Mr. Y enter treatment for alcohol abuse was crafted, along with the consequence if he refused. In this instance, the consequence was two-fold: first, Mrs. X would orchestrate and implement a second confrontation involving family members and friends, and second, she would state that she would take further serious but unspecified action.

Rehearsal of the Presentation

The therapist played the role of Mr. X so that Mrs. X could practice the script. Rehearsal focused on appropriate posture, eye contact, tone and strength of voice, naturalness in delivery, and following the script. Feedback was provided through audio recordings and the therapist's comments during and after rehearsals. Refinements in the script were made as necessary at various points in the rehearsals.

Staging the Confrontation

Planning for the confrontation included the following: what to say to Mr. X to request his presence at the session ("we need your help at the next session and would like to have you attend"), when and how to make the request for his attendance, the time and date for the confrontation, how to maximize the likelihood that Mr. X would attend the confrontation and be sober, and seating arrangements to decrease the likelihood of Mr. X walking out during the confrontation.

Postconfrontation Planning

Planning for the period after the confrontation included prearranging treatment for Mr. X, the recommendation that Mrs. X not enter into any discussion of the content of the script or revert to her old system of influences after the confrontation occurred, and preparation for her to follow through on the consequences in the event that Mr. X failed to follow through with agreements made at the time of the confrontation.

Conduct of the Confrontation

After meeting Mr. X and seating everyone according to the plan, the therapist introduced the session, thanked Mr. X for coming, and indicated that Mrs. X would do most of the talking. While maintaining eye contact with Mr. X and only occasionally glancing down at the script, Mrs. X delivered the confrontation. Mr. X interrupted his wife on several occasions, but Mrs. X was well prepared, was not diverted, and continued on with the delivery as planned. Mr. X was uncomfortable during the confrontation and was visibly angry. He refused to accept any alcohol-related treatment. Instead, he indicated firmly that he would gradually reduce his alcohol consumption by two ounces per week until he was at the level of 6-8 ounces per day.[8] The therapist then closed the session, encouraging both spouses not to discuss the matter further at this point.

Postconfrontation Monitoring and Follow-Through

At a subsequent treatment session scheduled soon after the confrontation, the graduated reduction plan proposed by Mr. X was discussed with Mrs. X in light of the fact that Mr. X had already started to implement the plan with success and still steadfastly refused to enter treatment. Because Mr. X did all of his drinking at home and Mrs. X had been shown to be a good observer of the amount of alcohol consumed, it was agreed that Mrs. X should go along with the graduated reduction plan. If Mr. X failed to follow through with the plan, she would invoke the contingencies.

Mr. X reduced his drinking as planned over a period of 9 weeks; alcohol consumption leveled off at approximately 6 ounces per day, where it remained until the end of treatment. Mrs. X reported that her husband was more pleasant, stayed up later in the evenings, was able to awaken on his own in the mornings, and was in better moods during the day.

With regard to maintenance, Mrs. X was helped to identify and avoid possible high-risk situations. She was also helped to identify and initiate alternative activities not related to alcohol. She began to praise Mr. X's reduction efforts and the resulting improvements in his behavior. She was advised to continue to engage in the new behaviors she had developed throughout the course of treatment after treatment ended. For example, she was advised to continue with her relationship enhancement and disenabling programs and with relapse-prevention behaviors. In the event that Mr. X resumed his previous level of drinking, she agreed to carry out the contingency actions developed earlier. Follow-up at 6 and 12 months indicated that Mr. X continued to drink at the moderate level of 6-8 ounces per day.

Programmed Request

Mr. and Mrs. Z were both in their forties, had been married for eighteen years, and had two children. Mrs. Z reported that her husband had drunk heavily since prior to his first marriage. Typically, Mr. Z began drinking upon arriving home from work at approximately 11:00 p.m., and generally drank 12 12-ounce cans of beer before going to bed at approximately 4:00 a.m. During the period of delay before treatment for Mrs. Z, Mr. Z continued to drink at the same high level.

The first 12 sessions of treatment for Mrs. Z were devoted to orientation, assessment, and establishing and maintaining the role-induction components. Concurrently, the programmed request, which was delivered between sessions 12 and 13, was planned. Mr. Z agreed to enter treatment; sessions 13 through 15 were focused on postrequest follow-up and maintenance.

The steps followed in preparing the programmed request are also those given in Table 2. The programmed request was chosen instead of a programmed confrontation because Mrs. Z was not prepared at this point to make any major changes in her life or marriage in the event that Mr. Z refused to stop drinking. She also indicated that Mr. Z might be receptive to a request that he receive alcohol treatment, if the request was properly presented. It was planned that if Mr. Z refused to obtain help, Mrs. Z was to state that the marital relationship would continue to deteriorate and distance between her and Mr. Z would increase (a "dire prognostication").

It was decided that the request would be delivered on Mr. Z's day off, in a familiar restaurant instead of at the Project office. Mrs. Z agreed to arrange seating at the back of the restaurant and to make her request after the meal. She reported that she delivered the presentation at the restaurant as scripted and rehearsed and that Mr. Z agreed to enter treatment. Although he objected to the treatment arrangements Mrs. Z suggested and insisted on finding his own therapist, he followed through with an appointment with a therapist and entered in-patient treatment as the therapist recommended. Work on maintenance following Mr. Z's entry into treatment was foreshortened because the couple also entered family treatment as part of Mr. Z's in-patient treatment program. However, Mrs. Z was advised to continue with treatment-based changes such as relationship enhancement, reduction of the customary drinking control efforts, and disenabling. Mr. Z was abstinent following treatment and continued to be abstinent at the 6- and 12-month follow-ups.

POSTSCRIPT

Entry into treatment and subsequent abstinence, as achieved with Mr. Z, are of course the preferred treatment outcomes. However, when working with and through a spouse to reach the uncooperative alcohol abuser, it is sometimes necessary to settle for less which, in the case of Mr. X, was a reduction to a level often called controlled drinking and no entry into treatment. Given the objectives of the treatment program, both cases were deemed successes, and demonstrate the effectiveness of the confrontive interventions used in that crossover experimental dyad. Considered more generally, positive outcomes of the treatment program were found for abusers and spouses in two studies, as indicated and cited earlier.

REFERENCE NOTES

1. Adapted with permission from Thomas, E. J., Adams, K. B., Yoshioka, M. R., and Ager, R. D. (1990), Unilateral relationship enhancement in the treatment of spouses of uncooperative alcohol abusers, *The American Journal of Family Therapy, 18,* 334-344 published by Brunner/Mazel, Inc., 19 Union Sq. West, New York, NY 10003.

2. A regular baseline could be obtained and may be desirable for some purposes, but the retrospective baseline has been found adequate for these clinical purposes.

3. This list and other material referred to here are available by request from the author.

4. Adapted with permission from Yoshioka, M. R., Thomas, E. J., and Ager, R. D. (1992), Nagging and other drinking control efforts of spouses of uncooperative alcohol abusers: Assessment and modification, *Journal of Substance Abuse, 4,* 309-318 published by Ablex Publishing Corp., 355 Chestnut St., Norwood, NJ 07648.

5. The SSII is a clinical and research instrument based on inductively derived instances of spouse influence. The items fall into one of two scales: (a) the Spouse Drinking Control Scale (45 items), which encompasses those actions intended to stop or to thwart abuser drinking and/or drinking opportunities; and (b) the Spouse Sobriety Support Scale (7 items), which consists of those actions intended to support non-drinking or sobriety behaviors. For each item, the spouse is asked to indicate how often he or she has engaged in that behavior over the past six months. Response options range from 5 (never) to 1 (always), and are reversed in direction for scoring. Psychometric properties of the SSII are to be reported elsewhere.

6. If the SSII is used, a list is prepared from the Inventory and is presented to

the spouse without indicating that these were the items the spouse responded to earlier as those having been moderately or highly endorsed. The list is described as some examples of the behaviors many spouses living with a problem drinker have employed to try to get the drinker to reduce or stop drinking.

7. Adapted with permission from Thomas, E. J., and Yoshioka, M. R. (1989), Spouse interventive confrontations in unilateral family therapy for alcohol abuse, *Social Casework,* 70, 340-347 published by Family Service America, 11700 W. Lake Park Dr., Milwaukee, WI 53224.

8. When the abuser insists on trying to reduce the drinking on his or her own, a "what if" agreement can be signed in which the abuser agrees to enter treatment if he or she cannot do it on his or her own.

REFERENCES

Leite, E. 1987. *Detachment: The Art Of Letting Go While Living With An Alcoholic, Rev. ed.* Minneapolis: Johnson Institute Books.

Thomas, E. J. (1989). Unilateral family therapy to reach the uncooperative alcohol abuser. In *Behavioral Family Therapy,* edited by B. A. Thyer, Springfield, IL: Charles C Thomas Publishers.

Thomas, E. J., K. B. Adams, M. R. Yoshioka, and R. D. Ager, 1990. Unilateral relationship enhancement in the treatment of spouses of uncooperative alcohol abusers. *American Journal of Family Therapy, 18,* 334-344.

Thomas, E. J. and R. D. Ager, 1992. Treatment mediation and the spouse as treatment mediator. *American Journal of Family Therapy, 19,* 315-326.

Thomas, E. J. and R. D. Ager, In *Marital and Family Therapy in Alcoholism Treatment,* Edited by T. O'Farrell New York: Guilford Press.

Thomas, E. J. and C. A. Santa, 1982. Unilateral family therapy for alcohol abuse: A working conception. *American Journal of Family Therapy, 10,* 49-58.

Thomas, E. J., C. A. Santa, D. Bronson, and D. Oyserman, 1987. Unilateral family therapy with the spouses of alcoholics. *Journal of Social Service Research, 10*(3), 145-162.

Thomas, E. J. and M. R. Yoshioka, 1989. Spouse interventive confrontations in unilateral family therapy for alcohol abuse. *Social Casework, 70,* 340-347.

Thomas, E. J., M. Yoshioka, R. D. Ager, and K. B. Adams, 1993. *Experimental Outcomes of Spouse Intervention to Reach the Uncooperative Alcohol Abuser: Preliminary Report.* Manuscript submitted for publication.

Yoshioka, M. R., E. J. Thomas, and R. D. Ager, 1992. Nagging and other drinking control efforts of spouses of uncooperative alcohol abusers: Assessment and modification. *Journal of Substance Abuse, 4,* 309-318.

Appendix C

Leading Effective Meetings– Encouraging Members to Listen Actively and Provide Support

Adrienne L. Paine
Yolanda Suarez-Balcazar
Stephen B. Fawcett
Leslie Borck Jameson

Good group members listen to each other. Listening is an active process. It lets individual group members know that people are interested in what they are saying and encourages them to continue talking.

People attending self-help groups tell each other about the problems they are facing, the things they are doing to address those problems, and the positive experiences they have had. Talking about these issues provides an opportunity for group members to provide support to one another. In a support statement, members communicate that they care, are interested, and perhaps share similar experiences. Take a minute, and think about how it feels when you talk about a problem, and friends listen carefully. What do they do and say that show you that they care?

In the space below, list some of the things that people do and say that make you feel good when you are talking to them:

Perhaps your friends sit quietly, look at you directly, and say things like "I understand," or "uh-huh," to let you know they are listening and understand how you are feeling. By their actions, your friends are letting you know that they are there for you and care about you. Listening actively and providing support go hand in hand.

This chapter discusses when and how to encourage members to listen actively and provide support. Examples and exercises are provided to give you practice in sharpening these skills. Here is an example of what listening actively and providing support would look like in a meeting of a self-help group for people with Multiple Sclerosis:

[Leader arranges room, reviews issues discussed at previous meeting, and prepares announcements.] [Members arrive for meeting on time.]

Leader: Hi. Joan, how are you? *(Exchange initial greetings)*

Joan: Fine, thanks.

[Members greet each other.]

Leader: [After a few minutes] If it's all right with everyone, let's get the meeting started. Well, at the last meeting we talked about feeling very fatigued. What would someone like to share with the group tonight? *(Refer to group topics)*

Joan: I'm really having a terrible time keeping up with school work this semester. I've been so tired lately, and I'm starting to lose my eyesight. *(Disclosure)*

Leader: [Eye contact, head nodding] Uh-huh. *(Active listening)*

[Members do not provide support.]

Leader: Oh no, that's really scary. *(Provide support)*

Joan: It's also getting more and more difficult to walk. I'm really having a hard time. *(Provide information)*

Leader: Uh-huh. *(Active listening)*

Julie: [Eye contact, lean forward] That must be real frustrating. *(Support)*

Let us look more closely at the activities involved in listening actively and providing support.

Listening Actively

How do we let someone know that we are listening? There are two parts to listening actively: using your body to show caring and support and providing brief statements to encourage talking.

To let someone know you are interested in what he or she is saying (For example, in a support group for family members of widows):
> *Member 1:* I'm having difficulty adjusting to my mother moving in with us.
> *Member 2:* [Eye contact, head nodding, concerned facial expression] Oh.

To encourage a member to continue talking
(For example, in a support group for stepparents):
> *Member 1:* I'm really worried about my stepson.
> *Member 2:* [Eye contact, head nodding, concerned facial expression] Uh-huh.

Body Actions

Think about all the things that people do to make you feel good while you are talking. Do they sit leaning slightly toward you? Do they look at you? Do they show a concerned facial expression? These body actions may be very simple, but they make a big difference.

While a group member is talking, other group members should look into the eyes of the person talking. Maintaining eye contact expresses interest, encourages the member to continue talking, and generally communicates that other members care.

Group members should also nod their heads occasionally. Good listening posture involves leaning slightly toward the member talking. Also important is what not to do while someone is talking. Try not to fidget with a pen or pencil; do not look at your watch or calendar; and don't look around the room. These things can be distracting and imply that you are not listening, even if you are.

Exercise: You are in a support group for single parents. List the body actions that you would make to show that you are listening.

1. _____
2. _____
3. _____
4. _____
5. _____

Brief Statements of Encouragement

Brief statements of encouragement might seem silly and unimportant, but they are helpful messages that communicate we are listening. Think about your list of things that people said and did to make you feel that they were really listening to you. Perhaps they said some of the following brief statements of encouragement:

"Uh-huh," "Yeah,"
"Mm-hm,"
"Yes," "I see," "Oh"

Exercise: A member of a support group for parents of troubled youths is talking about problems with her son. List four different brief statements of encouragement that you could make while she is talking:

1. _____
2. _____
3. _____
4. _____

Providing Support

Support statements offer approval of feelings, provide hope, express confidence that reaching a goal is possible, or just let you know that it's O.K. Some statements of support convey empathy or understanding from group members who share similar experiences. When providing support statements, direct them to the person talking about his or her personal experience.

Following a member's statement of a personal experience
(For example, in a support group for victims of a stroke):
> *Member 1:* I have decided to start swimming 3 times a week.
> *Member 2:* [While making eye contact] Good, I think you're doing the right thing.

Following a member's statement of a goal
(For example, in a support group for cancer patients):
> *Member 1:* I will make an appointment to see the doctor this week.
> *Member 2:* Great, I think that's terrific.

To the following statements of personal experiences, list examples of supportive statements.

Exercise: Assume you are part of a self-help group for teen-age mothers. A member says, "I'm going to make an appointment to talk to a career counselor this week."

1. _____
2. _____

(Some examples include: "Great, glad to hear it." "Good for you. I think it's a good idea.")

Exercise: Assume you are a leader of a self-help group for low-income women. One member says, "I don't know what to do. I don't think I'm going to get the job. I'm very worried."

1. _____
2. _____

(Some examples include: "I can relate. I know just how you feel." "I understand.")

Leader's Skills

To facilitate good self-help group meetings in which all members participate, leaders must not only be supportive members themselves, they must also help sharpen other members' abilities to listen actively and provide support. To help group members, leaders should demonstrate listening actively, providing support, and encouraging others to do the same.

Providing Support Yourself

When a member talks about a problem or positive experience and group members do not show that they are listening or are not providing support, it is important for the leader to do so. If, after a pause of approximately 10 seconds, with no group members providing statements of support, the leader should make a statement, while leaning forward and making eye contact with the person talking. Waiting a bit before providing support gives other group members an opportunity to provide support themselves. Below are two examples of a leader listening actively and providing support.

Example: You are part of a self-help group for people with Muscular Dystrophy. Assume a member has been talking for a few minutes, and the other group members have not yet provided support. In this situation, the leader should demonstrate support by providing it to group members.

> *Martha:* I've been feeling really sick lately, I hate going to the doctor. It's such a hassle to get there.
> *Leader:* [Eye contact, nodding, facial expression, posture] Uh-huh. [Pause].
> *Leader:* I know what you mean. *(Support)*

Example: In a support group for widows, a member has been talking for a few minutes, and the leader just provided support. In this situation, the leader should pause again, and give the other members an opportunity to provide support.

Margie: I really hate sleeping by myself every night. I haven't slept alone in 35 years. I miss my husband very much.
Leader: Yeah. *(Active listening)*
[Pause].
Member 2: I know just how you feel. *(Support)*

Below are some examples of members talking about personal experiences. After each statement, provide an example of how a leader would demonstrate active listening and support. Also, provide other examples of members listening actively and providing support.

Exercise: You are part of a self-help group for alcoholics.

> *Member 1:* I haven't had a drink in two days. I really feel good about it.

Leader: _____

Member 2: _____

(Some examples include: *Leader:* "Great, that's good to hear."
Member: "That's terrific.")

Exercise: You are a member of a self-help group for abusive parents.

> *Member 1:* I hate to come home and hear all the kids screaming
> at the same time. It drives me crazy!
> *Leader:* _____
> *Member 2:* _____

(Some examples include: *Leader:* "I can understand why you
didn't like it. I don't like it either" *Member 2:* "It's hard to
control ourselves sometimes, but we really have to try hard.")

Encouraging Others to Provide Support

Suppose the group still fails to provide support, even after the
leader demonstrated it. In such circumstances, it may be necessary
to encourage, instruct, or otherwise get statements of support from
members. To do so, the leader should ask group members how they
are affected by the discloser's experience. Asking one (or all) of the
members such questions should result in statements of support. The
following are examples of the leader encouraging group members
to provide support:

Example: Assume that members of a breast cancer support group
have not provided support to the person talking about a personal
experience. The leader has demonstrated statements of support
twice hoping that other group members would also give support to
the speaker. In this situation, the leader should encourage support
from the group members by asking them questions.

> *Member 1:* I've been feeling really sick lately from the weekly
> radiation treatments.
> *Leader:* [Eye contact, nodding, facial expression, posture] I see.
> [Pause].
> *Leader:* Sue, what can you say to Mary that might help? *(Encourage support)*
> *Sue:* I'm sorry to hear that. I've been there, too. *(Support)*

Example:

> *Member 1:* I'm feeling much better this week about keeping up with school.
>
> [Pause].
>
> *Leader:* [Turning to other group members] What do you think about that? *(Encourage support)*
>
> *Member 2:* I think it's terrific. *(Support)*
>
> *Member 3:* Yeah.

Below are some examples of members' statements about personal experiences. After each statement, provide an example of how a leader would ask for or encourage support.

Exercise: In a self-help group for people who are overweight, assume that the member talking has not been provided with support, and the leader has demonstrated support. After each statement, provide an example of a leader encouraging support. Also, provide an example of other members providing support.

> *Member 1:* I haven't been able to stick to my diet. I feel terrible about it.
>
> *Leader:* _____
>
> *Member 2:* _____
>
> (Some examples include: *Leader:* "How can we give some support now?" *Member 2:* "I know its tough. Just keep trying.")

Exercise: A self-help group for people with arthritis.

> *Member 1:* I will make an appointment to see Dr. Moore.
>
> *Leader:* _____
>
> *Member 2:* _____
>
> (Some examples include: *Leader:* "What do you think about that?" *Member 2:* "I think that's terrific.")

Summary

This chapter described what is involved in listening actively and providing support. Specific activities in encouraging members to listen actively and provide support include:

1. Body actions
   a. Eye contact
   b. Head nodding
   c. Facial expressions
   d. Body posture
2. Brief statements of encouragement
3. Providing support
4. Encouraging support

Review Questions

Review the following questions, making sure you can answer all of them. If you can't answer a question, refer back to the chapter before moving on to the skills practice.

1. What are the activities involved in listening actively and providing support? Describe and give an example of each.

2. Why is it important to listen actively and provide support?

3. Describe and give an example of each of the two leader skills involved in encouraging members to provide support.

Suggested Answers for Chapter 2 Review Questions

1. The activities involved in listening actively and providing support are: making eye contact, nodding your head, having a pleasant facial expression, leaning toward the person talking, making brief statements of encouragement, and providing statements of support.
2. It is important to listen actively and provide support to communicate listening and interest in what the person is saying. It lets the person know you care and understand.
3. The two leader skills involved in encouraging members to listen actively and provide support are providing the support yourself and asking questions to encourage other members to provide support.

Performance Checklist

A performance checklist can be used for role playing situations in which a person sharpening their leader skills and two partners can practice. One of the two partners should use the checklist to note how each skill was done for each situation. For each situation, use a checkmark to note each leader skill done well and a zero to note each activity that needs improvement. Each leader should practice until all leader skills are shown perfectly for three consecutive situations.

Chapter 2 Checklist:
Encouraging Members to Listen and Provide Support

Skill   Practice Session

	1	2	3	4	5	6
1. Body actions						
a. Eye contact						
b. Head nodding						
c. Facial expression						
d. Body posture						
2. Brief statements of encouragement						
3. Provide support / If members do not provide support:						
4. Encourage support						

_____ Okay   _____ Needs improvement

Note: We have provided a sample of how the checklist is completed for a hypothetical situation. The checkmarks note the activities that were completed according to the instructions. In this example, the leader needs to practice item #3. These activities should be practiced until the leader skills are perfect for three consecutive role play situations.

Suggestions for Role Play Situations

Role Play Situation 1: You are involved in a support group for parents of children with hearing impairments. A member is talking about having problems getting her child into a classroom closer to their home. She has talked with several schools nearby with no success. She is feeling very frustrated.

Role Play Situation 2: You are involved in a support group for teenage mothers. A member is talking about having trouble finding a babysitter. She has tried several options discussed in the group meeting and seems very frustrated.

Role Play Situation 3: During a support group meeting for people who are experiencing stress at work, a member has been talking about having difficulty dealing with her supervisor.

Role Play Situation 4: During a support group meeting for people who want to lose weight, a member has just told the group members that she has lost 5 pounds since the last meeting. She had been unable to lose weight for several weeks. She is feeling anxious about keeping the weight off.

Role Play Situation 5: You are involved in a support group for single women, over 35, who have decided to have a child. The members have been talking about how their family and friends accepted their decision to have a child.

Role Play Situation 6: You are involved in a support group for individuals who have recently retired. One of the members is talking about being depressed.

Role Play Situation 7: You are involved in a support group for adult adoptees in search of their biological parents. Members are discussing their frustrations about finding their biological parents.

Role Play Situation 8: During a support group meeting for men who have recently been divorced and have children, one of the members is talking about the stress he is feeling at home.

Role Play Situation 9: You are involved in a support group for people who have had polio. A member, who uses a wheelchair, is talking about finding an apartment in town that is accessible.

Role Play Situation 10: You are involved in a support group for people under 30 years old who have recently been diagnosed with breast cancer. A member is talking about feeling very depressed and frustrated.

Role Play Situation 11: During a support group meeting for people who are partially sighted, a member has been talking about being afraid that she may lose all of her vision.

Role Play Situation 12: You are involved in a support group for women who were pregnant as teenagers and gave up their babies for adoption. One of the members has been talking about her attempts to locate her child.

Role Play Situation 13: During a support group meeting for parents of teenagers, one of the members is talking about feeling very good about the improvements he has seen in his son over the last few weeks.

Role Play Situation 14: You are involved in a support group for single parents. One of the members just told the group that she had a great weekend with her daughter.

Role Play Situation 15: You are involved in a support group for students with Multiple Sclerosis. John is talking about having trouble keeping up with school. The other members have not provided support. The leader should encourage that member to continue talking about a personal experience. Start the role play at the beginning of the meeting.

Role Play Situation 16: During a support group meeting for recently divorced men, Jeff is talking about having trouble disciplining the children since his wife left. The other group members have provided suggestions about what he might do about It. He has decided to try one of the suggestions. The other members have not started to talk about themselves.

Role Play Situation 17: During a self-help group meeting for people who have lost a child to a severe illness, one of the members is having trouble dealing with his son's death. The other members have provided support, but have not started to talk about themselves. The leader has directed questions to the member talking as well as to the group. Start the role play at the beginning of the meeting.

Role Play Situation 18: In a support group for children of alcoholics, Sue tells the group that her mother has not had a drink in two weeks. Because of that, things at home have really improved. The other members have provided support, but have not started to talk about their own personal experiences. The leader has already asked questions of the group and a quiet member.

Subject Index

Name Index

DATE